The Hidden Affliction

Rochester Studies in Medical History

Series Editor: Christopher Crenner
Robert Hudson and Ralph Major Professor and Chair
Department of History and Philosophy of Medicine
University of Kansas School of Medicine

Additional Titles of Interest

China and the Globalization of Biomedicine
Edited by David Luesink, William H. Schneider, and Zhang Daqing

Explorations in Baltic Medical History, 1850–2015
Edited by Nils Hansson and Jonatan Wistrand

Health Education Films in the Twentieth Century
Edited by Christian Bonah, David Cantor, and Anja Laukötter

The History of the Brain and Mind Sciences: Technique, Technology, Therapy
Edited by Stephen T. Casper and Delia Gavrus

Technological Change in Modern Surgery: Historical Perspectives on Innovation
Edited by Thomas Schlich and Christopher Crenner

Setting Nutritional Standards: Theory, Policies, Practices
Edited by Elizabeth Neswald, David F. Smith, and Ulrike Thoms

Fit to Practice: Empire, Race, Gender, and the Making of British Medicine, 1850–1980
Douglas M. Haynes

Reasoning against Madness: Psychiatry and the State in Rio de Janeiro, 1830–1944
Manuella Meyer

Psychiatry and Racial Liberalism in Harlem, 1936–1968
Dennis A. Doyle

Childbirth, Maternity, and Medical Pluralism in French Colonial Vietnam, 1880–1945
Thuy Linh Nguyen

A complete list of titles in the Rochester Studies in Medical History series may be found on our website, www.urpress.com.

The Hidden Affliction

Sexually Transmitted Infections and Infertility in History

Edited by Simon Szreter

University of Rochester Press

 Chapter 9, "'A Wise Provision of Nature for the Prevention of Too Many Children': Evidence from the Australian Colonies," by Janet McCalman and Rebecca Kippen, was funded in part by the Australian Research Council.

First published 2019

University of Rochester Press
668 Mt. Hope Avenue, Rochester, NY 14620, USA
www.urpress.com
and Boydell & Brewer Limited
PO Box 9, Woodbridge, Suffolk IP12 3DF, UK
www.boydellandbrewer.com

ISBN-13: 978-1-58046-961-6
ISSN: 1526-2715

Library of Congress Cataloging-in-Publication Data

Names: Szreter, Simon, editor.
Title: The hidden affliction : sexually transmitted infections and infertility in history / edited by Simon Szreter.
Other titles: Rochester studies in medical history. 1526–2715 ; v. 46.
Description: Rochester, NY : University of Rochester Press, 2019. | Series: Rochester studies in medical history, 1526-2715 ; v. 46 | Includes bibliographical references and index.
Identifiers: LCCN 2019023514 | ISBN 9781580469616 (hardcover : alk. paper) | ISBN 9781787445826
Subjects: MESH: Sexually Transmitted Diseases—history | Infertility—history | Sexually Transmitted Diseases—complications | Infertility—etiology
Classification: LCC RC200 | NLM WC 140 | DDC 616.95/1—dc23
LC record available at https://lccn.loc.gov/2019023514

This publication is printed on acid-free paper.
Printed and bound in Great Britain by TJ International Ltd, Padstow, Cornwall

MIX
Paper from responsible sources
FSC® C013056
FSC
www.fsc.org

Contents

Acknowledgments

The chapters published here were given their first airing at a conference held at the Centre for Research in the Arts, Social Sciences and Humanities (CRASSH) in Cambridge, on September 28–30, 2015, made possible through funding from CRASSH; Pembroke College, Cambridge; St. John's College, Cambridge; the Cambridge Faculty of Classics; and the five-year Wellcome Trust Strategic Award, Generation to Reproduction, held at Cambridge's History and Philosophy of Science Department. The conference was part of the interdisciplinary research program initiated under Wellcome Strategic Award 088708, ably directed throughout by Nick Hopwood. The director, Simon Goldhill, and the staff of CRASSH and St. John's College provided much-appreciated support for the conference.

I wish to thank my Cambridge colleagues, Rebecca Flemming and Lauren Kassell, who co-organized the conference and also gave subsequent editorial advice; in particular I wish to acknowledge the editorial assistance of Tim Bayliss-Smith and Michael Worboys. I additionally am grateful to Boyd Brogan for an online published record of the conference on *Notches*, which well conveys the excitement of this interdisciplinary meeting (http://notchesblog.com/2016/01/28/sex-disease-and-fertility-in-history). My thanks are also extended to the two student helpers, Lauren Withall and Agnes Arnold-Foster.

Other colleagues who participated in the conference and added enormously to its vitality were Jeremy Boulton, Romola Davenport, Mary Dobson, Aleka Gurel, Susan Hakenbeck, Anne Hanley, Anne Hardy, Victoria Harvey, Nick Hopwood, Sheila Kohring, Rich McKay, Caroline Rusterholz, Kevin Siena, Richard Smith, Claudia Stein, Lutz Sauerteig, Katy Turner, Michelle Wallis, Samantha Williams, and Gabriella Zuccolin.

As to this volume's publication, I would like to say a personal word of thanks to Ted Brown, the founding editor of this excellent series, who initially encouraged me, as he did with my previous volume, *Health and Wealth: Studies in History and Policy*, to submit the original book proposal. I hope he finds his final commission a worthy addition to the series. Also, thanks go to his successor as series editor, Chris Crenner, and to Sonia Kane, Julia Cook, Jackie Heinzelmann, Susan Silver, Tracey Engel and the production team at the University of Rochester Press. Additionally, thanks to Graham CopeKoga for vital assistance with several of the images, to Pip Austin for the index, to the two anonymous referees for their most helpful and improving comments, and, as always, to Hilary Cooper.

Finally, I would like to dedicate this volume to the memory of Stephen J. Kunitz (1938–2018). He would have contributed to the conference and the volume if his health had permitted. It was a privilege to be able to count Steve as a good friend. He was a model scholar, equally generous with his wide knowledge, his wisdom, and his wonderful, dry wit.

Simon Szreter, Cambridge, May 1, 2019

Introduction

Simon Szreter

"A Riddle, Wrapped in a Mystery, inside an Enigma"

This volume is a necessarily multidisciplinary collection dedicated to the extremely difficult task of uncovering and exploring what can be reconstructed of the dimensions and the scale of the historical impact of sexually transmitted infections (STIs) on human infertility.[1] As a subject for inquiry, this comes close to Winston Churchill's celebrated phrase, "a riddle, wrapped in a mystery, inside an enigma." The riddle, which remains for medical and epidemiological science today, is how to quantify just how much the different STI organisms have affected female and male infertility. The mystery is how to find sufficient evidence to reveal how far different populations in the past were afflicted by these potentially sterilizing social diseases. The enigma is the question of whether any of the STIs have afflicted human populations from time immemorial, or whether there is evidence of more specific dating of the emergence of any STIs in historical, archaeological, or biogenomic records and, if so, when? The pandemic of HIV/AIDS in the late twentieth century demonstrated unequivocally not only that STDs are culturally refracted and technologically defined, which we already knew, but also that the infective microorganisms—being socially constructed through human activity—can themselves have a history and a potentially discoverable origin date in their entry into their human hosts. Therefore, there is a meaningful historical debate to be had over their origins.[2]

Owing to the conjectural state of both scientific and historical knowledge in all three of these areas—the riddle, the mystery, and the enigma—for us to make intellectual progress with uncovering the infertility implications of the historical STIs, *The Hidden Affliction* is burdened with simultaneously pursuing several related but distinct tasks—none of them easy. In particular, the study of venereal syphilis, caused by *Treponema pallidum* (subspecies *pallidum*), and its contested history has an important part to play in this volume.[3] Syphilis does not directly cause an incapacity to conceive, as gonorrhea and chlamydia both do, though it can certainly result in effective infertility for individual women due to fetal morbidity, multiple miscarriages, and early infant mortality, as chapter 9 harrowingly demonstrates.[4] However, its primary value for historians who wish to evaluate the likely role of historical STIs in causing infertility among past populations lies in the far greater visibility of syphilis in the documentary record. It is rarely completely asymptomatic, unlike both gonorrhea and chlamydia. There is consequently a much greater range of opportunities available for historians to study various, quite detailed, medical, legal, military, and other institutional records concerning affliction with syphilis.[5]

This can be of assistance because, in a number of circumstances, the incidence of syphilis may be able to provide a proxy indicator for the scale of gonorrhea likely to have been experienced in a population in the past. In relatively well-documented official studies, it was found that during the early twentieth century in Europe the rates of reported gonorrhea infection tended to be three to four times more prevalent than syphilis in unprotected populations lacking effective treatment.[6] Such a ratio is to be expected, since gonorrhea not only is much more infectious than syphilis but also confers no immunity to reinfection.[7] This could, then, enable informed estimates of the extent to which infertility, due to secondary sterility from gonorrhea, may have affected various temperate zone societies in the past, even where we have little or no surviving direct evidence for either gonorrhea or chlamydia (the restriction of such a method to temperate zone populations follows from the prevalence of the other three non-venereal species of *Treponema pallidum* in more tropical climates, each of which confers immunities against venereal syphilis). The application of this method, using historical epidemiological data on syphilis incidence to provide an estimate of STI-induced infertility, is discussed and presented in the final chapter in this volume, in a study of the modern demographic history of England and Wales during its initial period of modern fertility decline in the decades just before the Great War. The results of this exercise indicate that STIs may, indeed, have played a substantial and hitherto unacknowledged contributory role in the low marital fertility recorded in that period, as a number of doctors and many feminists claimed at the time.

To what extent might this approach be more widely usable for other times and places in European history, supposing appropriate data were available? There may be no possibility at all before the sixteenth century—or perhaps even before the seventeenth century. There has been a justly famous debate, itself over a century old, reviewed in chapter 3, positing a date of origin for venereal syphilis, at least as far as European populations are concerned, following the return of Columbus and his crew from the Americas in 1493. And what of gonorrhea—was it already extant in Europe in 1493? There are currently live debates about the origins of gonorrhea, and of chlamydia too, which each draw on a fascinating range of sources and scientific methods, and which are reviewed here in chapters 1, 3, 4, and 7.

Unveiling the Hidden Affliction

Infertility is now a high-profile contemporary public policy issue around the world.[8] A 2017 major literature review has reconfirmed that, even with today's public health surveillance systems and treatment facilities, gonorrhea and chlamydia remain the main cause of the most preventable condition, tubal factor infertility (TFI). In the United States chlamydia is the most common reportable disease (1.5 million annually), and gonorrhea is the second most common, while 30 percent of female infertility is attributed to tubal factor infertility.[9]

Nevertheless, it is appropriate in many ways to describe the historical infertility consequences of the "venereal diseases" as the *hidden affliction*, for at least five distinct reasons. There has been some recent attention given to infertility by historians.[10] Nevertheless, there has been remarkably little systematic and comparative historiography addressing the infertility aspects of historical STIs.[11] With the infectiousness of both gonorrhea and chlamydia and their known sequelae of secondary sterility, it is clear that infertility due to what were called in the past "venereal diseases," and today STIs, must have been a repeated occurrence among many populations. There has been a very considerable output of excellent studies of various aspects of such historical STIs.[12] However, the impact of STIs on reproduction has surfaced only rarely in historians' work as an explicit focus of attention.[13] Until Shane Doyle's important monograph, there have been relatively few extended treatments by historians: Michael Worboys's and Elliott Bowen's excellent social constructionist studies of gonorrhea bacteriology; the exemplary study by Megan Vaughan of the shared "panic" about sterility and venereal disease among both some colonial medical officers and indigenous chiefs in sub-Saharan Africa in the early part of the twentieth century; and the work of Noel Butlin on aboriginal population decline in Australia.[14]

As chapters 10, 11, and 12 explain, this historiographic inattention largely reproduces a constructed neglect by politicians, demographers, and medical epidemiology in the interwar decades, emerging, albeit in quite distinctive ways, in Germany, France, and Britain (and also in the United States and elsewhere). Consequently, historians, led by the availability of the primary sources, have produced excellent studies of venereal diseases and eugenics, feminism, social purity, prostitution, and public health policy, but no studies specifically in relation to infertility. Contemporary eugenicists and others focused their fears on their conviction (later shown to be an impossibility) that "congenital syphilis" showed it was a heritable taint (reflected in the title of Edvard Munch's 1897 painting *The Inheritance*, which adorns this volume's cover). They ignored the evidence already available—until feminists forcefully brought it to their attention—that gonorrhea caused infertility.[15] Not until the 1890s and 1900s (and initially only in Germany and Austro-Hungary) was there a growing acceptance of Emil Noeggerath's pioneering evidence and thesis, originally published in 1872, regarding the importance of latent (i.e., symptomless) gonorrhea, which was crucial to his claim that this STI was a major cause of sterility in both sexes.[16]

Gradual international acceptance of this link followed the publication in 1891 of Ernst Wertheim's conclusive supporting evidence from the university hospital in Prague (see chapter 10). In the United States Margaret Marsh and Wanda Ronner concur with Allan Brandt's pioneering study showing that, while there was medical consideration of gonorrhea as a cause of marital infertility in the first decade of the twentieth century, thanks to the medicomoral campaigning of Prince Albert Morrow (since 1884 professor of genitourinary diseases at New York University), nevertheless little practical attention was given to it, probably in part because doctors could not offer any revenue-generating treatment.[17] Brandt has documented how, even as late as the 1930s in the United States under surgeon general Thomas Parran's personal crusade, syphilis and its amenability to prenuptial Wassermann testing remained the primary focus of attention, not gonorrhea, despite the latter's known capacity to render marriages sterile.[18] Thus, this lack of historiographic attention reflects the fact that contemporary biomedical, demographic, and epidemiological science has consistently paid only intermittent attention to the infertility consequences of the pre-HIV STIs, and this has broadly continued into the second half of the twentieth century.

However, from the 1950s onward, biomedical science developed increasing interest in a newly recognized disease entity with infertility implications: chlamydia. In chapter 5 Worboys provides the first historical account available of the complex story of its emergence from the range of imprecisely termed conditions known variously as blennorrhea, Waelsch's urethritis, then NGU and NSU (nongonorrheal and nonspecific urethritis, respectively). Worboys shows that during the 1980s and 1990s the newly created NHS specialism of GUM (genital and urinary medicine) effectively used the perceived fertility threat of the recently identified disease entity of chlamydia to justify professional claims for expanding resources for new, improved microscopy tests. Professionally, this was a highly successful strategy, in the sense that each new test identified more and more chlamydia in the population, requiring more resources to treat it.[19] However, Worboys points out that, despite this, both the public's and medical science's primary attention by the mid-1980s was rapidly becoming much more exclusively focused on combating the threat of the frightening and even newer STI of HIV/AIDS, pushing chlamydia onto the sidelines until the very late 1990s, when a partial national screening approach was launched in the United Kingdom. This intervening period of predominant attention to HIV, in both the global North and South, perhaps partly explains why there has been no general account specifically addressed to the subject of infertility and pre-HIV STIs since 1984.[20]

A second general reason for neglect of the subject is that the relationship between sex, disease, and infertility has often, as a matter of behavioral, cultural, and associated medical practice, been imperfectly understood throughout most of history. Sociologists have insightfully explored the cultural, medical, and technological constructions of the contemporary positive concept of "in-fertility" as one scientific form of "disrupted reproduction."[21] But in the past, where such disrupted reproduction was actually due to an individual contracting an often-asymptomatic STI, childlessness—or the inability to conceive further children—was experienced as something far less well defined: something that simply did not happen, and for no manifest, physical reason. It has comprised for many such sufferers, not the certainty of an act of commission, nor even a focused regret, but the amorphous and imprecise uncertainty of an absence, of being denied something available to others, but for no apparent reasons.

It is entirely rational in those circumstances that the search for meaning and attribution of responsibility for their inexplicable misfortune might often have taken the form of superstition and suspicion of malevolence or witchcraft on the part of others.[22] Another explanation was divine punishment for wrongful behavior, especially since miscarriages, disfigured stillbirths, or sickly infants, as depicted in Munch's 1897 composition, would also occur in communities where syphilis as well as gonorrhea was rife. Often both illicit sexual acts and disease manifestations were involved in this infertility. In such cases chapters 1 and 2 both discuss explanations invoked in the European ancient and early modern past, in terms of the morally "wrong" kind of sex (too much, too little, "impure"). Closely associated with such transgressive notions, further levels of deliberate concealment have often been added in many cultures by those afflicted. It is therefore a fundamental premise of research on the association between infertility and STIs in the past that scholars and scientists must actively engage with the clandestine nature of the subject. Even the name *Chlamydia*, adopted by science for the organism responsible, *C. trachomatis*, as recounted in chapter 5, translates from the Greek original as "cloaked."

The third reason for the historically hidden nature of the affliction is that the other main pre-HIV STIs with implications for human infertility, gonorrhea and syphilis, were also relatively opaque to the medical gaze until late in the nineteenth century. Previously gonorrhea and syphilis had often been considered as manifestations of a single affliction varying in severity, the clap and the pox in early modern English vernacular. In contrast, today, following the shift from a physiological to the ontological conception of disease, we see them as the product of two quite distinct microorganisms.[23] The gonococcus was first seen under the microscope by Albert Neisser in 1879, and the transparent spirochete of syphilis was only finally visually identified as recently as 1905.[24] Furthermore, even the potentially lethal nature of each of the two diseases was long hidden from medical knowledge. It is now well known that syphilis, after a varying duration of deceptive latency amounting even to several decades, has the capacity to kill a significant proportion of its victims of both sexes in various ways, mainly through damage to the brain, the nervous system, or the aorta. This was increasingly suspected by specialist medical professionals in the late nineteenth century, particularly those working in asylums with those suffering from conditions given the medial names of "locomotor ataxy" and "GPI" (general paralysis of the insane), but it could not be finally proven until several years after identification of the spirochete.[25] Gonorrhea can result in acute pelvic inflammatory disease in women. It is certainly a cause of secondary sterility for a proportion of those infected, through blockage of the fallopian tubes (salpingitis), but it can also be fatal, not least due to associated ectopic pregnancies.

Fourth, gendered power relations have undoubtedly played a formative role, not simply in the most obvious sense of the behaviors involved in transmitting the diseases, but more insidiously, on account of the patriarchal lens and interests through which the diseases have been viewed by the medical profession. As Worboys has shown, both gonorrhea and then chlamydia, the two most serious sterilizing diseases of women, were each initially treated indulgently by the medical profession in the nineteenth and again in the mid-twentieth centuries, respectively, as minor nuisance conditions afflicting only young men "sowing their wild oats." It took scientific breakthroughs, which in each case were not initially believed, before the medical patriarchy came to acknowledge each disease as a serious threat to female fertility.

As J. D. Oriel pointed out, Noeggerath challenged the patriarchal legal assumptions and cultural practices of the male medical profession as much as he challenged medical science. He caused a furor when presenting his research to the inaugural meeting of the American Gynecologic Society in 1876. The reaction there was less because of any discussion of the validity of his research methods and findings and more because of a claim he made that over half of men in large US cities had been infected with gonorrhea at some point and that because of his latency theory this meant that over half of the wives of such men would then be infected. Consequently, "the president of the society said that he regarded these estimates as not only offensive but an unwarranted attack on the moral standards of the American male."[26] The evasive disposition of the predominantly male medical profession toward this morally challenging disease continued for decades to exert insidious effects, including perpetuating its own ignorance of best practices, with harmful consequences. Half a century later, Dr. Percy Pelouze claimed, in the preface to the 1928 first edition of his commercially successful practical handbook on gonorrhea, aimed at informing American practitioners, that "at least 90 per cent of those afflicted are treated by men who frankly confess to themselves, and to their medical companions, that they really have but very meager knowledge of the scientific facts of the disease and of the precise methods of its most effective treatment."[27]

Fifth, the venereal diseases, and their manifestations and consequences, were not only passively hidden by the limitations and biases of male medical science and knowledge until well into the twentieth century but also often actively hidden by the sufferers themselves, as explored in chapter 2 by Olivia Weisser, where early modern medical practitioners are shown to have prided themselves on coaxing accounts of clandestine sexual encounters out of unwilling patients presenting with certain symptoms. In many societies sexual behavior is subject to widely observed restrictive customs or laws, often associated with the prevailing religious codes, whose transgressions are sources of shame or guilt, though in some cultures there is wider latitude, as today in many "Western" societies and also in some other communities in the past, such as in the "Aphrodisian" cultures encountered in certain Pacific Islands, which are discussed in Tim Bayliss-Smith's chapter 6. In the rather more numerous cultures, including those subscribing to Christianity, Judaism, and Islam, which proscribe sex outside marriage or its equivalent, to contract a disease that appears, from the bodily location of the manifest lesions and sources of discomfort, to be associated with sexual intercourse, is problematic for the affected individuals. Indeed, in a model chaste and nuptial society, in which sexual activity only ever occurred between legally married adults, the microorganisms of STIs would invariably fail to spread and would not exist, nor manifest themselves as disease entities. This would be as true of polygamous as of monogamous societies, regardless of sexual orientation.

However, given that human sexual behavior in most known populations of any size has often been conducted by some, at least, outside the moral prescriptions and even the strictest, formal legal codes governing sexual expression, to hide their shame such individuals have frequently sought in many societies to deny and to conceal the disease from themselves, from their spouses, and from the community in which they were living.[28] In the self-publicizing accounts of their curative prowess published by the early modern medical practitioners (all men) that Weisser examines in chapter 2, they dwelled on the importance of their skill in extracting a secular "confession" of the clandestine and transgressive extramarital liaison that accounted for their patients' conditions—the confession was itself a morally purgative part of their cure. Echoing this clandestine situation, but in an inverted fashion two centuries later in the closing decades of the nineteenth century, it seems likely that it was common practice among many male medical practitioners in western Europe and North America to collude with the wealthy men who formed much of their clientele to save them from the embarrassment of informing their wives of evidence of the venereal disease that their husbands had given them.[29] This zealous adherence to the notion of patient confidentiality interestingly paralleled the code governing priestly receipt of confessions in the Catholic Church. There were cases where the evidence of the disease was clearly manifest in the bodies of the clients' wives, who might be kept in ignorance by medical practitioners of a condition transmitted to them by their husbands that could on occasions prove fatal to them.[30]

Such patriarchal collusion against the health of the women of their own class became a major provocation to outrage expressed by the more courageous and iconoclastic figures within the early twentieth-century feminist movement, in the United States, Britain, and elsewhere. This was most famously expounded in Christabel Pankhurst's coruscating polemic, *The Great Scourge and How to End It*, published in 1913.[31]

As chapters 10 and 11 contrastingly explore, across the channel in France and also in Germany at this time, both the medical science of the infertility threats posed by the venereal diseases and the politicized interpretations of those threats took somewhat different public and political manifestations. A male bias was certainly common to the medical professions and the political classes in all these western European national cultures. In Britain, as in the United States, this bias manifested itself as discretion and public silence until feminists forced it onto the public agenda. In Germany it was expressed in positive encouragement to men to use the condom by German medical authorities because of the precocious acceptance there by the early 1890s that gonorrhea could cause *male* infertility.[32] Christina Benninghaus finds a widening acceptance among the educated class of laboratory microscopy to test for male azoospermia among infertile couples as early as the 1890s. By contrast, French medical practitioners remained skeptical and uninterested in subjecting their fee-paying clients to semen tests.

There may be larger historical and institutional influences at work here. Whereas the tradition of *Medizinpolizei* in German-speaking states had long linked issues defined as being of national medical interest with obedience to officially sanctioned medical authority (and Robert Koch's officially funded Prussian bacteriological science was flying high in this period), the practice of medicine in France has been characterized as the most dominated by private interests in Europe.[33] In pre-1914 Britain and the United States, there was preparedness to consider psychological conditions such as neurasthenia or masturbation in relation to impotence, but male infertility as a consequence of STIs went almost completely undiscussed, as in France.[34]

As Benninghaus shows, approbation for prophylactic condom use in Germany went alongside a relaxed attitude to demography. With its national birthrate remaining high for several decades after the United States', France's, and Britain's declined, political anxiety in Germany about the nation's falling fertility did not appear until after the 1910 census first showed an incipient fall. However, subsequent attention in the Weimar era was primarily focused on voluntary childlessness attributed to the supposed selfishness of women of luxury, not to STIs. This was despite the fact that throughout this period it was widely accepted in Germany that STIs accounted for about half of the 10 percent of couples that official statistics showed to be experiencing childlessness. In low-fertility France, by contrast, Fabrice Cahen and

Adrien Minard find in chapter 11 that the long-standing, official pronatalist obsession dating back to defeat in the Franco-Prussian War, along with pronounced Catholic influence, ensured aversion to any public sanctioning of condom use in marriage, formalized by legal prohibition in 1920. This was also despite widespread venereal infection due to the acceptability of the custom of initiation of young men through visits to prostitutes and the associated "manly" badge of the experience, in the form of a ritual bout of gonorrhea ("chaude-pisse" in the French colloquialism). Even after the Great War, and despite an evident rise in gonorrhea infections among the wives of poilus who served at the front, chapter 11 shows that French official, medical, and public opinion and indignation was focused on a campaign against female-procured abortions as the great social evil in the patriotic battle to raise the French birthrate, not on male responsibility for gonorrhea-induced sterility. In the 1960s French men were apparently still highly averse to using condoms, even when engaging—as a great many still did—in commercial sex. So the only time when condoms have been widely used in France was probably by the Wehrmacht during the Nazi occupation in World War II.

Thus, the chapters in part 4 show how in Germany, France, and Britain by the 1920s all public, political, and scientific attention was devoted to the voluntary and sociocultural sources of reduced national birthrates, not to the involuntary infertility due to STIs. Chapters 6 and 7 show that such a view also prevailed where Europeans studied population decline in the Pacific, which was attributed to "culture shock" after contact with the West. Only in parts of sub-Saharan Africa, as chapter 8 shows, was there any focus by the colonial authorities at this time on STIs as a remediable cause of infertility, but even here that interest evaporated once antibiotics appeared to solve the problem from the later 1940s onward.

This brings us back full circle to the five reasons why infertility due to STIs has remained mostly a hidden affliction, both in history and in historiography, such that even in a 2017 multiauthored volume devoted to childlessness, the chapter offering a historical survey of European trends since the beginning of the twentieth century makes no reference at all to STIs.[35]

The Benefits of a Multidisciplinary Approach

How, then, to reveal the concealed infertility due to STIs in the past? To give ourselves the maximum opportunity to learn as much as possible, we need to study carefully the various reports of the experiences of the afflicted.

We should certainly study the humanly constructed and recorded history of the disease entities, which have gone under various names in the past before coming to be known today as syphilis, gonorrhea, and chlamydia. But we also need to study and integrate into our historical understanding the most up-to-date scientific knowledge available regarding the three bacterial microorganisms principally responsible: *Treponema pallidum* (*pallidum*), *Neisseria gonococcus*, and *Chlamydia trachomatis*.

A purist historicist approach might insist that, especially given the clandestine nature of the subject, all we can uncover from the past are our attempts to capture various meanings that contemporaries in different eras and places attributed to a range of disputed and negotiated disease conditions observed to affect the genital organs. Such contemporaries may or may not have believed these conditions affected fecundity in some way. Certainly, the recovery of these diverse perceptions, anxieties, and understandings is of primary significance for any history of the meanings of sex, disease, and infertility.[36] Such an approach informs much of the subject matter presented in the chapters in this volume: by Rebecca Flemming, relating to the ancient world; by Weisser, on early modern Britain; by Cahen and Minard and by Benninghaus, relating to later nineteenth-century and early twentieth-century France and Germany; and by Worboys, relating to the evolving understandings of what we now call the disease category of chlamydia during the course of the early and mid-twentieth-century decades.

However, to restrict our curiosity and range of inquiry solely to approaches fashioned to investigate literary, medico-scientific, and representational texts is to adopt an unnecessarily circumscribed and limited approach, even to the effort of understanding those texts and signifiers themselves. Dimensions of meaning concealed within and evaded by the surviving texts, along with understanding of the anxieties and wider social and economic pressures that were conducive to texts being framed in the ways that they were in the diverse cultures of the past, will ultimately be accessible to us as historians only by juxtaposing against these texts all the range of insights from the other forms of evidence available to us. This includes such archaeological and paleopathological evidence as is presented and discussed in the chapter by Charlotte Roberts and Rebecca Redfern; the fascinating new genomic reconstructions of the evolutionary history of the currently extant range of disease organisms, discussed by Ian N. Clarke and Hugh R. Taylor in chapter 4; and whatever other scientific or historical evidence we can assemble and compare. Depending on what kind of sources have survived, some of this evidence may even be rendered into epidemiological and quantifiable form for certain populations in different times and places, such as that which is presented in chapters 6, 7, 8, 9, and 12, relating to diverse populations in Oceania and Africa, Britain and Australia.

All these different dimensions of evidence need to be understood by reference to the most up-to-date scientific knowledge we have today about the medical manifestations and the social and biological transmissibility of such clandestine diseases. It is extremely important to know, for example, that many men and most women infected with gonorrhea (and chlamydia) are symptomless.[37] The power of these diseases to cause infertility is not dependent on their capacity to manifest symptoms, especially in women. Therefore, many women in many cultures psychologically suffering the curse of barren sterility would have had no perceptible bodily signs or symptoms of the likely reasons for their affliction.[38]

To take another crucial example of the importance of applying current scientific knowledge to our historical researches, the historical STI that has left most evidence for us to study, both of a written form and in the archaeological bone record, as discussed in chapter 3, has been syphilis. However, an understanding of the research and transmission models of contemporary clinical epidemiologists, reviewed in the next section, informs us that, among the historical STDs, syphilis was characterized by a relatively low prevalence and low incidence compared with both gonorrhea and chlamydia. Thus, it is of cardinal importance for us as historians to understand that syphilis, the disease most highly visible in the available historical record from both textual and paleopathological sources of evidence, is not the one that most afflicted various populations in the past, nor of course is it the disease that has most directly impacted both female and male infertility in history. If we want to infer something of value about the hidden affliction of infertility from the surviving historical sources of evidence documenting either past perceptions or other surviving markers of the venereal diseases, it is vital also to know as much as we can from today's biological, evolutionary, and epidemiological sciences about the differential visibility and infertility consequences of the distinct STIs, and it is crucial not to restrict ourselves only to texts from the past but to embrace all available forms of relevant evidence.

Science—both expert and lay understandings of it—along with belief, morality, public policy, ideology and politics, medicine, education, gender relations, reproductive customs, familial property, and survival strategies have all been involved, often in a highly integrated fashion, in determining the experience and the patterns of STI-related infertility in the past.[39] We need a multiplicity of disciplinary approaches to grasp the interrelations among all these aspects to understand how sexuality, disease, and fertility have had an often hidden but nevertheless influential history in different times and places. For instance, in Western societies, though medical scientists were discussing new findings about the STIs and influencing government policies throughout the first half of the twentieth century, the communication of such knowledge to the general public through sex education in schools or via the mass media remained evasive, sporadic, moralizing, and crudely admonitory at best.[40] It did very little, except in Germany, to publicize the one measure that would have made a difference to communicability of the microorganisms: condom usage.[41] Indeed, in both France and the United States legislation supposed to promote the sanctity and fruitfulness of marriage prohibited the sale of contraceptives.

Among the Haya people in Uganda, as Doyle's chapter 8 documents, the constellation of factors conducive to the spread of fertility-impeding STIs was of course quite different from that in Europe, but it did share the feature of, in part, springing from self-defeating publicly articulated motives. Both popular belief and practical economic considerations dictated that childlessness must be avoided at all costs because it could spell the loss of vital landed property. Consequently, high rates of STIs were exacerbated by a range of contributory practices: impatient, rapid divorce of "barren" wives even within a year of marriage, young wives advised by canny older women to ensure their fertility by going with other supposedly potent men as well as their husbands, older infertile men repeatedly trying to produce an heir with untaken young teenage girls.

Integration with the cultural history of the emotions is important, too. The capacity of biological sterility due to STIs to inflict both physical pain and emotional suffering on women and men is currently still a largely hidden aspect of their history. Nevertheless, it is a crucial aspect of this volume's goals, embracing not only medical, epidemiological, and demographic history but also sexual, gender, social, and emotional history, to acknowledge that lives are damaged by STIs. This is most clearly conveyed in chapter 9 and also in chapters 1 and 2. A public clarion call for historians to embrace and learn from the rapidly changing biological sciences with their new agenda of epigenetics has come in 2014 from Lynn Hunt, the leading cultural historian. Hunt acknowledges that in fact demographic, epidemiological, and environmental historians have been continually engaging with biology since at least the 1960s (and indeed even before that, in French historiography of the Annales school and among Anglophone economic historians and historical geographers). Her call, however, is addressed to the mainstream body of historians who have tended to pursue more exclusively literary, cultural, and intellectual history approaches during the past several decades. It is through a focus on furthering the history of the emotions, to which her own seminal work on *Inventing Human Rights* has made a major contribution, that Hunt has extolled the virtues of all historians engaging with biological sciences and their findings.[42]

The approach adopted in *The Hidden Affliction* fully endorses that call for multidisciplinarity and sharing of knowledge across the humanities and the sciences.[43] Combining diverse knowledge bases helps us to begin to make more sense of the relationship between STIs and infertility in the past, opening-up many illuminating comparative insights.

How Important Have STIs Been as a Cause of Infertility in History?

The simple answer to this question is that currently we do not have extensive documented evidence. Owing to what is understood today by medical science of the capacity of the three main STIs present in the pre-HIV/AIDS era—gonorrhea, syphilis, and chlamydia—to affect fertility negatively, it is certainly eminently plausible that these diseases, especially gonorrhea, may at times have had a very substantial impact, not only on individuals and couples but on the fertility of whole populations, societies, and their cultures, as Roy Scragg argues in chapter 7. Other chapters here also document this.

The biological pathways through which each of these three STIs affect fertility is different. The two most important STIs that, if untreated, are known today to each exert a direct negative impact on the fertility of a proportion of their human hosts are gonorrhea and chlamydia, caused by *Neisseria gonococcus* and the genital serovars of *Chlamydia trachomatis*, respectively. Gonorrhea is epidemiologically the more important of the two, in terms of its quantitative capacity to cause permanent sterility in women through salpingitis, which is the form of pelvic inflammatory disease (PID) specific to the fallopian tubes, resulting in tubal factor infertility (TFI). It causes sterility in women by attaching to the epithelial mucosal cells lining the fallopian tubes, which then results in the destruction of the associated ciliated cells, which provide the hair-like structures that transport the egg from the ovary down the fallopian tube.[44] Damage may be either in the initial section before fertilization can happen or in the final section of the tube before delivery of the fertilized egg to the uterus. In the latter case an ectopic pregnancy can ensue, though of course in the past this would invariably have resulted not in infertility but in the death of the would-be mother. Gonorrhea additionally has a far from insignificant capacity to render infected males infertile through epididymitis: infection and inflammation of the long, coiled tube where sperm matures after initial production in the testes and before ejaculation; the physical blocking of this tube, as shown in Figure 10.3 below (page 320), impedes healthy sperm production.

The principal mechanism through which an infection by chlamydia can damage the fallopian tubes in such a way as ultimately to cause either infertility or ectopic pregnancy is fundamentally different. It occurs as a side effect of the body's immunologic response causing tissue scarring and fibrosis of the tube walls due to an inflammatory cytokine response.[45] Unlike gonorrhea, it seems that the scarring does not progress to the same sterilizing degree in the male epididymitis. A likely reason for this is the lack of a reservoir of indole in the male urogenital system, which is abundantly available among the vaginal microbiota. As is explained in chapter 4, *C. trachomatis* is dependent on tryptophan (an amino acid), which it biosynthesizes from indole. Therefore, a single original episode of infection into the female urogenital system can produce a much longer-lasting episode of disease with continual scarring while *C. trachomatis* remains present, whereas in a male any single episode of infection will run out of tryptophan much sooner, and so scarring will cease until another infection is acquired, introducing a new colony of *C. trachomatis*.

Syphilis, by contrast, has no direct effect on the capacity of either sex to conceive. It probably exerts, overall, a relatively neutral net effect on a population's apparent, observed fertility rate, if simply measured in narrow demographic terms as the collective rate of childbearing. It causes miscarriages, stillbirths, and early deaths among infants, who can contract the disease from infectious mothers either in utero or during parturition shortly after childbirth. This increase in fetal and premature deaths tends, in those many populations throughout history that have practiced breastfeeding for many months after birth, to reduce the average time elapsed before the next conception due to the earlier cessation of lactational amenorrhea and the return of ovulatory cycles. An individual woman's capacity to bear healthy live-born children may be interrupted for a period by an infection with syphilis, but her capacity to conceive is not permanently curtailed. Once the syphilitic infection has been fully contained by her immune system, she will usually be able to take healthy fetuses to term again, provided she has no other illnesses.[46] However, it should be noted that in a population suffering extensively from syphilis, other STIs are always also present along, often, with a range of other vectors of morbidity. Thus, the net effect of syphilis on any real population's capacity to reproduce may not be positive, especially if the disease is widespread in the community, since it exerts a toll of serious morbidity and therefore vulnerability to coinfections on adults of both sexes and also especially on the health and survival of infants, who may register as live births but fail to survive childhood. In chapter 9 Janet McCalman and Rebecca Kippen document such infertility and premature mortality problems of oppressed populations suffering from a heavy burden of syphilis infections in association with other STIs.

The potential of STIs to endanger even the very survival of some island populations was first conclusively demonstrated by the extraordinary pioneering study conducted during the early 1950s by Roy Scragg.[47] In his chapter below, he revisits these findings among the dwindling population of the island of Tabar in New Ireland (today a province of Papua New Guinea). Combining demographic survey and clinical medical histories with rigorous diagnostic investigations including semen microscopy and pelvic X-rays of the fallopian tubes, Scragg overturned the previous dominant view of Pacific Islanders' infertility. This view was derived from the fieldwork and interpretation of the eminent anthropologist and psychiatrist, William H. R. Rivers (sometimes known as the "English Freud"), who held that the islanders were suffering from enervating "culture-shock" following contact with the West.[48]

Scragg found from his medical histories of the infertile that, far from having given up in despair, the islanders' plight was made worse by the behavior of childless, infected older males, desperate to have heirs, who sought young virginal partners, a practice facilitated by the island's sexual culture and rituals. Scragg found very high rates both of double-tubal blockage and male sterility and subfertility (caused mainly by the male gonorrheal sequelae of epididymitis, also known as epididymo-orchitis, or by stricture of the urethra).

Bayliss-Smith's chapter explores this theme further with a comparative historical demographic study of four different island societies of Oceania in the Solomon Islands. On Simbo and Vella Lavella there was a sexually libertarian "Aphrodisian" culture, not dissimilar to Tabar in New Ireland. Bayliss-Smith presents evidence that gonorrhea became prevalent there following first contact in the nineteenth century with Western sailors, whalers and traders, resulting in low birthrates and a documented shrinking population in the subsequent generations. By contrast, he shows that the inhabitants of Malaita and Guadalcanal subscribed to an entirely distinct sexual code of strict virgin marriage—this contrast was also noted historically by maritime visitors. On Malaita and Guadalcanal, Bayliss-Smith is able to document stable high birthrates and a sustained population on the island throughout the period of contact with the West.

Thus, as both Scragg's and Bayliss-Smith's chapters make clear, the gonococcus—biology alone, in other words—does not have the autonomous power to cause the decline of a population. This depends critically also on the moral codes, cultural practices, and accepted behaviors of a society and how these interact with the presence of other diseases in the population. Where such practices combine to positively encourage the coupling of infected individuals with a large proportion of the young females in the community, the most extensive diffusion of the gonococcus among women with an early reproductive age is assured, and this is likely to have the greatest impact on the entire community's infertility, even to the point of threatening the survival of the population.

STIs are, of course, not the only widespread historical afflictions that could have caused populations to experience infertility. Although this volume does not focus its attention on nonsexual sources of infertility, they should be mentioned.[49] Puerperal fever or sepsis after giving birth due to streptococcus infection, can result in secondary sterility (and can also cause loss of the mother's life), as Worboys notes in his chapter. Tragically, as Irvine Loudon has shown, the dangers of puerperal fever were exacerbated during the late nineteenth and early twentieth centuries, due to the increased willingness of (mostly male) doctors to intervene in various ways during childbirth while paying insufficient attention to their own hygienic practices.[50] McCalman and Kippen's chapter 9 presents distressing evidence of some of the unfortunate consequences and of others, too, due to additional shortcomings of medical practices, which can be reconstructed from the preserved case records of the Melbourne Lying-In Hospital from 1883 to 1909.

Two other diseases are also potentially demographically significant. Tuberculosis bacilli can spread to the genital organs among some of those infected and cause consequent sterility (which, unlike gonorrhea, typically takes the form of primary sterility in both sexes, since tuberculosis is usually acquired in childhood, and it is most likely that its nodules will develop to block the fallopian tubes or the epididymis in males during adolescence).[51] Certainly, tuberculosis has been prevalent in many crowded and impoverished populations throughout much of history, and there is some clinical evidence that it could be a cause of infertility at least among a fraction of those manifesting illness and seeking treatment.[52]

The high fevers of the falciparum variant of malaria is the other major nonsexually transmitted disease with infertility implications: these can cause both impaired sperm production for up to two months after the fevers and the possibility of pregnancy loss. Its possible contribution has been evaluated in another major, well-known and well-documented case of the suspected extensive impact of historical STIs on human fertility, the so-called equatorial African infertility belt. This has been the subject of some debate and a sequence of influential studies, which began with those of colonial medical officers raising the alarm in the early twentieth century, as studied by Megan Vaughan.[53] In chapter 8 Doyle reviews this debate and offers a new contribution derived from some of his own researches on the Bahaya and Baganda peoples in contemporary Tanzania and Uganda. By studying the subsequent mid-twentieth-century rise in fertility in these communities Doyle concludes that reduced STIs were probably the most important single factor contributing to a prior decline in infertility but that a range of other influences were also involved, related to the arrival of a much enhanced and more accessible primary health care system during the midcentury decades, itself in part due to the mobilization of resources to deal with the STI threat. This delivered, in addition, falling rates of malarial infection, postpartum infection, and malnutrition. In Tabar, by contrast, Scragg has presented compelling evidence that female gonorrhea infection at early ages was probably the sole cause of the high rates of early twentieth-century infertility, since there was such a spectacular positive effect on fertility of an unusual initiative in Tabar, which saw the universal administration of penicillin to the whole population in the early 1950s. This tells strongly, in that case at least, against the importance of tuberculosis, malaria, or indeed chlamydia, since none of these, unlike gonorrhea (at that time), respond to penicillin.

Thus, the patterns that can be uncovered, where the rare opportunity of the availability of the right evidence occurs, show a strong relationship between gonorrhea and threateningly high levels of infertility in some societies in the past. This comparative historical evidence can be productively juxtaposed with the analytic insights and predictions that have been developed by contemporary epidemiological models of the transmissibility and infectiousness of STIs. This shows that the spread of an STI through a population can be analyzed as the product of three factors: the transmission probability of each specific STI organism; multiplied by the contact rate between those currently infected and those currently uninfected (the "susceptible" population, which technically excludes those enjoying immunity due to a past infection); and further multiplied by the duration a current sufferer remains infectious (before death or recovery).[54]

Evidently, each of these three components of the model has a purely biological but also an equally integral sociocultural and sociomedical aspect to its determination, especially where sexually transmitted diseases are concerned. On the one hand, the different microorganisms have quite distinctive biological properties. The syphilitic spirochete typically elicits a strong symptomatic reaction and antibodies, which makes it unlikely that an infected individual will be unaware of their state of illness and which also means they are highly unlikely to be subsequently reinfected; so a single infection removes most individuals permanently from the pool of susceptibles. It is also an organism that requires access to the bloodstream of a new host via a small abrasion, and so it is not routinely caught from a single sexual encounter with an infectious individual; hence its overall transmission probability is relatively low unless a susceptible individual is exposed regularly to an infected individual (as could happen in a stable relationship, but where one of the two parties has "cheated"). Due to immunity among its ex-victims and relative difficulty of transmission, syphilis tends to exhibit a relatively low prevalence (defined as the proportion of currently infectious cases in the population) and also a relatively low rate of incidence (number of newly infected cases reporting the disease).

Neisseriae gonorrheae, by contrast, eludes the body's immunological defenses and therefore often produces no apparent symptoms in its victims, who may infect others without realizing. With no protective immunity, individuals can continually reinfect one another, and the pool of susceptibles is continuously close to maximum. Thus, in modern populations with sophisticated public health surveillance and laboratory diagnostics, gonorrhea tends to exhibit the epidemiological characteristics of higher prevalence than incidence, within the terms of the epidemiologists' transmission models.

Finally, the several genital serovars of *Chlamydia trachomatis* are also often symptomless because they evade the immunological system by residing within the cytoplasm of body cells for a large part of the life cycle (hence Chlamydia is termed an "obligate intracellular pathogen"). Chlamydia has two developmental stages: the elementary body and the reticulate body. Reticulate bodies are the noninfectious intracellular-dwelling form and they make up the metabolically active replicating stage of the life cycle, through binary fission. After this division the resultant elementary body exits the host cell (through reverse endocytosis), and it is only these elementary bodies that are susceptible to antibiotics in the period before they enter new cell hosts (through endocytosis). Chlamydia therefore has the additional distinctive property that hosts can remain infectious for a very long time, even with modern treatments. Not all the active organisms are eliminated by any one single course of antibiotics, and so treatment has to be repeated several times before a victim is entirely clear. Consequently, in modern populations its incidence level is approximately as high as its very high prevalence level.

On the other hand, all of the three dimensions of the epidemiologists' transmission model are also subject to sociocultural, as well as biological, codetermination. This involves malleable beliefs and behaviors, as well as scientific understandings and diffused medical practices in relation to the STIs. The different sexual and gendered attitudes and behavioral norms of different societies and of their various subcultures—often reflecting ethnicity and past migration and current mobility patterns as well as socioeconomic inequalities—can all influence patterns of contact and transmission of the STIs and, consequently, their capacity to affect overall fertility. For instance, Doyle's research reported in chapter 8 includes interview evidence that reveals not only levels of infertility but also the family-size aspirations of potential parents. Both factors adapted across generations in East Africa, as people attempted to respond both to the implications of secondary sterility and to the consequent perceived economic predicaments for the family unit of fewer children. Conversely, Doyle also documents the cultural responses following the arrival of penicillin, which was perceived to have substantially lifted the threat. As a result, aspirations for family size now increased significantly, showing how rising fertility was not simply an involuntary product of the lifting of a biological restraint but also reflected the cultural values and changing desires of the populace. Similarly, as the earlier reference to modern populations with modern laboratory diagnostics makes abundantly clear, changes in medical technology and associated public education propaganda can alter a population's symptom-recognition capabilities and so can influence voluntarily preferred patterns of sexual contact. As Doyle also shows, the arrival of penicillin in East Africa had similar impact to that seen in the Pacific, but with widely differing effects on sexual behavior. In Buganda it was viewed as a license for a rise in male promiscuity without fear, whereas in neighboring Buhaya marriage became more stable once STI-related infertility was reduced because wives were more likely to be able to produce the heir that married men desperately wanted (for land-inheritance purposes).

The clinical epidemiological transmission model very helpfully identifies the key factors and their interrelationships that produce different rates of the spread of different STIs. It has been developed primarily to assist contemporary public health analysts, with access to the appropriate data, to design prevention and treatment strategies through understanding the dynamics of rates of transmission between infectious sections of the population, usually of course a minority at any point in time, and the uninfected "susceptibles"—the rest of the population. However, the framework of understanding that the model offers can equally provide historians with a critical resource to help them place in epidemiological context the forms of evidence available to them on the incidence and the prevalence of STIs in past populations, even though they will not necessarily have all the range of information available to fully operationalize the model empirically.

For instance, Turner and colleagues report a 1990s study finding gonorrhea rates strongly correlated with poverty both nationally and in a more detailed study in South London, where incidence was ten to twenty times higher among black Caribbean ethnic groups than among whites, reflecting similar, earlier findings in the distinct circumstances of black poverty in United States.[55] In London black males were identified as also performing a "bridging" function, since black women tended to have only black male partners, but black males also had white female partners. Obviously, the further explanation for this particular pattern lies in the intersectionality of cultural and socioeconomic relationships of gendered power and inequality.

By comparison, McCalman and Kippen in chapter 9 investigate in illuminating detail the health and infertility problems of an impoverished section of the British and Irish population 150 years earlier than Turner et al.'s study. Without the prospect of treatment in the pre-antibiotic era, a proportion of those infected were also marked by the sequelae of infertility. The primary sources relate to nine thousand female and sixteen thousand male convicts arriving in Van Diemen's Land (Tasmania) between the 1840s and 1860s. These documents allow exploration of the infertility consequences for some of these most unfortunate individuals, those whose lives were lived within the eye of the storm of the structural violence perpetrated on the poor of Britain during the early decades of expansionary industrial capitalism. They find 80 percent of the transported males remaining in Tasmania were recorded as fathering no more than one child, while over 35 percent of the females were subsequently infertile, notably those originating from the streets (literally) of London—and of Britain's industrial cities. The designation "on the town" in their transportation record signified a previous life in Britain of survival through commercial sex, which was probably part of the coping strategies for many very poor women in urban Britain, especially after the withdrawal of long-standing sources of social security and the new practice of stigmatizing unmarried mothers brought in with the draconian, moralizing reforms of the New Poor Law of 1834.[56]

The details the authors have elicited from their various Australian sources also include the information that in Melbourne in the 1870s there was a child sex trade related to the folk superstition (brought from Britain) that sex with a virgin was a cure for the pox. This, then, is a practice that links, with a common cause, the infertility of some of the urban poor in Australia with that of the Haya in Tanzania and the Melanesian island of Tabar, where it was also found by Doyle and by Scragg that the patriarchal power of infertile or infected elderly males to command the sexual services of younger females was a significant cause of STI transmission. Those transactions formed a bridge, in the terminology of the epidemiologists' transmission model, between the infected and the susceptible sections of the population and thereby accounted significantly for a wider prevalence of gonorrhea among young females than would otherwise have been the case, so maximizing its sterilizing consequences.

Thus, several of the chapters here show that historic STIs significantly impacted fertility, often associated with the dynamics of power and inequality between the sexes, the races, and different individuals in imperialist and capitalist contexts.[57] In helping us to understand more fully the hidden history of infertility and sexual disease, this volume exposes a further aspect of the structured violence that characterizes the patterns of health in human history.[58]

When Was Infertility Caused by STIs, and When Did They Originate?

The vital importance of drawing on multidisciplinary knowledge is nowhere more evident than in relation to the most fundamental of questions for a volume devoted to the history of sex, disease, and infertility: when did the STIs causing infertility first appear in human history?

The easy assumption that the "venereal diseases" must surely have always been with human society, since time immemorial, rests in fact on rather slender evidence. In chapter 1 Flemming discusses anew the long-running debate over whether the disease first named as gonorrhea in texts of ancient Greek medicine should be equated with the disease currently recognized by that term. She concludes that skepticism on this point is the more justifiable position, because a careful rereading of the texts of antiquity reveals that the two conjoined symptoms that are today recognized as diagnostic of likely gonorrhea—pain in urination combined with a discharge—never in fact occur together in those texts. Flemming's view is that these texts, referring for instance to an involuntary flowing of seed, are more reliable for informing us about sexual behavior and attitudes in Hellenistic society: in particular, a commonly held view that lack of moderation and self-control might impair fertility. This opening chapter in the volume thereby provides an intriguing echo of the furious debate in Germany just over a century ago over the same intellectual turf of classical texts, also in relation to the then-new findings of laboratory science, in this case over the issue of the disputed origins of syphilis rather than gonorrhea.[59] That debate still remains an unsettled matter between the thesis of a European or American "origin" of syphilis, also addressed here in chapter 3 by Roberts and Redfern.

It may well be that the classical texts are in fact more consistent with reportage on manifestations of chlamydial, not gonorrheal, infection. As Flemming notes, that would also be consistent with the argument that the pronatalist Roman state would have been hard-pressed to maintain its demographic vigor if the gonococcus of modern clinical experience had been present, given the socially extensive scale of Rome's commercial sex industry. One of the conclusions of the research reviewed in this volume is that chlamydia does not appear to have quite the same potential as gonorrhea for causing widespread, community sterility and that it would not, alone, have caused population decline. There are certainly a number of symptoms in the classical sources that are much more consistent with chlamydia (such as bleeding between periods and increased vaginal discharge in conjunction with low, abdominal pain).

Chlamydia's ancient lineage would be a striking reversal of previous assumptions. Chlamydia has had the superficial appearance of being, rather like HIV/AIDs, a brand new epidemic sweeping through the populations of the world in the past few decades. However, Worboys's interpretation, shared by Clarke and Taylor in their review, contributory to chapter 4, of the long-term history of both the ocular and genital trachoma clades is that this has been primarily an illusionary statistical artifact. It is the result of dramatic improvements in the observational instruments developed to track a widely prevalent organism, which, it has been progressively found, has at least fifteen distinct serovars, some of which are adapted to ocular epithelial cells, while the original variants colonized genital tract tissues.[60]

As chapter 4 by Clarke and Taylor shows, it is highly probable that chlamydia, the most newly identified of the three major pre-HIV STIs, is in fact the longest-lived unwanted companion of the human species among all the currently known STIs. This follows from the fact that it has a particularly complex parasitic life cycle, living within the mucous membrane cells of its host for a considerable portion of its life cycle, a pattern that cannot have evolved at all rapidly. Second, *C. trachomatis* variants are commonly found across so many diverse species, famously including koalas, but also reptiles.[61] (It is a so far unexplained oddity that all other large primates—except *Homo sapiens*—are among the minority of vertebrates that are apparently not afflicted by chlamydia.)

A newly available and rapidly developing scientific approach for examining the historical provenance of disease organisms derives from gene-sequencing technologies applied to the study of genomes and their evolutionary ancestry (in terms of Bayesian phylogenetics). As Clarke explains in his contribution to the joint chapter with Taylor, these techniques permit bounds to be placed around the likely timescale of existence of different organisms, in terms of reproductive generations. These are estimates from the knowledge of the complexity of the organism's genetic structure and calculations of its associated "molecular clock." This technique uses the mutation rate of biomolecules—that is, molecules involved in the maintenance and metabolic processes of living organisms—to deduce the point in their prehistory when two or more current life forms diverged, termed their "time to most recent common ancestor," tMCRA (the biomolecular data used for such calculations are usually nucleotide sequences for DNA or amino acid sequences for proteins). This line of research confirms that the human variants of *C. trachomatis* have almost certainly accompanied humankind at least throughout the era of recorded written history and, furthermore, that the urogenital trachoma clade (T1), transmitted sexually, is the earlier variant, from which the ocular clade (T2) mutated.

The latest findings using these new scientific techniques currently indicate that gonorrhea, by contrast, may be a relative newcomer, emerging circa 1544–1622, thus provisionally confirming Flemming's skeptical reading of the ancient texts.[62] However, gonorrhea has a well-attested capacity in the twentieth century to adapt and coevolve rapidly in the presence of antibiotic threats, which has resulted in a classic "Red Queen" dogfight between medical science and gonorrhea. The sulfonamides were first successfully applied to cure gonorrhea in the late 1930s but were then quickly found before the end of the 1940s to be less effective than initially hoped for and were then replaced by penicillin—for a while.[63] Indeed, renewed concern over antibiotic-resistant gonorrhea has in part stimulated the current research on its genome.[64] We cannot therefore be sure, as Scragg avers, that earlier mutational variants of the gonococcus did not previously exist and then disappear before the mid-twentieth century making them now unavailable for the genomic back-projection dating technique.

If correct, however, then this latest biogenomic research interestingly suggests that the form of gonorrhea with which modern medical science is familiar and which carries its threat to fertility may have an approximately similar, relatively short, history of afflicting humankind to that of syphilis. That would be the case if, also, a version of the old "Columbian" theory was proved to be correct, namely, that sexually transmitted syphilis first erupted in western Europe shortly after the return of Columbus from the Americas. Indeed, Piers Mitchell proposes a variant of this theory, arguging that a less harmful, non-venereal treponemal disease, widely prevalent in the pre-Columbian Americas (i.e., yaws or endemic syphilis, which, in sufficiently warm climates, can be passed merely by skin and surface contact) was brought back to temperate Europe, where in the climatically different and more urban environment it rapidly mutated into the devastating venereal form, dependent in these temperate climates on access to the temperature-controlled environment internal to the human body.[65] If the provenance of both syphilis and gonorrhea, each originating sometime in the late fifteenth and sixteenth centuries, were, indeed, to be proved correct, this would of course bring up the intriguing possibility that the emergence of venereal syphilis in comparatively recent human history may have also had something to do with the emergence, at the same time or shortly thereafter, of gonorrhea (or possibly even vice versa, or some form of coevolution), further illustrating the significance of Emmanuel Le Roy Ladurie's celebrated thesis of the importance of the microbial unification of the world in these early modern centuries of transoceanic contact.[66]

However, there is much yet to be further researched about the putative origins and history of syphilis itself, before any such speculations about possible early modern coevolution with gonorrhea can be further entertained. As the chapter by Roberts and Redfern indicates, bioarchaeology remains divided over the interpretation of major finds of skeletal remains, notably those recovered from the St. Mary Spital site in London, which has permitted analysis by chronological phasing of large numbers of European remains going back to the eleventh century, long before the Columbian encounter with the Americas. This evidence, placed alongside that from other Eurasian excavated sites and also from the Americas, is critically reviewed in their chapter. The evidence is tantalizing in suggesting the possible—but unfortunately not entirely conclusive—presence of venereal syphilis in Europe before 1492. For the data to be entirely convincing, there would need to be a good number of intact, whole skeletons, definitely dated to pre-1492 and exhibiting the unambiguous syphilitic combination of both long-bone tibia deformities (sabre shins) and frontal, cranial pitting of the skull in the same individual. There are very few such attested cases pre-1492, but a relative abundance for the following century. Thus, the archaeological evidence currently available would also be consistent with the proposition that even if venereal syphilis did exist in pre-Columbian Europe, for some reason it may not have existed very extensively. Its infectious or its pathological—or both—characteristics may have been transformed shortly after the return of Columbus and his crew. This could have been due to coincident changes in the socioecological environment and sexual behavior of urban communities in Europe at this time. Alternatively, the archaeological evidence may be picking up on the effects of something else entirely in pre-1492 Europe, including perhaps the skeletal marks of disease-causing microorganisms no longer extant. In that case the sexually transmitted *Treponema pallidum* may have been genuinely new to Europe after 1492, hence its well-documented rapid and frightening impact in that virgin population and the apparent absence of pre-1500 evidence for it elsewhere in Eurasia.[67]

Treponema pallidum pallidum, which causes venereal syphilis, is, like the other treponemes—*Treponema pallidum endemicum* (bejel) and *Treponema pallidum carateum* (pinta)—both morphologically and serologically identical to *Treponema pallidum pertenue*, which causes yaws. Phylogenetic analysis has established that yaws is the oldest of the four treponemes and that there are minute genetic differences between each of them.[68] Yaws, pinta, and bejel (sometimes called "Arab" syphilis) are all endemic to rural populations and are relatively easily passed by simple, physical contact. Yaws is prevalent in humid, warm conditions and the other two in less humid and even arid (bejel) but also warm conditions.[69] Venereal syphilis appears to be adapted more exclusively to a sexual transmission path and is therefore not dependent on any specific climatic conditions but is dependent on intimate human contact. It is therefore likely to be strongly human density–dependent and to flourish in urban settings, especially if there are no strict codes of restricted sexual interaction—or if such codes are not observed (as for instance in wartime by armies, which are considered to have been a principal agent in the frightening proliferation of syphilis in Europe during the protracted wars on the Italian peninsula between 1494 and 1559). Yaws was quite definitely endemic in South America when Columbus arrived, and it would have conferred cross-immunity against syphilis on the indigenous population.[70] Venereal syphilis could therefore also have been present in the pre-Columbian Americas, but, if so, it would have been at relatively low levels of incidence due to cross-immunities and also it would not have appeared as a distinctive health threat to the community, since quite a number of dermatological symptoms are common between yaws and venereal syphilis (though only syphilis exerts the potentially fatal tertiary-stage effects on a proportion of its victims).[71] Its manifestation as a widespread and apparently new illness would then have become possible only when *Treponema pallidum pallidum* was brought back by Columbus's crew to temperate Europe, where it could spread within urban populations with no cross-immunities, since there was no yaws in Europe.

It currently remains unclear whether either venereal syphilis or gonorrhea in fact afflicted any human populations in the world before the 1490s and differences of opinion on this are expressed by different contributors to this volume. The latest genomics research would back a post-Columbian dating for Treponema pallidum.[72] Similar research methods would also appear to suggest that the strains of gonorrhea available to science for study today probably were not present before the sixteenth century. However, as noted, the gonococcus, unlike Treponema pallidum, is a formidably adaptive and mutable microorganism.[73] Other now-extinct variants may well have preexisted, though whether posing the same threat to human fertility we may never know. Equally, research also suggests that, independently of either syphilis or gonorrhea, due to the enduring presence of genital serovars of *Chlamydia trachomatis*, the capacity of sexual behavior to transmit infections that cause infertility has been a hidden affliction of long provenance among human populations. The more visible and well-studied history of human affliction from the ocular variants of *C. trachomatis*, documented by Taylor in chapter 4, suggests that chlamydia may have become a serious threat to the infertility of human groups only when living for long periods in conditions that were crowded, unhygienic, and stressed. Such conditions probably became a regular experience in the course of human history only after the domestication of plants and animals led to increasingly dense settlement patterns, as in the urban centers of past empires and more generally across the globe after the industrial revolution's intensification of densely crowded forms of urbanization and the expansion of the transoceanic communications, whose effects ultimately even on island populations in the Pacific are so fascinatingly documented in chapters 6 and 7.

The chapters in parts 3 and 4 of this volume show that the history of STIs and their perceived capacity to cause infertility—even to the point of "race suicide," as a eugenics-inflected language over fears of depopulation or "degeneration" portrayed these issues in the early twentieth-century decades—was thoroughly integrated in diverse ways into imperial, and postimperial political economy and its accompanying racial discourses and medico-scientific practices. As chapters 7 and 9 document in certain Pacific islands and in outback Australia, indigenous populations occupying territory with little strategic or economic value were perceived fatalistically as "dying races" by the occupying European powers. Yet, in East Africa, where military control of territory was competitive between the imperial powers and where tax revenue was wanted from the local population to pay for their "protection," proactive medical policies were pursued, in collaboration with local leaders, in the attempt to forestall unwanted depopulation. Intriguing and unexpected parallels occured: government-sponsored health policies to control the fertility-threatening STIs emerged as an early universalist, free health care system to protect the military and industrial effectiveness of the British working class in the interwar United Kingdom and, almost simultaneously, was also instigated in colonial East Africa to protect Africans. Furthermore, while in both the Pacific and in East Africa, gonorrhea may well have been brought to these indigenous populations by outsiders, venereal syphilis may also have been inadvertently exacerbated by European doctors. They often misdiagnosed, as venereal syphilis, various symptoms of the non-venereal tropical treponemes, which in fact conferred immunity against syphilis; when the latter were "cured" by Western antibiotics, venereal syphilis could become a greater problem in such tropical populations.

Behind the Veil

To make progress with the study of sex, disease, and infertility, we need the combined—not separated—insights of very different disciplines and their approaches, embracing history and the life sciences. We need to study texts and all other relevant sources of information on the interactions in different times and places between humans and the relevant microorganisms—those that we today recognize as causing the diseases of syphilis, gonorrhea, and chlamydia but that have had revealingly different designations (or none at all) in the past and in other cultures. We need to relate this to changing cultures of the perception of these diseases and also to our contemporary, increasing, and quite rapidly changing scientific and epidemiological understanding of the characteristics and the likely natural histories of the relevant microorganisms, which we today identity as *T. pallidum*, *N. gonorrheae*, and

C. trachomatis. This introduction can only hope to provide a survey and some summary—but necessarily provisional—thoughts, which reflect the current state of knowledge at this point in time.

Each of these three major historical STIs was capable of preventing or prematurely destroying human life. Each has its unique characteristics of concealment as a hidden affliction, both at the microbial level and as manifest disease. Syphilis, though often evident and sometimes quite hideous in its bodily manifestations, could also hide in plain sight as the "great imitator," causing a wide range of symptoms similar to many other diseases, while its entirely transparent spirochete, the pale treponeme, eluded microscopic identification for decades.[74]

Gonorrhea was the great deceiver. It was thought of as "merely" the clap, *Tripper* (in German) or the jocular *chaude pisse*, which remained the subject of manly banter in France as recently as the mid-twentieth century, as chapter 11 mentions. It was also often completely asymptomatic for many women. Yet, of the three, it was the most deceptive in its destructive powers, being the most ferocious sterilizer of both sexes.

Chlamydia, however, was the most clandestine of all. It was the last to be literally uncloaked by science, not emerging as a clinical entity—an identified microorganism officially considered definitely responsible for a defined disease—until as recently as the 1970s, as chapter 5 recounts. Yet in all probability it has abided with its human host in its several genital serovar forms, for many millennia. Like gonorrhea, it silently sterilizes a proportion of women infected, with the majority of them unaware of the danger they are in, and it is consequently the subject of massive screening efforts today.

However, unlike gonorrhea, which has been documented to have brought some island populations to their knees, it seems unlikely that chlamydia, alone, has exerted such a virulent sterilizing power on an entire population. As would be predicted from evolutionary theory, such a very long-term and ubiquitous, if largely unsuspected, parasite accompanying the human species through much of its history would be highly adaptive and therefore unlikely to exert the kind of scale of effect on its host's reproductive capacities as to threaten their mutual survival. But that does not of course mean that it has not also been responsible for much individual psychological pain and suffering for the many individuals who found themselves inexplicably infertile, as most searingly brought to life for theater audiences in Federico García Lorca's stage masterpiece of 1934, *Yerma*.

The essays in this volume cannot realistically aspire to move us in a single leap from a state of dimly perceived ignorance to a comprehensive solution to the riddle at the volume's heart, the history of pre-HIV STIs and their manifold consequences for human infertility. For instance, there are no chapters here focused on evidence relating to either Asia or the Americas. Though the geographic and temporal coverage may be finite and only partial, there has been a more comprehensive effort to draw together a sufficiently wide, if not quite "global," range of relevant disciplinary knowledges with which to approach an understanding of the riddle. We may perhaps, with the appearance of this volume, no longer be under the spell of the enigma, and, though we may yet have much to contend with, it is hoped that we have at least made a helpful start with unwrapping some of the mystery.

Notes

1. Google Ngrams indicates that since 1994 the abbreviation *STI* has been increasingly replacing *STD* (sexually transmitted disease), in recognition of the clinical importance of the asymptomatic nature, especially in women, of both gonorrhea and chlamydia. Ngrams also indicates that previously the collective noun, *venereal disease*, was about twice as commonly used as *venereal diseases* throughout the twentieth century, until both were overtaken around 1983 by the abbreviation *STD*, which had been on the rise since the early 1950s. https://books.google.com/ngrams/graph?content=STDs%2CSTIs%2Cvenereal+disease%2Cvenereal+diseases&year_start=1900&year_end=2008&corpus=18&smoothing=5&share=&direct_url=t1%3B%2CSTDs%3B%2Cc0%3B.t1%3B%2CSTIs%3B%2Cc0%3B.t1%3B%2Cvenereal%20disease%3B%2Cc0%3B.t1%3B%2Cvenereal%20diseases%3B%2Cc0, accessed February 14, 2019. Readers will note that in the text of this chapter and elsewhere in the volume the terms *venereal disease(s)* and *STI* are both in use (and sometimes *STD*), with the usage dependent on context.

2. For the pioneering study demonstrating the early twentieth-century origins of HIV/AIDs in Africa, see John Iliffe, *The African AIDS Epidemic: A History* (Athens: Ohio University Press, 2006).

3. The three other variants are *Treponema pallidum pertenue* (yaws), *Treponema pallidum endemicum* (endemic syphilis or bejel), and *Treponema pallidum carateum* (pinta), none of which are specifically sexually transmitted or cause fertility-related problems.

4. Lauren Arnesen, Suzanne Serruya, and Pablo Duran, "Gestational Syphilis and Stillbirth in the Americas: A Systematic Review and Meta-analysis," *Revista Panamericana de Salud Pública* 37, no. 6 (2015): 422–29.

5. For an example, see Simon Szreter, "Treatment Rates for the Pox in Early Modern England: A Comparative Estimate of the Prevalence of Syphilis in the City of Chester and Its Rural Vicinity in the 1770s," *Continuity and Change* 32, no. 2 (2017): 183–223.

6. See Simon Szreter, "The Prevalence of Syphilis in England and Wales on the Eve of the Great War: Re-visiting the Estimates of the Royal Commission on Venereal Diseases, 1913–1916," *Social History of Medicine* 27, no. 3 (2014): 508–29; see page 528 on Swedish and British evidence.

7. Richard Pattman et al., eds., *Oxford Handbook of Genitourinary Medicine, HIV, and Sexual Health*, 2nd ed. (Oxford: Oxford University Press, 2010).

8. Ulla Larsen et al., "Suffering Infertility: The Impact of Infertility on Women's Life Experiences in Two Nigerian Communities," *Journal of Biosocial Science* 42 (2010): 787–814; Aditya Bharadwaj, *Conceptions: Infertility and Procreative Technologies in India* (Oxford: Berghahn 2016); Michaela Kreyenfeld and Dirk Konietzka, eds., *Childlessness in Europe: Contexts, Causes and Consequences* (Cham, Switzerland: Springer Open, 2017). However, this is a relatively new development, with the first substantial global academic focus on the subject appearing as recently as 2002: Marcia C. Inhorn and Frank van Balen, eds., *Infertility around the Globe: New Thinking on Childlessness, Gender and Reproductive Technologies* (Berkeley: University of California Press, 2002).

9. Danielle G. Tsevat et al., "Sexually Transmitted Diseases and Infertility," *American Journal of Obstetrics and Gynecology* 216 (2017): 1–9, https://doi.org/10.1016/j.ajog.2016.08.008.

10. See the many contributions to Gayle Davis and Tracey Loughran, eds., *The Palgrave Handbook of Infertility in History: Approaches, Contexts, Perspectives* (London: Palgrave Macmillan 2017). The editors discuss in their introduction the limited attention historians have previously given to the subject, identifying the only dedicated previous study as Naomi Pfeffer's polemic, *The Stork and the Syringe: A Political History of Reproductive Medicine* (Cambridge: Polity, 1993). There is also now a historical monograph: Daphna Oren-Magidor, *Infertility in Early Modern England* (London: Palgrave Macmillan 2017); and a journal special issue on medical understandings: Daphna Oren-Magidor and Catherine Rider, "Infertility in Medieval and Early Modern Medicine," *Social History of Medicine* 29 (2016): 211–23. See also Rebecca Flemming, "The Invention of Infertility in the Classical Greek World: Medicine, Divinity, and Gender," *Bulletin of the History of Medicine* 87 (2013): 565–90, https://doi.org/10.1353/bhm.2013.0064.

11. This is a statement about the output of historians. There has of course been plenty of significant attention given by clinicians, demographers, and public health epidemiologists to infertility aspects of gonorrhea and more recently chlamydia and HIV/AIDS. In his extensive history of STDs, Milton Lewis restricts his discussion of the relationship with infertility to a review of the Butlin-Gray debate (see below, note 14): *Thorns on the Rose: The History of Sexually Transmitted Diseases in Australia in International Perspective* (Canberra: Australian Government, 1998): 34–37, 365–67. A historical survey volume of STDs in Asia and the Pacific, though generally informative, does not appear to mention infertility at any point, and there is only one point in a companion survey volume on Africa where the subject is mentioned, which is briefly in relation to Uganda in the 1950s and 1960s:

Milton Lewis, Scott Bamber, and Michael Waugh, eds., *Sex, Disease and Society: A Comparative History of Sexually Transmitted Diseases and HIV/AIDS in Asia and the Pacific* (London: Greenwood, 1997); Philip W. Setel, Milton Lewis, and Maryinez Lyons, eds., *Histories of Sexually Transmitted Diseases and HIV/AIDS in Sub-Saharan Africa* (London: Greenwood, 1997), 108–9, 115.

12. A selection, only, of such studies includes Alain Corbin, *Women for Hire: Prostitution and Sexuality in France after 1850* (1978; repr., Cambridge, MA: Harvard University Press, 1990); Judith R. Walkowitz, *Prostitution and Victorian Society: Women, Class and the State* (Cambridge: Cambridge University Press, 1980); Kenneth Ballhatchet, *Race, Sex, and Class under the Raj: Imperial Attitudes and Policies and Their Critics, 1793–1905* (London: Weidenfeld and Nicholson 1980); Claude Quétel, *History of Syphilis* (1986; repr., Cambridge: Polity, 1990); Allan M. Brandt, *No Magic Bullet: A Social History of Venereal Disease in the United States since 1880* (Oxford: Oxford University Press, 1987); Lesley A. Hall, *Hidden Anxieties: Male Sexuality, 1900–1950* (Cambridge: Polity, 1991); Jon Arrizabalga, John Henderson and Roger French, eds., *The Great Pox in Renaissance Europe* (New Haven: Yale University Press, 1997); Mary Spongberg, *Feminizing Venereal Disease: the Body of the Prostitute in Nineteenth-Century Medical Discourse* (New York: New York University Press 1997); J. David Oriel, *The Scars of Venus: A History of Venereology* (London: Springer, 1998); Randolph Trumbach, *Sex and the Gender Revolution. Volume One.* (Chicago, University of Chicago Press, 1998), chap.7 "The Foul Disease"; Peter Baldwin, *Contagion and the State in Europe, 1830–1930* (Cambridge: Cambridge University Press, 1999), chap. 5; Lutz Sauerteig, *Krankheit, Sexualität, Gesellschaft: Geschlechtskrankheiten und Gesundheitspolitik in Deutschland im 19. und frühen 20. Jahrhundert* (Stuttgart: Steiner, 1999); Roger Davidson, *Dangerous Liaisons: A Social History of Venereal Disease in Twentieth-Century Scotland* (Amsterdam: Rodopi, 2000); Roger Davidson and Lesley A. Hall, eds., *Sex, Sin and Suffering: Venereal Disease and European Society since 1870* (London: Routledge, 2001); Philippa Levine, *Prostitution, Race and Politics: Policing Venereal Disease in the British Empire* (London: Routledge, 2003); Kevin Siena, ed., *Sins of the Flesh: Responding to Sexual Disease in Early Modern Europe* (Toronto: Centre for Reformation and Renaissance Studies, 2005); Kevin Siena, *Venereal Disease, Hospitals and the Urban Poor: London's "Foul Wards," 1600–1800* (Rochester, NY: University of Rochester Press, 2004); Antje Kampf, *Mapping Out the Venereal Wilderness: Public Health and STD in New Zealand, 1920–1980* (Berlin: LIT Verlag 2007); Gayle Davis, *The Cruel Madness of Love: Sex, Syphilis and Psychiatry in Scotland, 1880–1930* (Amsterdam: Rodopi, 2008); Claudia Stein, *Negotiating the French Pox in Early Modern Germany* (Farnham: Ashgate, 2009); Philip Howell, *Geographies of Regulation: Policing Prostitution in Nineteenth-Century Britain and the Empire* (Cambridge: Cambridge University Press, 2009); Laura J. McGough, *Gender, Sexuality and Syphilis in Early Modern Venice: The Disease That Came to Stay* (London: Palgrave Macmillan, 2011); Julia Laite, *Common Prostitutes and Ordinary Citizens: Commercial Sex in London, 1885–1960* (Basingstoke: Palgrave Macmillan, 2011); Lisa Featherstone, *Let's Talk*

about Sex: Histories of Sexuality in Australia from Federation to the Pill (Newcastle-on-Tyne: Cambridge Scholars 2011), chap. 4; Christian Bonah and Anja Laukötter, eds., "Screening Diseases: Films on Sex Hygiene in Germany and France in the First Half of the 20th Century," special issue, *Gesnerus* 72, no. 1 (2015): 5–158; Monika Pietrzak-Franger, *Syphilis in Victorian Literature and Culture: Medicine, Knowledge and the Spectacle of Victorian Invisibility* (Cham: Palgrave Macmillan 2017); Kari Nixon and Lorenzo Servitje, eds, *Syphilis and Subjectivity: From the Victorians to the Present* (Cham: Palgrave Macmillan, 2018); Noelle Gallagher, *Itch, Clap, Pox: Venereal Disease in the Eighteenth-Century Imagination* (Yale University Press 2018). For two overviews, see Kevin Siena, "'The Venereal Disease,' 1500–1800," and Lesley A. Hall, "Sexual Disease since 1750," both in *The Routledge History of Sex and the Body 1500 to the Present*, ed. Sarah Toulalan and Kate Fisher (New York: Routledge, 2013), 463–78, 479–92.

13. But see Donna T. Andrew, *Philanthropy and the Police: London Charity in the Eighteenth Century* (Princeton: Princeton University Press, 1989), 98–134; and Anne Hanley, "'The Great Foe to the Reproduction of the Race': Changing Medical Knowledge and Practice; Diagnosing and Treating Infertility Caused by Venereal Diseases, 1880–1914," in Davis and Loughran, *Palgrave Handbook of Infertility*, 335–58. There is no mention of the link with infertility in Ornella Moscucci's pioneering study, *The Science of Woman: Gynecology and Gender in England, 1800–1929* (Cambridge: Cambridge University Press, 1990).

14. Shane Doyle, *Before HIV: Sexuality, Fertility and Mortality in East Africa, 1900–1980* (Oxford: Oxford University Press, 2013); Mick Worboys, "Unsexing Gonorrhea: Bacteriologists, Gynaecologists and Suffragists in Britain, 1860–1920," *Social History of Medicine* 17, no. 1 (2004): 31–59; Elliott Bowen, "Limits of the Lab: Diagnosing 'Latent Gonorrhea,' 1872–1910," *Bulletin of the History of Medicine* 87 (2013): 63–85; Megan Vaughan, *Curing Their Ills: Colonial Power and African Illness* (Stanford, CA: Stanford University Press, 1991), chap. 6. The thesis of aboriginal decline due to STI infertility was championed by Butlin and contested by Gray: Noel Butlin, *Our Original Aggression: Aboriginal Populations of Southeastern Australia, 1788–1850* (Sydney: Allen and Unwin, 1983); Alan Gray, "Some Myths in the Demography of Aboriginal Australia," *Journal of Australian Population Association* 2 (1985): 136–49; see also Hanley, "Great Foe."

15. Art and literature at this time was much preoccupied with fears of syphilis and particularly its supposed hereditary nature. Meegan Kennedy, "Syphilis and the Hysterical Female: The Limits of Realism in Sarah Grand's *The Heavenly Twins*," *Women's Writing* 11 (2004): 259–80.

16. On the slow and reluctant reception of "latent" gonorrhea in Britain, see Worboys, "Unsexing Gonorrhea," who notes that William Japp Sinclair, professor of obstetrics and gynecology at the University of Manchester, was an exceptional early advocate of Noeggrath's findings; see also Bowen, "Limits of the Lab" and, more generally, Hanley, "Great Foe."

17. Margaret Marsh and Wanda Ronner, *The Empty Cradle: Infertility in America from Colonial Times to the Present* (Baltimore: Johns Hopkins University Press, 1996), 89–92, 116–18; Brandt, *No Magic Bullet*, 11–17.

18. Brandt, *No Magic Bullet*, chap. 4; Thomas Parran, *Shadow on the Land: Syphilis* (New York: Reynald and Hitchcock 1937).

19. As chapter 4 details, the species *Chlamydia trachomatis* comprises at least eight variants—serovars—that cause the fertility-threatening genital infections with which this volume is primarily interested, as well as four that cause ocular disease and three LGV variants producing lymphogranuloma venerum.

20. Joseph A. McFalls and Marguerite H. McFalls, *Disease and Fertility* (London: Academic Press, 1984), pt. 3. The literature on HIV and AIDS is legion, especially for sub-Saharan Africa. For the best single historical account of the disease, see Iliffe, *African AIDs Epidemic*; and for an example of the work of a leading analyst of HIV and infertility in Africa, see Larsen, "Suffering Infertility." On the timing of evolving public perceptions of the international AIDS threat, see Virginia Berridge, *AIDS in the UK: The Making of Policy, 1981–1994* (Oxford: Oxford University Press, 1996); and Rich A. McKay, *Patient Zero and the Making of the AIDS Epidemics* (Chicago: University of Chicago Press, 2017).

21. Inhorn and van Balen, *Infertility around the Globe*, pt. 1, esp chap. 2; Marcia C. Inhorn, ed., *Reproductive Disruptions: Gender, Technology and Biopolitics in the New Millennium* (London: Berghahn 2007). For the prior elucidation of the politics of reproduction and the associated concept of "stratified reproduction," see Faye D. Ginsburg and Rayna Rapp, eds., *Conceiving the New World Order: The Global Politics of Reproduction* (Berkeley: University of California Press, 1995).

22. Caroline Bledsoe, *Contingent Lives: Fertility, Time and Ageing in West Africa* (Chicago: University of Chicago Press, 2002), 228.

23. Worboys has noted that it was gonorrhea itself that was the first disease seen to satisfy Koch's four postulates for proving a specific bacteriological etiology for a communicable disease and thereby heralding this shift from doctors defining disease according to symptoms and effects on the body's functioning and instead increasingly turning to the laboratory for microscopic or serological identification of the presence of specific microbes: "Unsexing Gonorrhea," 41–42; and see K. M. Flegel, "Changing Concepts of the Nosology of Gonorrhea and Syphilis," *Bulletin of the History of Medicine* 48, no. 4 (1974): 571–88, 576–84.

24. Oriel, *Scars of Venus*, 73; see also Bowen, "Limits of the Lab." For documentation of the difficulties, confusions, and crude racial stereotyping that even doctors trained in Germany, where the science of the diseases was most advanced, continued to experience in the period before the Great War in dealing with the practicalities of attempting to treat the disease, see Daniel J. Walther, *Sex and Control: Venereal Disease, Colonial Physicians and Indigenous Agency in German Colonialism, 1884–1914* (New York: Beghahn 2015), especially 60–72, 80–84, 104–7, 122–24.

25. Davis, *Cruel Madness*. On Sir Frederick W. Mott's work on GPI, see J. D. Hurn, "The History of General Paralysis of the Insane in Britain, 1830 to 1950"

(PhD diss., University of London, 1998), chap. 3; and S. Matthews, "Matter of Mind: The Contributions of Neuropathologist Sir Frederick Walker Mott to British Psychiatry, c. 1895–1923" (PhD diss., University of Manchester, 2006), esp. chap. 6.

26. Oriel, *Scars of Venus*, 126.

27. Percy S. Pelouze, *Gonorrhea in the Male and Female: A Book for Practitioners*, 3rd ed. (Philadelphia: Saunders, 1941), 9–10 ("Preface to the First Edition").

28. Linda E. Merians, ed, *The Secret Malady: Venereal Disease in Eighteenth-Century Britain and France* (Lexington: University Press of Kentucky 1996).

29. See the contemporary critical discussion by the reforming US doctor Prince A. Morrow: *Social Disease and Marriage: Social Prophylaxis* (New York: Lea Brothers, 1904), chap. 3. For a relatively brief comparative historical study, see Andreas-Holger Maehle, *Contesting Medical Confidentiality: Origins of the Debate in the United States, Britain, and Germany* (Chicago: University of Chicago Press, 2016), esp. chap. 2. Victoria Bates, *Sexual Forensics in Victorian and Edwardian England Age, Crime and Consent in the Courts* (London: Palgrave 2016) is also of relevance.

30. Jill Harsin, "Syphilis, Wives, and Physicians: Medical Ethics and the Family in Late Nineteenth-Century France," *French Historical Studies* 16 (1989): 72–95.

31. Christabel Pankhurst, *The Great Scourge and How to End It* (London: E. Pankhurst, 1913). See also Susan K. Kent, *Sex and Suffrage in Britain, 1860–1914* (London: Routledge, 1990). In the United States Charlotte Perkins Gilman's short novel of 1911, *The Crux*, also mounted an influential feminist denunciation. Perkins Gilman, *The Crux: A Novel*, edited with an introduction by Jennifer S. Tuttle (Newark: University of Delaware Press, 2002).

32. Lutz Sauerteig, "'The Fatherland Is in Danger: Save the Fatherland!' Venereal Disease, Sexuality and Gender in Imperial and Weimar Germany," in Davidson and Hall, *Sex, Sin and Suffering*, 76–92, 82.

33. Matthew Ramsey, "Public Health in France," in *The History of Public Health and the Modern State*, ed. Dorothy Porter (Amsterdam: Rodolpi 1994), 99–102; on Johann Peter Frank's famous doctrine of *Medicinische Polizey*, see George Rosen, *A History of Public Health* (Baltimore: Johns Hopkins University Press, 1993), 137–43.

34. Angus McLaren, *Impotence: A Cultural History* (Chicago: University of Chicago Press, 2007), chap. 5; and see Hanley, "Great Foe."

35. Tomas Sobotka, "Childlessness in Europe: Reconstructing Long-Term Trends among Women Born in 1900–1972," in Kreyenfeld and Konietzka, *Childlessness in Europe*, 17–53. Other historical studies of childlessness have similarly only mentioned STIs, if at all, as one of a list of possible causal factors: Dudley L. Poston and Katherine Trent, "International Variability in Childlessness: A Descriptive and Analytical Study," *Journal of Family Issues* 3 (1982): 573–91; S. Philip Morgan, "Late Nineteenth and Early Twentieth-Century Childlessness," *American Journal of Sociology* 97, no. 3 (1991): 779–807; Donlad T. Rowland, "Historical Trends in Childlessness," *Journal of Family Issues* 28, no. 10 (2007): 1311–37; Sandra Brée, Thierry Eggerickx, and Jean-Paul Sanderson, "Low Fertility, Childlessness and

Family Changes in the First Half of the 20th Century in France and Belgium," *Revue Quetelet Journal* 5, no. 1 (2017): 7–31, https://doi.org/10.14428/rqj2017.05.01.01.

36. For an exemplary study adopting this approach, see Stein, *Negotiating the French Pox*.

37. The estimates are 40–50 percent of men and 70–80 percent of women: Pattman et al., *Oxford Handbook*, 150.

38. Arthur L. Greil, Kathleen Slauson-Blevins, and Julia McQuillan, "The Experience of Infertility: A Review of Recent Literature," *Sociology of Health and Illness* 32, no. 1 (2010): 140–62, https://doi.org/10.1111/j.1467-9566.2009.01213.x. On the English-language etymology of the key terms *barren, sterile* and *infertile*, see Tracey Loughran and Gayle Davis, "Introduction: Defining the 'Problem'; Perspectives on Infertility," in Loughran and Davis, *Palgrave Handbook of Infertility*, 29–35, 30.

39. Grmek's capacious 1969 concept of pathocenosis may be particularly applicable to STIs, as he himself has argued. Mirko D. Grmek, *History of AIDS: Emergence and Origin of a Modern Pandemic* (Princeton, NJ: Princeton University Press, 1990), esp. 156–60.

40. See Lutz Sauerteig and Roger Davidson, eds., *Shaping Sexual Knowledge A Cultural History of Sex Education in Twentieth Century Europe* (London: Routledge, 2012), 40–43, 56–58, 76–92, 176–83, 218–27, on interwar Britain, Sweden, and Poland; Angela Davis, "'Oh No, Nothing, We Didn't Learn Anything': Sex Education and the Preparation of Girls for Motherhood, c. 1930–1970," *Journal of the History of Education* 37 (2008): 661–77; and Simon Szreter and Kate Fisher, *Sex before the Sexual Revolution: Intimate Life in England, 1918–1963* (Cambridge: Cambridge University Press, 2010), chaps. 2–3, 6. More generally on the media in Britain, see Adrian Bingham, *Family Newspapers? Sex, Private Life and the British Popular Press, 1918–1978* (Oxford: Oxford University Press, 2009).

41. A rare example in English of such direct public advice given in the context of a fully informative guide was available only at the very end of the interwar period and was in fact a translation of a German text: Fritz Kahn, *Our Sex Life: A Guide and Counsellor for Everyone*, trans. George Rosen (London: Heinemann Medical Books, 1939), chap. 21.

42. Lynn Hunt, "AHR Roundtable: The Self and Its History," *American Historical Review* 119 (2014): 1576–86; Hunt, *Inventing Human Rights: A History* (New York: Norton, 2007).

43. For another volume explicitly committed to this approach, see Philip Kreager et al., eds., *Population in the Human Sciences 2015: Concepts, Models, Evidence* (Oxford: Oxford University Press, 2015).

44. Harold C. Wiesenfeld and Willard Cates Jr, "Sexually Transmitted Diseases and Infertility," in *Sexually Transmitted Diseases*, ed. King K. Holmes et al., 4th ed. (New York: McGraw-Hill Medical, 2008), chap. 79, pp. 1511–27, 1514–15.

45. Wiesenfeld and Cates, "Sexually Transmitted Diseases," in Holmes et al., *Sexually Transmitted Diseases*, chap. 79, pp. 1511–27, 1514–15. However, while the mechanism of damage is known, the relationship between chlamydial infection and

infertility remains a complex matter open to considerable current scientific debate over the pathways involved, in part because of the difficulty in defining a discrete episode of infection. Even among clinical populations receiving monitored treatment, a single initial infection can result in an inflammation continuing for many weeks, if not months, because a single course of antibiotics will not completely clear the infection. See chapter 12, appendix E, in this volume, for further discussion and references to current research.

46. This pattern of repeated syphilitic miscarriage and stillbirths followed by sickly and then healthy live births was sufficiently evident to nineteenth-century medical observers that it was termed Kassowitz's Law and considered diagnostic of syphilitic infection: Hanley, "Great Foe," 343. For a summary, see McFalls and McFalls, *Disease and Fertility*, 333–40.

47. Roy F. R. Scragg, *Depopulation in New Ireland* (Port Moresby: Administration of Papua and New Guinea, 1957).

48. William H. R. Rivers, 1864–1922, an eminent anthropologist and early psychiatrist, was much involved in treating shell-shocked troops (including Robert Graves and Siegfried Sassoon) during World War I, and the concept of shell shock was collectively developed through this clinical experience. Peter Leese, *Shell Shock: Traumatic Neurosis and the British Soldiers of the First World War* (London: Palgrave Macmillan, 2002); Tracey Loughran, *Shell-Shock and Medical Culture in First World War Britain* (Cambridge: Cambridge University Press, 2016).

49. On tuberculosis, malaria, and postpartum infection, see McFalls and McFalls, *Disease and Fertility*, chaps. 3, 4, 16. Other, less widely prevalent, infectious diseases that can cause infertility are also considered at length in other chapters by the McFalls: Filiarsis (chap. 5), Schistosomiasis (chap. 6), African Sleeping Sickness (chap. 7), and Chagas Disease (chap. 8).

50. Irvine Loudon, *Death in Childbirth: An International Study of Maternal Care and Maternal Mortality, 1800–1950* (Oxford: Clarendon, 1992), chaps. 12–15.

51. McFalls and McFalls, *Disease and Fertility*, 484.

52. Tsevat et al., "Sexually Transmitted Diseases," 9. A rare report on clinical research reported that 1.32 percent of 3,088 female cases registered and treated for TB during 1989–99 in Fars Health Center (Iran), were diagnosed with genital tract TB, and 76 percent were infertile. This would imply that about 1 percent of women sufficiently unwell to come to this clinic and who were then diagnosed with TB had a sterilizing case of infertility. B. Namavar Jahromi, M. E. Parsanezhada, and R. Ghane-Shirazib, "Female Genital Tuberculosis and Infertility," *International Journal of Gynecology and Obstetrics* 75 (2001): 269–72. It is not possible, however, to draw any inference from the information contained in this article about the extent to which TB, alone, was responsible for the sterility, nor what proportion the population of the Fars province (population 4.6 million in 2011) was affected. It has been argued, though not on the basis of any robust clinical epidemiological evidence, that TB was a significant cause of rising infertility among the US black population during the period 1880–1960, where its impact has even been claimed to have been

comparable to that of gonorrhea. However, that claim was a self-generated one due to the authors' unwarranted assumption that genital TB rates in 1880 would have been one-fifth the rate found in 1940: McFalls and McFalls, *Disease and Fertility*, 484–500, esp. 498.

53. Vaughan, *Curing Their Ills*, chap. 6.

54. The epidemiologists' transmission model is expressed mathematically in the equation $R_0 = \beta * c * D$ (where R_0 is the basic reproductive rate of a parasite or an infectious disease agent, measured in terms of the ability of an infection to produce a secondary case (or a second-generation parasite) before it dies or enters a persistent (dormant) state due to the host's immunological response. The Greek letter β is the transmission probability (how likely the microorganism is to pass from one host to another per discrete contact episode); *c* is the contact rate between infectious and susceptible (noninfected) individual members of the host population; and *D* is the duration of infectiousness (how long an infected individual can pass on the disease). When $R_0 = 1$ a disease is just maintaining itself within a host population with, on average, each case of infection leading to just one further case of infection. For public health preventive epidemiology the measurement of the value of R_0 is extremely useful to estimate the proportion of a closed population needing to be immunized or treated either to eradicate or to reduce a disease's prevalence to a desired minimal level. For a classic full exposition, see Roy M. Anderson and Robert M. May, *Infectious Diseases of Humans: Dynamic and Control* (Oxford: Oxford University Press, 1991).

55. Katy M. E. Turner et al., "Investigating Ethnic Inequalities in the Incidence of Sexually Transmitted Infections: Mathematical Modelling Study," *Sexually Transmitted Infections* 80 (2004): 379–85, https://doi.org/10.1136/sti.2003.007575; on the United States, see McFalls and McFalls, *Disease and Fertility*, chap. 19.

56. Thomas Nutt, "Illegitimacy, Paternal Financial Responsibility, and the 1834 Poor Law Commission Reports: The Myth of the Old Poor Law and the Making of the New," *Economic History Review* 63 (2010): 335–61. On the plight of poor women in London, see Lynn MacKay, *Respectability and the London Poor, 1780–1870* (London: Pickering and Chatto 2013); and Samantha Williams, *Unmarried Motherhood in the Metropolis, 1700–1850: Pregnancy, the Poor Law and Provision* (London: Palgrave 2018).

57. For a wide-ranging cultural and historical consideration of many of these issues in relation to medicine, biology, race, and social stigma, see Sander L. Gilman, *Diseases and Diagnoses: The Second Age of Biology*, 2nd ed. (New York: Routledge, 2017), notably chapter 2 in relation to STIs.

58. See Paul Farmer on the concept of structured violence: *Pathologies of Power* (Berkeley: University of California Press, 2003), chap. 1. More generally, see Richard Wilkinson and Kate Picket, *The Spirit Level* (London: Lane 2009).

59. Claudia Stein, "Divining and Knowing: Karl Sudhoff's Historical Method," *Bulletin of the History of Medicine* 87 (2013): 198–224.

60. See also Hugh Taylor, *Trachoma: A Blinding Scourge from the Bronze Age to the Twenty-First Century* (Melbourne: Centre for Eye Research Australia, 2008).

61. Indeed, there is considerable current public concern over koala susceptibility to chlamydia. Mindy Weisberger, "Why the Heck Do So Many Koalas Have Chlamydia?," *Live Science*, May 9, 2018, https://www.livescience.com/62517-how-koalas-get-chlamydia.html.

62. Leonor Sánchez-Busó et al., "Antimicrobial Exposure in Sexual Networks Drives Divergent Evolution in Modern Gonococci," *bioRxiv*, preprint posted May 31, 2018, https://doi.org/10.1101/334847.

63. Leigh Van Valen, "A New Evolutionary Law," *Evolutionary Theory* 1 (1973): 1–30.

64. Magnus Unemo and William M. Shafer, "Antimicrobial Resistance in Neisseria Gonorrheae in the 21st Century: Past, Evolution, and Future," *Clinical Microbiology Reviews* 27, no. 3 (2014): 587–613, https://doi.org/10.1128/CMR.00010-14; Alan P. Johnson and Gwenda Hughes, "The Prospect of Untreatable Gonorrhea: An International Threat That Requires a Coordinated International Response," *BMJ* 358, no. 3973 (2017), https://doi.org/10.1136/bmj.j3973.

65. Piers Mitchell, "Pre-Columbian Treponemal Disease from 14th Century AD Safed, Israel, and Implications for the Medieval Eastern Mediterranean," *American Journal of Physical Anthropology* 121, no. 2 (2003): 117–24.

66. Emmanuel Le Roy Ladurie, "Un concept: L'unification microbienne du monde (XIVe–XVIIe siecles)," *Revue suisse d'histoire* 23, no. 4 (1973): 627–96.

67. As Peter Boomgardt has remarked in his review of the scattered evidence relating to South and East Asia, "After all, most regions of Eurasia had been part of a common disease pool for a long time. . . . The fact that syphilis was apparently new in Asia around 1500 is a confirmation of the notion that it was new to Europe, too, thus supporting the Columbian hypothesis." "Syphilis, Gonorrhea, Leprosy and Yaws in the Indonesian Archipelago, 1500–1950," special issue, *MANUSYA: Journal of Humanities* 14 (2007): 20–41, 36. On related evidence for an upsurge in global demand, including in China and Japan, for a range of cures from sarsaparilla and guiacum to mercury and China root (*tu fu ling*) in the sixteenth century and after, see Anna E. Winterbottom, "Of the China Root: A Case Study of the Early Modern Circulation of *Materia Medica*," *Social History of Medicine* 28 (2014): 22–44.

68. Oriol Mitjà, Kingsley Asiedu, and David Mabey, "Yaws," *Lancet* 381, no. 9868 (2013): 763–73, http://dx.doi.org/10.1016/S0140-6736(12)62130-8.

69. Peter L. Perine et al., *Handbook of Endemic Treponematoses: Yaws, Endemic Syphilis and Pinta* (Geneva: World Health Organization, 1984), table 1.

70. Bayliss-Smith, in chapter 6 in this volume, notes that in the Solomon Islands endemic yaws minimized the impact of syphilis but could not, of course, protect against gonorrhea when both diseases were brought to the islands through Western contact.

71. Doyle, in chapter 8, and Cahen and Minard, in chapter 11, note that European observers often mistook yaws or endemic syphilis (bejel) for venereal

syphilis or "Arab syphilis" among sub-Saharan and North African populations, respectively.

72. N. Arora et al., "Origin of Modern Syphilis and Emergence of a Pandemic *Treponema pallidum* Cluster," *Nature Microbiology* 2 (December 5, 2016), article number 16245, https://www.nature.com/articles/nmicrobiol2016245.pdf. For a wide-ranging review pre-dating the 2016 research results, see Lorenzo Giacini and Sheila A. Lukehart, "The Endemic Treponematoses," *Clinical Microbiology Reviews* 27 (2014), 89–115.

73. Richard B. Rothenberg, "Gonorrhea," in *The Cambridge World History of Human Disease*, ed. Kenneth F. Kiple (Cambridge: Cambridge University Press, 1993), 756–63.

74. It was the great turn-of-the-century physician Sir William Osler (1849–1919), founding professor of medicine at Johns Hopkins and concluding his career as regius professor of medicine at Oxford, 1905–19, who was the source of the description of syphilis as the "great imitator."

Part One

The Hidden Pitfalls in the Early Documentary Record

Chapter One

(The Wrong Kind of) Gonorrhea in Antiquity

Rebecca Flemming

Historiography and Methodology

Studying the relationship between disease and fertility in antiquity is challenging. The first difficulty is establishing the presence, and then prevalence, of any particular condition before an assessment can be made of its demographic impact. In the case of what are now called sexually transmitted infections (STIs), the empirical obstacles to identifying such infections in the classical world are exacerbated by the moralizing that attends discussions of sexual practice and that has so strongly characterized the ways sexual behavior and pathology have been, and continue to be, conceptually conjoined. Julius Rosenbaum's influential and exhaustive nineteenth-century exploration of the ancient history of syphilis (broadly construed), for example, is based on the assumption that venereal diseases are caused by the "abuse" of the genital organs for nonprocreative purposes. Their history is, therefore, the history of human "lasciviousness and debauchery," and there was so much of that in classical Greece and Rome that syphilis and all kinds of genital afflictions necessarily followed.[1]

More methodologically reputable approaches to the problem of past disease presence are threefold.[2] The first is retrospective diagnosis, based primarily on the written sources surviving from a historical society, in which the descriptions of various ailments are critically assessed against modern clinical accounts and understandings. Paleopathology provides the second, focused on the analysis of the biological remains of that society, mostly on osteological scrutiny of skeletal evidence, but also increasingly on the study of ancient DNA (aDNA). Third, the development of next-generation gene-sequencing technologies and advances in Bayesian phylogenetics over the past decade have led to a dramatic increase in molecular clock–dating studies, including various key pathogens: it is now possible to produce a reasonably robust evolutionary timeline for present populations of microbes from genomic data about those populations, and more historical samples are now available.[3] All these techniques and approaches have their strengths and weaknesses; they are best combined and, of course, ultimately reliant on the availability and quality of the evidence itself.

In terms of retrospective diagnosis from ancient texts, there has been much debate among medical historians and physicians, often with a classical education and interests, about whether modern syphilis, gonorrhea, or any other genital affliction was present in antiquity. In the early years of the twentieth century, syphilis found no champions, but views were more divided on gonorrhea, which is the focus here.[4] Parisian urologist Georges Luys opened the first substantial general medical treatise on gonorrhea to be published following the discovery of its causative agent by Albert Neisser in 1879 with the bold statement that "gonorrhoea is as old as mankind," but others were more doubtful.[5] British doctors Henry St. Hill Vertue and J. David Oriel rejected this assertion most strongly, finding no evidence for any venereal disease (except genital warts) in classical literature, medical or otherwise, and concluding that the often-cited passage from Leviticus about the "uncleanness" of a man with "running issue" completely lacked the necessary diagnostic specificity.[6] Toward the end of the past century, Mirko Grmek, in his groundbreaking, truly interdisciplinary, *Diseases in the Ancient Greek World*, was more circumspect. The ancient literary sources are inconclusive: "On the one hand, the diagnosis of gonorrhea is compatible with certain ancient descriptions, and on the other, for none of these descriptions is it the sole interpretation possible." But he preferred to think that the relevant pathogen was present in the classical Mediterranean world, as this provides a better fit, he suggested, with both the ancient texts and the "biological properties of the germ itself."[7]

Paleopathology has yet to contribute much to these discussions, except in relation to syphilis.[8] Gonorrhea and other STIs do not leave decisive skeletal traces, nor have these diseases been identified in any mummified tissue, and it is unlikely (though not impossible) they will be in the future.[9] One aDNA study of the medieval oral microbiome, in which analysis was conducted on calcified dental plaque from four adult human skeletons buried at a cemetery associated with the monastic site at Dalheim, Germany, has produced indications of the presence of both *Neisseria meningitidis* and *Neisseria gonorrhoeae* (also known as gonococcus)—that is, the bacteria that can cause meningitis and gonorrhea, respectively.[10] However, not only is this evidence probably from the eleventh century at the earliest, but the application of shotgun DNA-sequencing techniques to this kind of material, even supported by other methods, generates sequences of variable length and thus identifications of variable security. The traces of *Neisseria gonorrhoeae* were too slight to inspire much confidence in this respect. The section on sexually transmitted diseases in the authoritative volume of Arthur Aufderheide and Conrado Rodríguez-Martín, *The Cambridge Encyclopedia of Human Paleopathology*, is entirely aporetic on the question of whether gonorrhea was an ancient disease.[11]

Phylogenetics, on the other hand, is becoming an increasingly significant player in debates about the history of STIs, including gonorrhea. Research on chlamydia, and especially on the serovars causing lymphoma granuloma venereum, has added to the general sense of the changeability and adaptability of pathogens over time, including over very short timespans.[12] This work strengthens the impression that, contrary to what used to be assumed, diseases are often historically unstable entities as much because their causative agents, the microbes themselves, turn out to be pretty unstable as because of any conceptual shifts or environmental alterations.[13] Gonorrhea is about to take center stage in these respects. The emergence and rapid spread of antibiotic-resistant gonococcus strains from the end of the twentieth century has set alarm bells ringing across the global public health community, and the collection and scrutiny of genomic data about *N. gonorrhoeae* is part of the internationally coordinated response to this situation.[14] Research is massively ratcheting up as a result.

Unfortunately, a properly historical dimension to these genetic and epidemiological investigations has so far been missing. When this present reengagement with STIs is framed with reference to their past, this is done rather poorly, with far less rigor than attends any comparable scientific claim. Luys's assertion that gonorrhea is as old as humanity is uncritically repeated, though without attribution, while all previous and subsequent debates and discussions on the subject are ignored.[15] If any evidence is supplied to support these statements, it is badly misrepresented, if not traduced; basic standards of scholarship are not attempted. It is clear, as Vertue bemoaned in the 1950s, that the actual texts themselves have not been read, or even looked at (whether in translation or the original languages); rather, it has been taken for granted that they say whatever the author wants.[16] The worry is, of course, that as well as spreading general misinformation, these unfounded assumptions about the long-term existence of *N. gonorrhoeae*, and therefore about the durability and nature of the pathogen-host relationship, impact the research agenda.

All this serves to underline, again, the importance of interdisciplinary historical projects such as represented by this volume, as well as adding some urgency to the content of this chapter. The evidence relating to the presence or absence of various STIs in the ancient Mediterranean world is rehearsed again, carefully scrutinized, with special attention paid to modern gonorrhea and chlamydia. After a brief brush with ancient Egyptian medicine from the second millennium BC, this analysis starts with the book of Leviticus from the Hebrew Bible (since this is perhaps the most often–cited ancient text in these respects), which probably took roughly its current form in the fifth century BC, though it casts the institution of the ritual laws it expounds back much further.[17] The Palestinian and diaspora Jewish communities were mostly part of the Persian Empire at that time, as were the Greek cities of Ionia, centers of early natural philosophical speculation and contributors to the explosion of Greek medical writing that began as the century drew to a close.[18] The many treatises generated in this outburst, later collected together as the Hippocratic Corpus, offer rather slight pickings for this discussion, however, and most weight falls on the abundant written remains of the Roman Empire. Learned medicine flourished in the imperial period, and a rich literature engaged with many aspects of social and erotic life. The ancient disease of *gonorrhoia* had acquired an established place in the pathological landscape. The term, an abstract noun formed from the Greek for seed (*gonos*) and flow (*rhoos*), was inherited, not—as commonly claimed—coined, by Galen of Pergamum, the great imperial physician of the second century AD.[19] While many Latin satirists enjoyed exposing all Rome's sexual foibles in explicit detail, if there is evidence of STIs to be found in antiquity, this is the best place to look.

The argument is, however, that no such evidence is to be found. The symptoms of painful urination and some kind of vaginal or penile discharge, perhaps with swelling of the foreskin or lower abdominal pain, the conjunction of which would be taken to indicate modern gonorrhea (and, indeed, chlamydia), do not appear together in any ancient medical text, nor in any other part of the ancient literary record.[20] This is a significant absence, given the dense coverage of human ailments, injuries, and cures in written material from classical Greece and Rome. Nor are notions of the sexual transmission of disease to be found in antiquity; sexual encounters were not considered sites of pathological danger. But that is not the only way that sex and disease can go together, and this chapter makes a positive argument as well as a negative one, tracing an ancient thematics of sexual sickness, shaped by contemporary understandings, values, and concerns, including around fertility. It is no accident that one of the main sexual diseases of the classical world—that is, conditions with a sexual dimension running through their causes, symptoms, and therapies—was *gonorrhoia*, with its focus on seed, the substance of human generation, and its management and control.

While work on the evolution of human pathogens in historical time might be considered to provide theoretical support for the possible absence of modern gonorrhea from the ancient Mediterranean world, such an absence may be, as it were, total or partial. It could be that *N. gonorrhoeae* had yet to come into being or had yet to reach this part of the globe. Perhaps it had yet to take its present form or was less virulent, producing a less symptomatic version of gonorrhea, which left little trace. This possibility will be examined in a bit more detail at the end of this discussion, with some new phylogenetic evidence from a more historically conscientious genomic study, but it is worth bearing in mind throughout, along with the problems caused by the generally asymptomatic character of modern chlamydia.[21]

Searching for Ancient Gonorrhea

Histories of STIs sometimes begin with a reference to the Ebers Papyrus, the longest of the surviving ancient Egyptian medical papyri, comprising a collection of different texts, written in hieratic and dating to the 1530s BC.[22] The precise translation of much of its contents remains uncertain, but they definitely include a set of therapies for urinary problems, for regulating the flow of urine.[23] John Nunn renders the "rather enigmatic Ebers 265" as "another [remedy] to eliminate heat (*tau*) in the bladder, when he suffers retention (*hedbu*) of urine."[24] He continues, "The first part suggests cystitis, and the second outflow obstruction due perhaps to urethral stricture or an enlarged prostate. Both parts would certainly apply to a urethritis." Nunn does not specify, but such a urethritis could obviously be gonococcal or nongonococcal, and today chlamydia is thought to be the cause of a substantial proportion of the latter. There are no references to nonurinary penile discharges, however, nor to any of the nonmenstrual forms of female flux that will become a feature of later Greek and Roman medical writings. There is a mysterious segment in the Ebers Papyrus that deals with sufferings in connection to "secretions" (*setja*), and the shorter Kahun Papyrus, from around 1825 BC, includes remedies for "*khaau* of the uterus," the verb *khaa* generally meaning "throw, cast off, eject, or excrete," though what sort of conditions are being treated here is entirely unclear.[25]

Passages in the book of Leviticus in the Hebrew Bible are more standard fare in these historical outlines. This book recounts the rules regarding ritual and priestly conduct, and purity and impurity, imposed by Yahweh on the Israelites through Moses and Aaron, and it covers male and female discharges as part of the regulatory system. Chapter 15 is the most important, though there are related references elsewhere in the book, and it follows a neat chiastic structure. First the impurity of a man with a discharge—"his discharge being from his member"—is dealt with, then the lesser impurity of a man who has a seminal emission.[26] The same status applies to a woman with whom the man has intercourse, which marks the shift to female impurity.[27] First up is a woman with a discharge—"her discharge being blood from her body"—that is, menstruation, which renders her impure for seven days, then a woman who has a significant discharge of blood outside or beyond the time of her menstrual impurity.[28] She is impure until seven days after she has been healed, at which point sacrifices are offered and rituals performed. The same is the case for the man who has a discharge: he remains impure for seven days after healing, and sacrifices are then offered and rituals performed. All these impurities are contagious, to different degrees, passed by direct or indirect contact with other people, animals, and objects. Mostly this secondhand impurity is discharged by cleansing or washing and lasts only until evening, but intercourse with a menstruating woman makes a man impure for seven days.

Much has been written about this passage in Leviticus: in the context of wider explorations of the overall purity and pollution system of the Hebrew Bible and the notions of purity and pollution more generally, as well as in the context of examining sex, sexuality, and gender.[29] Here, however, the question is rather different and more specific: is there an STI in this text? There is disease, it seems. Both the man with a discharge from his member and the woman with the nonmenstrual discharge of blood are "healed" of their condition: the Hebrew verb *tâhar* here denoting physical, not ritual, purification.[30] The first, and to some extent the second, symptoms are compatible with modern gonorrhea (and chlamydia) as well as a range of other conditions; the gender differentiation of the character of the discharge is part of a wider pattern of equivalence but not symmetry between male and female impurities across the regulatory scheme.[31] Whether these are meant to be viewed as the same ailment in men and women or not is left uncertain.

There is a sexual and generative dimension, at least on the male side. It is assumed that his discharge is seed, since its normal, healthy but still impure, equivalent in the sequence is a seminal emission such as during intercourse. The same pattern occurs in the pairing of normal, healthy and abnormal, diseased discharges of the same substance—blood—on the female side. The point is made explicit in the Septuagint, the Greek translation of the Hebrew Bible produced in early Hellenistic Alexandria, which speaks specifically of "seed" (*gonos*) in this sequence and even renders the phrase "man with a discharge" as *ho gonorrhuês*, literally, "the seed-flowing-man."[32] And, of course, the sexual transmission of impurity is possible, though mentioned only in cases of normal discharge, where there is a particular gender asymmetry, but the general danger of physical touch is present in the aberrant situations too. There is, however, nothing other than impurity under discussion in this passage—that is, ritual impurity, where being impure is a ritual status, entailing exclusion from certain ritual acts and sacred spaces. There is, indeed, no sense of prohibition implied here. Yahweh is simply setting out the rules that must be obeyed, but that obedience is where the force of religious and thus moral obligation falls, not in the content.[33]

Symptoms such as the flow of seed, urinary problems, and a range of vaginal discharges, both sanguineous and otherwise, also feature in the earliest surviving Greek medical writings, which emerged in the late fifth and early fourth century BC, less than a hundred years after Leviticus took its final form and in a more northerly sector of the Mediterranean world. Later collected under the name of Hippocrates of Cos, the legendary founding father of learned Greek medicine, the roughly sixty treatises that compose the Hippocratic Corpus include those that focus on describing diseases and their cures as well as those engaged with more abstract matters of causation and somatic composition, practical matters of regimen, surgery, and prognosis, not to mention the nature of the medical art itself.[34] The extant material is, then, rich and varied, but the cosigns of modern gonorrhea never appear together; rather, they each form part of their own pathological packages, some recognizable in current medical terms, others less so. The question is, again, how to interpret this pattern, shaped as it is by the particular commitments and concerns, assumptions and objectives, of Hippocratic physicians as much as by their disease environment.

The fact that the individual symptoms of modern gonorrhea (and chlamydia) were identified in classical Greece, roughly where they would otherwise be expected, but never described together, is telling. Painful urination, along with sharp pains in the kidney, loins, flank, and testicle on one side of the body is a sign of kidney stones, for example, in the Hippocratic treatise *Internal Affections*, where it forms part of a diagnosis that would be recognized in modern medicine too.[35] Bladder stones and strangury (*strangouriê*)—the latter being a condition in which urine is passed a little at a time—can also conjoin pain and urination.[36] Flow of seed, during the night and even when out walking, also appears in *Internal Affections*, but as a characteristic of a kind of *tuphos*, caused by compaction and drying out of the moisture in the body.[37] Emaciation, weakness, a change of somatic color, excessive hunger, and enjoyment of the smell of extinguished lamps count among the other symptoms of this disease, which, if not effectively treated at the outset, will continue for twenty years.

Seminal flux is also associated with *phthisis*—consumption—a different type of wasting away. The fullest description is provided by the Hippocratic author of *Diseases 2*, in relation to *phthisis* of the back, arising from the spinal marrow, a substance strongly associated with seed by the philosopher Plato and some Hippocratic writers.[38]

> It most frequently seizes those who are newly-married and fond of sexual intercourse (*philolagnos*). They are without fever, and eat well, but still waste away. And if you ask the patient, he will say that it feels as if, starting from his head, something is tiptoeing down his spine, like ants. And whenever he passes urine or stools, much watery seed comes forth. He produces no offspring, and has nocturnal emissions, whether he has intercourse with his wife or not. Whenever he walks or runs, especially uphill, he suffers breathlessness and weakness, and heaviness of the head, with ringing in the ears. When, eventually, violent fevers take hold, he will die from an intermitting fever.[39]

So early medical intervention is advisable, beginning with upward and downward purging, then a diet of milk and a little gruel, followed by more substantial sustenance; the patient should abstain from drunkenness, sexual activity, and any exercise except walking (but not in the cold or sun) for a year.

Women can also suffer from a flow of seed, since, as Hippocratic writers variously presume and explain, both men and women produce seed that is necessary for the generation of offspring.[40] Issues of fertility are thus implicated, as a passage in *Diseases of Women 1* makes clear, one of the so-called gynecological texts in the Hippocratic Corpus in which female health and procreation are essentially aligned.[41] Thus, in this passage a situation that favors conception in terms of a woman's wishes, seed, sexual activity, and uterine configuration is contrasted with one in which her seed runs out in a continual flow, without stopping; she does not welcome intercourse with her husband and does not become pregnant.[42] She is also afflicted with pain in her loins, a slight fever, weakness, and fainting, and her womb is not in its proper place.

The flow of seed is, however, just one of a whole range of unhealthy female fluxes that feature in Hippocratic writings. The opening sequence of *Diseases of Women 2* describes therapies for eleven different flows (*rhooi*): two of blood, one red, one yellow red (*purros*, that is, fire or flame colored), two white, one like sheep's urine, two like egg, and two like the juice from roasted meat.[43] All are accompanied by a shifting set of other symptoms: often fever, pains, swelling, breathlessness, ulcers, and pustules; several are explicitly the result of miscarriage, a problematic birth, or incomplete purging thereafter, though general bodily imbalances can also cause such ailments. It is one of the "white fluxes" that is usually identified as modern gonorrhea by those inclined to do so. Neither bears much resemblance to the current condition, but perhaps closest is the case where "what is purged is a yellow-green white, and whenever she urinates it bites and stings, and the uterus is ulcerated, and she has acute fever, is very hot, thirsty and unable to sleep, and becomes delirious, and whenever she hurries, she has difficulty breathing, and her limbs loosen."[44] There is no indication here, or elsewhere in this sequence, that the flux is in any sense seminal, just as none of them are menstrual; if there is blood, it is not from menstruation.[45]

Learned Greek medicine took a more orderly form in the Hellenistic period, in the expanded Greek world created by the conquests of Alexander the Great, contested and then consolidated after his death in 322 BC.[46] Almost none of the extensive and highly influential medical writings produced in this time survive, however, so the developments they enacted have to be reconstructed from later works, which variously absorbed, elaborated, and debated them. One such development was in the field of pathology, where the Hippocratic proliferation of symptoms and their intermingling with diseases was reined in and organized into a roughly shared categorical framework. A more or less settled catalog of diseases was established, each constituted by an essentially agreed-on set of symptoms, though their causes and cures remained more contentious.

Gonorrhoia emerged as one of these established diseases. Its first extant appearance as such is probably in an anonymous medical handbook from the first century AD—that is, after the Hellenistic kingdoms themselves had fallen to Rome, while Greek medicine and culture had been absorbed into the Roman Empire, which now encompassed the whole of the Mediterranean world and more.[47] This is, however, a synoptic text, summarizing existing ideas and practices. So *gonorrhoia* already had a history, though one that seems not to have reached back as far as Hippocrates, Diocles, Praxagoras, or Erasistratus, the four key medical authorities whose views on the causes of each disease the author liked to cite if he could.[48] The latest of them, the great Alexandrian anatomist Erasistratus of Ceos was active in the early third century BC, so *gonorrhoia* was a late Hellenistic product, of the second or perhaps first century BC. It had, moreover, already been translated into Latin in the early first century AD. Around the AD 30s, the Roman gentleman Aulus Cornelius Celsus included mention of *profusio seminis*, "the flux of seed," in the medical books of his great encyclopedia—his collection, organization, and presentation in Latin of all the technical knowledge a member of the Roman elite like himself should possess, knowledge often derived from Greek sources.[49]

That these are the same disease can be confirmed by comparing their descriptions. Celsus spoke about a complaint located in the genital region, of excessive flow of seed, "which occurs without sexual intercourse, and without nocturnal imaginings, so that over time the sufferer is consumed by wasting."[50] The anonymous Greek author provided a slightly fuller account: "In those suffering from *gonorrhoia* there is an involuntary, permanent flow (*rhein*) of seed (*gonos*), without pleasure. They waste away, lose their colour and strength; they become fevered, with loss of appetite, and even their pulse fades."[51] This is a chronic disease, which arises from paralysis of the seminal vessels, both issues Celsus avoids, since the most important division for him is between affections arising from the whole, or a specific part, of the body, and he is not much interested in etiology at all.[52] There is more overlap again in respect to their therapeutic prescriptions, though the anonymous author offered a much longer, more detailed set of instructions. These begin with rest, fasting, and the application of cold sponges and vinegar to the lower abdomen, groin, and hips and end many days later with vomiting from radishes. He suggested that the patient should lie on a hard bed with a sheet of lead under his loins, while Celsus advises the patient against sleeping on their back.

Other Greek medical texts from the first and second century AD discuss *gonorrhoia* in very similar terms. All describe it as an ongoing, uncontrolled flow of seed, without desire, which results in loss of strength and color, a general wasting away. If the immediate cause is identified, it involves impairment of the seminal vessels, and there is also some repetition, as well as variation, in respect of therapeutic recommendations. Soranus of Ephesus, a prominent authority in the methodic school of medicine, active in Rome around AD 100, made it clear in his *Gynecology* that "*gonorrhoia* occurs not only in men but also in women," a point echoed by the less renowned medical writer, Aretaeus of Cappadocia, in his work *On Acute and Chronic Diseases*, composed about the same time.[53] Other authors offer no real indications as to whether this is a disease affecting both sexes or not.[54] Galen of

Pergamum, for instance, the most influential physician and medical writer of the imperial period, operating later in the second century AD, provided such a male-focused discussion of the topic that the implication would seem that females are not affected, though he is deeply committed both to a universal human pathology and to female seed production across his oeuvre.[55]

For Soranus *gonorrhoia* was essentially the same in men and women, but Aretaeus took a different view, part of a distinctive approach to the condition more broadly. His chapter opens with the statement that "*gonorrhoia* is not deadly, but it is unpleasant, and disgusting even to hear about," in contrast to the neutral tone adopted in all the other surviving accounts. The distastefulness of the disease resides mostly in its emasculating effect on men, which is where the emphasis of his account falls: the condition specifically undermines key male qualities, such as courage, strength, and decisiveness, as well as being more generally enfeebling. Also repellent is its assault on female sexual restraint, since in women "the seed is poured forth by them with titillation of the parts and pleasure, and in shameless intercourse with men, but men are not at all irritated in this way." Their loss of virtue was thus manifested in quite a different form.

A late antique latinization of Soranus's work *On Acute and Chronic Diseases* preserves only a fragmentary version of the chapter on "discharge of seed (*lapsus seminis*), which the Greeks call *gonorria*." It includes the statement that bodies affected by long-term weakness or impacted by sexual overactivity are particularly susceptible. Though no such claim appears in Soranus's *Gynecology*, that sexual excess might be implicated is hinted at by the therapies prescribed. Not only is it recommended that the woman sleep with a lead sheet under her loins; but they also enjoin the avoidance of anything sexually "provocative." The patient is not to be shown erotic paintings or told stories about sexual encounters; rather, her entertainment is to be somber and austere in tone and content.[56] This emphasis on sexual restraint, on closing down the production of seed as means to regain control of the processes of seminal manufacture, accumulation, and emission, is certainly suggestive of the opposite as a possible underlying cause of the disease.

Aretaeus concurred, in a more gendered way. The cure of *gonorrhoia* is an urgent matter, for the affection is unpleasant and the consumption dangerous. There is the lack of offspring to consider, the threat to the continuation of humanity, so the flow of seed must be stopped immediately.[57] Along the same lines as other authors, cooling and astringent applications to the genital region are accompanied by efforts to dry out the body more broadly and gradually restore strength. But manliness and self-mastery are what is most at stake in all this: "If he is self-controlled in sexual matters and takes cold baths, the hope is that the patient quickly returns to manhood."

The same texts and authors continued to record painful urination as a symptom of various kidney and bladder diseases, most especially bladder stones.[58] Soranus provided a full discussion of different typologies of female flux, mentioned more briefly elsewhere.[59] The general appearance of male and female genitals also received some sustained attention, with issues around the foreskin and some testicular swellings noted, explicated, and treated, as well as a variety of ulcerations and growths.[60] All these signs and conditions can then be traced, on their separate tracks, through the surviving medical writings of the later Roman Empire and beyond. Versions of these same accounts of *gonorrhoia* appear, for instance, in Greek medical encyclopedias from the fourth into the seventh centuries AD and, calqued as *lapsus* or *fluxus seminis* and *effusio spermatis* (that is, "flow of seed" or just transliterated as *gonorrhea*) feature in Latin medical texts over the same period and thereafter.[61] There is some variation of emphasis, of anatomical and etiological detail or precise therapies, but also more repetition and compaction.

It is clear, then, that while *gonorrhoia* became, and persisted as, a well-established disease in classical medical discourse, it was not modern gonorrhea, either in concept or actuality. The ideas and understandings that shaped and drove *gonorrhoia* were quite distinct, and the symptomatic match with any modern STI is poor. From the messy beginnings of Hippocratic medicine to the well-structured contents of late antique medical encyclopedias, though all the individual symptoms of gonorrhea and chlamydia were recorded, they never appear in combination. Indeed, there is a sense in which the basic point about absence can be pushed back to the medical papyri of ancient Egypt, but the omission becomes increasingly significant as the amount of surviving evidence increases, and its type and focus shift, in classical Greece and especially the Roman Empire. Now there is reasonable expectation that if modern STIs were present, they would be recognizable in the texts in some form. But, despite the richness of pathological descriptions, the wealth of detail, painful urination was never associated with any kind of penile or vaginal emission. Moreover, while there are historical reasons to think that the discursive focus would be on seed in these settings, there is nothing that would prevent genital discharge and urinary troubles from occurring together in writing if they did in life. Signs more rarely seen in modern gonorrhea or chlamydia, such as various swellings, lower abdominal and testicular pain, or bleeding between periods, are all duly noted in their places, but these are by and large separate from one another and from *gonorrhoia*.

There were what might be called "sexual diseases" in classical medicine: diseases in which sexual behavior might play a causal role and that had effects on sexual activity and manifested sexual symptoms. But this is sexual behavior in a quantitative sense: who with and of what kind is irrelevant, and no single encounter can be damaging. Moreover, this is part of a wider package of moderation, a world in which any excess or imbalance threatens health, and for *gonorrhoia* the symptoms and effects are as much about generation as about sex.

Still Searching

Medical writers have, of course, no monopoly on ancient discourses of either sex or disease. There are many other descriptions of bodies that survive from the classical world and especially from Rome. Members of the Roman elite wrote to one another about their ailments and treatments, and those of their friends and family, and offered advice and encouragement, while satirists scrutinized the social and sexual comportment of a wider segment of the city's population in more hostile fashion. This was a world of public nakedness, in the baths, gymnasium, and brothels, in which power and status determined the rules of sexual conduct, so there was always something at stake in any erotic activity. It produced an array of art and poetry, visual and literary representations, which later viewers and readers would label pornographic and obscene, cover up and confine to the "secret cabinets" of museums, and bowdlerize and refuse to translate: from the typology of sex acts depicted in the frescos from the Suburban Baths of Pompeii to the so-called *Carmina Priapea*, the collection of verses dedicated to Priapus, the phallic god.[62]

Women were regularly attacked for wrinkled flesh and withered breasts; for cut, worn, and lumpy genitals; and, most persistently, for their spacious and sagging cunts (the Latin *cunnus* bears no other translation).[63] They were blamed for sexual overactivity, for a lasciviousness that became embedded in their anatomy, and for a desire that long outstripped their desirability to men.[64] "Lydia is as roomy as the arse of a bronze horseman" is the first of ten such similes in an epigram of Martial, composed toward the end of the first century AD, the last being her anatomical alignment with the "ugly throat of a pelican from Ravenna."[65] The poem closes with the couplet: "I am said to have fucked her in a fishpond. I don't know, I think I fucked the fishpond." Smooth and worn anuses and buttocks were the main male failing, the signs of a man who enjoyed being penetrated in anal intercourse rather than doing the penetrating, as he should.[66] Martial had Charinus go one step further:

his anus is ripped up to his middle, but he still wants more; the point of entry is destroyed, but Charinus still needs to be entered.[67] Circumcised and infibulated penises were also alluded to, hidden or revealed in the baths or gymnasium, along with the genital proportions of slave attendants in some of the same contexts.[68]

Disease occasionally strikes as part of this mocking supervision of Roman gender and sexual norms, mostly orally. For Roman citizen men to make sexual use of their mouths was not only unmanly but also polluting, and all kinds of odium followed. An "unseemly disease" took hold of Nannius's "fornicating tongue" while he was deep in the act, Martial explained, and he can no longer get it up.[69] More has been made of the "figs" that blight several satirical bodies, variously understood as hemorrhoids, warts, or other anal growths.[70] The verses are unclear, but there is certainly emphasis on the lack of fertility signified by the human version of a fruit that otherwise symbolizes fecundity and abundance and a corresponding implication that certain sexual activities, as well as bareback horse riding, might be a cause.[71] Testicular hernias and hydroceles were also derided, at least until their poetic assailant caught sight of himself in Nero's baths, so the joke was on him.[72]

Assorted genital afflictions appear beyond the realms of satire. The Roman senator Pliny the Younger wrote, at the end of the first century AD, to his colleague Calpurnius Macer about a couple from his hometown of Como, in northern Italy, who had thrown themselves into the lake together.[73] The husband had been suffering from a rotting ulcer in "those parts which modesty conceals" for a long time before his wife prevailed on him to allow her to examine the sore and provide an honest opinion on its curability. Upon inspection she determined that the case was hopeless, and so, since his ability to live a good life was thus irrevocably compromised, he should bring his existence to a close. She helped her husband achieve that goal by tying herself to him before they both leaped into the water, a deed as laudable as the better-known actions of Arria, who famously led her husband to a noble end.[74] The story is mainly about the rules of Roman death, but it also indicates that, while rotting genitals impeded marital intimacy, this was essentially a pragmatic issue. There is no mention of cause or blame, the discussion between husband and wife was full and frank, and Pliny willingly shared the details with a fellow senator and indeed the world.[75] He used a circumlocution to refer to the parts in question, but there is no hint that this disease itself was judged any differently from any other. Around the middle of the second century AD, the future emperor Marcus Aurelius wrote to his tutor and friend, Fronto, that his sister had been "seized with such a pain in her female parts that it was horrible to see."[76]

Once again, therefore, the point is that the silence about genital discharges and the lack of reference to the symptoms of modern gonorrhea and chlamydia comes not as part of a wider set of silences or neighboring omissions but rather the reverse. Genital afflictions were by no means off-limits in polite conversation, and they were pretty central to the concerns of those whose verses operated in a different register. The size, shape, texture, integrity, and elasticity of both male and female genitals were all recurrent themes in Roman satire, all evoked to comic and censorious effect, without any mention of drips. It is hard not to agree with, and expand on, Vertue's verdict on Juvenal, a younger contemporary of Martial, whose longer poems covered essentially the same ground: he (and his fellow social critics) "would have been by no means ignorant of a contagious urethritis if it had been beneath his eyes, and he would have made eloquent use of his knowledge in exposing what was abhorrent to him and obnoxious."[77]

But what about *gonorrhoia*? These omissions also cover the symptoms of the ancient disease, which must raise questions about relations between descriptions and reality on one side or the other, if not both. Nor indeed is *gonorrhoia* itself to be found outside medical texts, with one exception. This expression does fit in with wider patterns, since Roman discussions about health and sickness not involving professionals tended to be vague and symptom-based rather than in terms of the specific diseases that appeared in medical handbooks—and the exception is instructive.[78]

In his Greek account of the first Judean revolt against Rome, the Jewish historian Josephus used *gonorrhoioi* and *gonorrhoiikoi*, both ways of referring to those suffering from *gonorrhoia*, as terms roughly equivalent to those with abnormal genital discharges in Leviticus.[79] There had been some wider reworking of the biblical regulations, at least as Josephus described the range of exclusions from sacred space and sacrifice that obtained before the sack of Jerusalem, which essentially ended the revolt in AD 70; as the scion of a priestly family he should have been cognizant of the rules. *Gonorrhoia* was then aligned with *lepra*, a generic Greek term for assorted skin diseases that translated the Hebrew *ṣâraʿat* (scale disease) of Leviticus chapter 13; affliction with either entailed exclusion from the whole city.[80] The abnormal female discharge of blood had dropped out of the equation, but menstruating women were barred from the Jerusalem Temple and had only limited access when they were not, like other impure men. It may be, therefore, that, in assimilating the biblical condition with the disease of *gonorrhoia*, Josephus takes this as something both men and women suffer from: both have seed and both can therefore be troubled by improper flows in this respect.

Still, even if Josephus provides evidence for awareness of *gonorrhoia* beyond medical writing, its symptoms remain missing from the sustained somatic scrutiny enacted by Roman satirists and letter writers. Or, at least, its eponymous permanent flow of seed is missing. The weakness and wasting, and loss of color and vigor, which were also fundamental to the condition, are more often reported to attend sexual overindulgence of various sorts. There are, moreover, reasons to think that the permanence of the seminal flux might well have been exaggerated in the medical accounts for definitional purposes: Soranus, indeed, offers a more episodic version of uncontrolled emission.[81] It might even be the case that the looser Hippocratic collection of signs including, but not organized around, lack of control over seed and its discharge was more accurate, and the emergence of *gonorrhoia* as a disease entity was driven by more structural and ideological concerns. It made sense to have an affection focused around the management of generative seed. The poetry reflected those concerns in its own ways and picked up more directly on the moralizing discourse around the necessary alignment of sexual behavior and social status and around fertility, the need to produce legitimate offspring for the good of the community.

Moreover, while Vertue's argument that the Roman moral system was "incompatible" with the presence of untreated, unregulated venereal infection may be somewhat optimistic, he made a valid pragmatic point that needs some attention to finish.[82] It is the Roman promotion of prostitution as an institution that protected marriage and the production of legitimate children that Vertue found most problematic in this respect.[83] Thus, the stern champion of traditional Roman values, Cato the Censor, is reported to have congratulated a well-known gentleman he met coming out of a brothel, for he had done the right thing with his lusts and kept well away from other men's wives.[84] It is also recorded that, after repeated encounters in the same location, Cato added that his approbation extended only to the occasional visit, not to making the brothel home: the man had obligations to his patrimony, to his family's fortunes as well as to the families of others, not to mention to his dignity and self-control.[85] Still, the easy recourse of men from all levels of society to prostitutes in Rome and the size and openness of the sex industry in the city is indisputable, and Vertue is surely right to raise the question of whether that free and favored position would have been sustainable in the face of unchecked gonococcal contagion, especially given the vigorous pronatalism of the Roman state.

He is surely wrong, however, in the categorical confidence of his negative answer. While it seems likely that some anxieties, debates, and even action would have been stirred in such a situation, the sex trade was so integral to the Roman sexual, social, and economic order that the barriers to any restrictions, reorganization, or rethinking would have been very powerful. Around AD 40 the emperor Gaius even brought in a prostitution tax that proved so lucrative that, centuries later, Christian emperors could not bring themselves to repeal it, despite now publicly abhorring the activities they were profiting from.[86] Vertue thus reverses Rosenbaum: the presence of such flagrant debauchery in a functioning society oblivious to the dangers of STIs proves the absence of those infections rather than mandating their proliferation. His thesis is no more valid than the original, though the objections are of a somewhat different order. Still, the fact that the Roman Empire enjoyed growth and prosperity over the period most under scrutiny here and that prostitution, power, and population flourished in the first two centuries AD does seem to favor a scenario without modern sexually transmitted diseases.[87]

Absence of Evidence Is Evidence of Absence

This chapter has argued that there is no evidence for modern gonorrhea in the ancient Mediterranean world, in a strong sense. In this case the absence of evidence does equate to evidence of absence. There are numerous places where, if the symptoms of modern gonorrhea had been present together, all the indications are they would have been recorded: there are extensive surviving medical, satirical, and epistolary writings from ancient Greece and especially Rome that describe and assess bodies, disease, and sexual activity. These themes are indeed conjoined on occasion, but disease plays a rather slight part in connections between the other two. Excess in any area of human behavior was considered potentially damaging to health and somatic fitness and function, with sex no exception, but nor was it particularly prominent; other aspects of life and the environment receive greater attention. Fertility was more of a medical concern; generative failure was a pathological as well as ideological problem. Again, sexual misconduct kept a low profile in these discussions, despite looming larger in wider moralizing discourses and indeed state action in the Roman world.

These findings, which follow the earlier arguments of Vertue and Oriel, gain further support from a much more current source. Results now emerging from genetic research driven by the renewed public health concerns around *N. gonorrhoeae*, and its antibiotic resistance strains in particular, include "time to most recent common ancestor" (tMRCA) estimates for the current bacterial population. The Pathogen Genomics group at the Wellcome Trust Sanger Institute sequenced as large a number of *gonorrhoeae* isolates as possible, drawn from more than fifty different countries and from roughly the past fifty years, and calculated a tMRCA of 1589, with a confidence interval of 1544 to 1622.[88] The sampling in this study is, of course, biased, selected through antibiotic usage, but, still, it is a significant new datum to consider: the most systematic investigation currently available into the emergence and rapid global spread of *N. gonorrhoeae*, using the most up-to-date methods of genomic sequencing and phylogenetic analysis, locates that emergence in the sixteenth century.

To return to the point made at the outset, this emergence is of the gonococcus in its present form. The current population of the microbe can apparently be traced back to a common ancestor around 1590, but the genetic lineage may continue further into the past. A more distant, divergent ancestor of *N. gonorrhoeae* may have existed prior to this juncture, even back as far as 500 BC, though it might have gone through several significant genetic shifts in the intervening period. Based on the historical evidence scrutinized here, any of these earlier bacteria around the Mediterranean would likely have been less virulent, producing fewer discernible symptoms or, at least, fewer distinctive symptoms; they might have been closer to chlamydia in their manifestations, about which it has been harder to be at all conclusive in the discussion so far. The impact of this proto-gonorrhea and any chlamydia on fertility remains deeply hidden and can thus only be guessed at. It seems quite possible that they had some detrimental effects in this respect, though there has been a retreat (including as reported in chapters in this volume) from some of the more extravagant claims linking STIs with infertility in the present day that characterized the field just a few decades ago.[89] All in all, then it seems most likely that other factors were more important in determining the size of Greek and Roman families.

Notes

Research for this paper has been undertaken within the framework of the Cambridge University Generation to Reproduction Project, supported by a strategic award from the Wellcome Trust (Grant no. WT 088708).

1. Julius Rosenbaum, *Geschichte der Lustseuche im Alterthume*, 5th ed. (Halle: Schmidt, 1892), 46–47; see also Mirko D. Grmek, *Diseases in the Ancient Greek World*, trans. Mireille and Leonard Muellner (Baltimore: Johns Hopkins University Press, 1989), 142–44; and Daniel Orrells, *Sex: Antiquity and Its Legacy* (London: Tauris, 2015), 83–89.

2. Piers Mitchell, "Retrospective Diagnosis and the Use of Historical Texts for Investigating Disease in the Past," *International Journal of Paleopathology* 1 (2011):

81–88; Evilena Anastasiou and Piers Mitchell, "Paleopathology and Genes: Investigating the Genetics of Infectious Diseases in Excavated Human Skeletal Remains and Mummies from Past Populations," *Gene* 528 (2013): 33–40.

3. Charlotte Roberts and Rebecca Redfern, chap. 3; and Ian N. Clarke and Hugh R. Taylor, chap. 4, both in this volume, provide case studies of the latter methods with respect to syphilis and chlamydia, respectively.

4. For summaries of these debates see, for example, Grmek, *Ancient Greek World*, 142–46; and J. D. Oriel, *The Scars of Venus: A History of Venereology* (London: Springer-Verlag, 1994), 4–6.

5. Georges Luys, *A Textbook on Gonorrhoea and Its Complications*, trans. Arthur Foerster (London: Baillière, Tindall and Cox, 1913). The first French edition—*Traité de la blennorragie et de ses complications*—was published in 1912. For a national overview of developments in the field in the decades after Neisser's discovery, see Michael Worboys, "Unsexing Gonorrhoea: Bacteriologists, Gynaecologists and Suffragists in Britain," *Social History of Medicine* 17 (2004): 41–59.

6. Henry St. Hill Vertue, "An Enquiry into Venereal Disease in Greece and Rome," *Guy's Hospital Reports* 102 (1953): 277–302; J. David Oriel, "Gonorrhoea in the Ancient World," *Paleopathology Newsletter* 4 (1973): 7; Oriel, *Scars of Venus*, 4–8; see also R. H. Boyd, "Origin of Gonorrhoea and Non-specific Urethritis," *British Journal of Venereal Diseases* 31 (1955): 246–48.

7. Grmek, *Ancient Greek World*, 144–45.

8. See Roberts and Redfern, chap. 3, in this volume.

9. Arthur C. Aufderheide and Conrado Rodríguez-Martín, *The Cambridge Encyclopedia of Human Paleopathology* (Cambridge: Cambridge University Press, 1998), 289. *N. gonorrhoeae* can, rarely (in less than 3 percent of cases), cause septic arthritis or the more diffuse "disseminated gonococcal infection," which may affect the joints as well as producing skin lesions. These conditions could, therefore, leave skeletal traces, but they would be the same as those resulting from septic arthritis produced by other pathogens. In the absence of genital symptoms, diagnosis requires that the pathogen be identified. See, for example, Peter A. Rice, "Gonococcal Arthritis (Disseminated Gonococcal Infection)," *Infectious Disease Clinics of North America* 19 (2005): 853–61.

10. Christina Warinner et al., "Pathogens and Host Immunity in the Ancient Human Oral Cavity," *Nature Genetics* 46 (2014): 336–46.

11. Aufderheide and Rodríguez-Martín, *Cambridge Encyclopedia*, 288–89.

12. See Clarke and Taylor, chap. 4, in this volume; though note that mutations may also revert back to the genotype consensus.

13. That pathogens evolve, is of course well known, even in the ancient historical community, but it was largely taken for granted that the amount of change likely between, say the Roman imperial period and today, was quite small, at least in comparison to what went before. But see J. C. F. Poole and A. J. Holladay, "Thucydides and the Plague of Athens," *Classical Quarterly* 29 (1979): 282–300.

14. See, for example, World Health Organization, *Global Health Sector Strategy on Sexually Transmitted Infections, 2016–2021*, June 2016, http://apps.who.int/iris/bitstream/10665/246296/1/WHO-RHR-16.09-eng.pdf?ua=1; and the US Centers for Disease Control, *Gonoccoccal Isolate Surveillance Program (GISP): Protocol*, May 2016, www.cdc.gov/std/gisp/gisp-protocol-may-2016.pdf.

15. The editorial introducing a special journal issue dedicated to STIs—Didac Carmona-Gutierrez, Katharina Kainz, and Frank Madeo, "Sexually Transmitted Infections: Old Foes on the Rise," *Microbial Cell* 3, no. 9 (2016): 361—claims that gonorrhea is found in the bible, for example, citing the same claim in William M. Shafer and Elizabeth A. Ohneck, "Taking the Gonococcus-Human Relationship to a Whole New Level: Implications for the Co-evolution of Microbes and Humans," *Microbiology* 2, no. 3 (2011): e00067-11. The article on gonorrhea in the same special issue—Stuart A. Hill, Thao L. Masters, and Jenny Wachter, "Gonorrhea: An Evolving Disease of the New Millennium," *Microbial Cell* 3, no. 9 (2016): 372—cites a hundred-year-old authority to the same end: C. J. Hastings, "Public Health Aspects of Venereal Diseases," *Public Health Journal* 8 (1917): 37–41.

16. Vertue, "Enquiry into Venereal Disease," 278.

17. For a summary of debates about the chronology of biblical composition, see, for example, John Van Seters, "Historiography in Ancient Israel," in *The Oxford History of Historical Writing*, vol. 1, *Beginnings to AD 600*, ed. Andrew Feldherr and Grant Hardy (Oxford: Oxford University Press, 2011), 76–96.

18. On the emergence of Hippocratic medicine, and much else, see Vivian Nutton, *Ancient Medicine*, rev. ed. (London: Routledge, 2013).

19. The claim that Galen invented the name is one of the most often repeated historical errors in the literature; see, for example, Richard B. Rothenberg, "Gonorrhea," in *The Cambridge World History of Human Disease*, ed. Kenneth F. Kiple (Cambridge: Cambridge University Press, 1993), 759; Shafer and Ohneck, "Gonococcus-Human Relationship"; and Carmona-Gutierrez, Kainz, and Madeo "Sexually Transmitted Infections," 361.

20. Despite its many historical errors, I have used Richard Pattman et al., eds., *Oxford Handbook of Genitourinary Medicine, HIV, and Sexual Health*, 2nd ed. (Oxford: Oxford University Press, 2010) as a guide to the modern manifestations of the diseases discussed here.

21. Current estimates are that 70–80 percent of women and 40–50 percent of men infected with chlamydia experience no symptoms; see, for example, Pattman et al., *Oxford Handbook*, 150. And for more on chlamydia, see Clarke and Taylor, chap. 4, and Michael Worboys, chap. 5, both in this volume.

22. See John F. Nunn, *Ancient Egyptian Medicine* (London: British Museum Press, 1996).

23. Ebers 261–83; Nunn, *Ancient Egyptian Medicine*, 91–92.

24. Nunn, *Ancient Egyptian Medicine*, 91–92.

25. Ebers 530–42 (*setja*); Kahane, 3, 7 and 10 (*khaau*); and Nunn, *Ancient Egyptian Medicine*, 197.

26. Leviticus 15:2–15 (discharge); and 15:16–17 (emission). Translations are by Joseph Milgrom: *Leviticus 1–16: A New Translation with Introduction and Commentary* (New York: Doubleday, 1991), 902–3, and I am indebted to the extensive commentary and discussion in his volume also.

27. Leviticus 15:18.

28. Leviticus 15:19–24 (menstruation) and 15:25–30 (nonmenstrual discharge of blood).

29. It was, of course, Mary Douglas's *Purity and Danger: An Analysis of Concepts of Pollution and Taboo* (London: Routledge and Paul, 1966) and then *Leviticus as Literature* (Oxford: Oxford University Press, 1999) that added a whole new dimension to biblical scholarship on purity and pollution. The theme was developed by, for example, Jonathan Klawans *Impurity and Sin in Ancient Judaism* (New York: Oxford University Press, 2000) and Thomas Kazen, *Issues of Impurity in Early Judaism* (Winona Lake, IN: Eisenbrauns, 2010). For more gendered approaches, see Tarja S. Philip, *Menstruation and Childbirth in the Bible: Fertility and Impurity* (New York: Lang, 2006); Dorothea Erbele-Küster, *Körper und Geschlecht: Studien zur Anthropologie von Leviticus 12 und 15* (Neukirchen-Vluyn: Neukirchener, 2008); and Eve Levavi Feinstein, *Sexual Pollution in the Hebrew Bible* (New York: Oxford University Press, 2014).

30. Milgrom, *Leviticus 1–16*, 921.

31. Bleeding between periods is a rare symptom of modern gonorrhea in women. It is more common in chlamydia, in the 20–30 percent of women who are symptomatic at all, but other causes of such bleeding are more likely.

32. LXX (Septuagint) Leviticus 15:3 (*gonos*) and 15:4, 6–9, 11–13 (*gonorrhuês*). The translation of the Hebrew *ṭâhar* by the Greek *kathairein*—purge, cleanse, or purify—rather than a more specific verb of healing, on the other hand, rather weakens the sense of physical disease.

33. The relationship between the moral system of the Hebrew Bible and its ritual regulation, between impurity and sin, pollution and prohibition, is one of the key topics in the scholarship; see, for example, Klawans, *Impurity and Sin*.

34. See Elizabeth M. Craik, *The Hippocratic Corpus: Content and Context* (London: Routledge, 2015).

35. *Internal Affections* 14. Greek text and English translations of works in the Hippocratic Corpus are most easily accessible in the eleven Hippocrates volumes of the Loeb Classical Library (Cambridge, MA: Harvard University Press, 1923–2018). Here 6:118–21 (Potter).

36. *Affections* 28: strangury (5:50–51 Potter); *Diseases 4* 24 (55L): bladder stones (10:172–75 Potter). Strangury has fallen out of favor as a disease, though it remains a symptom; bladder stones are still considered to cause painful urination.

37. *Internal Affections* 43 (6:214–9 Potter). Ancient Greek *tuphos*, from which the modern disease name of typhus is misleadingly derived, covers a range of acute diseases involving fever and eventually delirium of some kind.

38. *Diseases 2* 51 (5:284–87 Potter); see also *Epidemics* 6.8.29 (7:286–89 Smith). On the spinal marrow as seed, or its immediate precursor, see, for example, Plato, *Timaeus* 91a–b; and the Hippocratic treatise *Generation* 2 (10:8–11 Potter).

39. This translation is adapted from that of Paul Potter, in Loeb, volume 5. Translations are my own unless otherwise noted.

40. This seed production is most famously explained at *Generation* 5–8 (10:14–21 Potter).

41. Ann Ellis Hanson, "The Medical Writers' Woman," in *Before Sexuality: The Construction of Erotic Experience in the Ancient Greek World*, ed. David M. Halperin, John J. Winkler, and Froma I. Zeitlin (London: Routledge, 1990), 309–38.

42. *Diseases of Women 1* 24 (Loeb 11: 64–67 Potter).

43. *Diseases of Women 2* 1, 3–13 (110, 112–22 L)(11:262–69 and 268–99 Potter).

44. *Diseases of Women 2* 8 (117 L) (11:282–8577 Potter).

45. The nonmenstrual nature of this blood is made clear at *Diseases of Women 2* 5 (114 L) (11:274–77 Potter).

46. See, for example, Nutton, *Ancient Medicine*, 130–59.

47. The author of this anonymous handbook is called, after the location of the main manuscript, Anonymus Parisinus. On this and the other Roman imperial medical texts to be discussed, see Rebecca Flemming, *Medicine and the Making of Roman Women: Gender, Nature, and Authority from Celsus to Galen* (Oxford: Oxford University Press, 2000).

48. See Philip van der Eijk, "The Anonymus Parisinus and the Doctrines of 'the Ancients,'" in *Ancient Histories of Medicine: Essays in Medical Doxography and Historiography in Classical Antiquity*, ed. Philip van der Eijk (Leiden: Brill, 1999), 295–331.

49. On Celsus and his translation project, see David Langslow, *Medical Latin in the Roman Empire* (Oxford: Oxford University Press, 1999).

50. Celsus, *On Medicine* 4.28. There is, again, an accessible, if somewhat dated Loeb edition and translation in three volumes (Cambridge, MA: Harvard University Press, 1935). The note on this section, provided by the translator, W. G. Spencer oddly asserts that "Greek and Roman medical writers refused to recognise this as an infection, in opposition to all popular knowledge," this "popular knowledge" apparently being contained in Leviticus (Loeb of Celsus 1:450).

51. Anonymus Parisinus 47: *Anonymi Medici De Morbis Acutis et Chroniis*, ed. Ivan Garofalo, trans. Brian Fuchs (Leiden: Brill, 1997), 240–43.

52. Celsus, *On Medicine* 3.1.3.

53. Soranus, *Gynecology* 3.45. The English translation by Owsei Temkin is easily accessible (Baltimore: Johns Hopkins University Press, 1965), with the chapter on what he renders as "Flux of semen" at 168–70. In note 80 Temkin seems to agree with a much earlier scholarly assertion to the effect that "the ancient concept of gonorrhea covered spermatorrhea, masturbation, and gonorrhea," though spermatorrhea had already ceased to be a disease recognized by modern Western medicine by the 1960s. Aretaeus, *Causes and Signs of Chronic Diseases* 2.5. Francis Adams's

(rather archaic) English translation is easily available, with the relevant chapter at pages 346–47 (London: Sydenham Society, 1856). On these texts and authors more generally, see Flemming, *Making of Roman Women*, 187–89, 228–46.

54. [Galen], *Medical Definitions* 288 (19:426 Kühn); Rufus of Ephesus, *On Satyriasis and Gonorrhoia* (Daremberg-Ruelle, 64–86); Flemming, *Making of Roman Women*, 186–91.

55. Galen, *On the Affected Parts* 6.6 (8:437–41 Kühn). The English translation of Rudolph E. Siegel (New York: Karger, 1976), though easily accessible, is very unreliable. See Flemming, *Making of Roman Women*, 336–37.

56. Soranus, *Gynecology* 3.46 (Temkin, 169–70).

57. Aretaeus, *On the Cure of Chronic Diseases* 2.5 (Adams, 488–89).

58. See, for example, Aretaeus's discussion of chronic bladder conditions, including the stone, in *Causes and Signs of Chronic Diseases* 2.4 (Adams, 344–46).

59. Soranus, *Gynecology* 3.43–44 (Temkin, 165–68).

60. Celsus is most fulsome on these matters, especially when discussing possible surgical interventions: *On Medicine* 7.18 (testicles and scrotum); 7.25 (penis and foreskin); 7.28 (ulceration of female genitals).

61. Greek: Oribasius, *Synopsis for Eustathius* 9.37; Aetius of Amida 11.33 and 16.68; Alexander of Tralles 11.7; Paul of Aegina 3.55. Latin: Caelius Aurelianus, *On Chronic Diseases* 5.6 and *Gynecology* 2.56–7; Muscio, *Gynecology* 138; Theodorus Priscianus, *Euporista* 2.11, 3.10.

62. See, for example, John R. Clarke, *Looking at Lovemaking: Constructions of Sexuality in Roman Art, 100 BC–AD 250* (Berkeley: University of California Press, 1998); and Christiane Goldberg, *Carmina Pripaea: Einleitung, Übersetzung, Interpretation und Kommentar* (Heidelberg: Winter, 1992).

63. See, for example, Horace, *Epode* 8; Martial, *Epigrams* 3.72, 9.37, 10.90; *Priapea* 12, 46.

64. See Amy Richlin, *The Garden of Priapus: Sexuality and Aggression in Roman Humor*, rev. ed. (New York: Oxford University Press, 1992).

65. Martial, *Epigrams* 11.21.

66. Martial, *Epigrams* 9.57 develops this theme along the same lines as 11.21; see also, for example, 9.27; and Juvenal, *Satires* 2.11–13.

67. Martial, *Epigrams* 6.37.

68. Martial, *Epigrams* 7.35, 82; 6.67; 11.63, 75; *Priapea* 77.

69. Martial, *Epigrams* 11.61, see also 11.85.

70. J. D. Oriel, "Anal and Genital Warts in the Ancient World," *Paleopathology Newsletter* 3 (1973): unnumbered pages; Judith Hallett, "Something in Excess? *Priapea* 50.2," *Mnemosyne* 31 (1978): 203–6. Fig terminology does wider sexual work in Latin (and Greek) too; see J. N. Adams, *The Latin Sexual Vocabulary* (London: Duckworth, 1982), 113–14.

71. Martial, *Epigrams* 1.65, 4.52, 7.71, 14.86; see also Juvenal 2.13; and *Priapea* 50.2.

72. Martial, *Epigrams* 12.83.

73. Pliny, *Letters* 6.24; for background, see Roy Gibson and Ruth Morello, *Reading the Letters of Pliny the Younger: An Introduction* (Cambridge: Cambridge University Press, 2012).

74. Arria features in Pliny, *Letters* 3.16; and see also 1.22 for another episode of serious illness that requires discussion of suicide, though with a different outcome.

75. Though styled as "private" letters, Pliny did "publish" this collection; see Gibson and Morello, *Reading the Letters*.

76. Fronto, *Letters to Marcus Caesar* (*Ad M. Caes.*) 5.23 (Loeb 1 196–97).

77. Vertue, "Enquiry into Venereal Disease," 288.

78. Marcus Aurelius and Fronto mainly tell each other about localized pain; see J. E. G. Whitehorne, "Was Marcus Aurelius a Hypochondriac?," *Latomus* 36 (1977), 416–18; and Rebecca Flemming, "Experience," in *A Cultural History of Medicine*, ed. Laurence M. V. Totelin, vol. 1 (London: Bloomsbury, forthcoming).

79. Josephus, *Jewish War* 5.227, 6.426; compare the slightly different formulations in his summary of Mosaic legislation at *Jewish Antiquities* 3.261–64.

80. *Lepra* translates to *ṣâraʿat* in the Septuagint (e.g., Leviticus 13:25, 27, 44 and 45) and, despite medieval usage of latinized versions, does not include leprosy (Hansen's disease) within its wide remit of skin blotches, patches, and encrustations—neither does *ṣâraʿat* (Milgrom, *Leviticus 1–16*, 816–20). There is some archaeological evidence for Hansen's disease in the ancient Mediterranean world; see, for example, Mauro Rubinia, Paola Zaiob, and Charlotte Roberts, "Tuberculosis and Leprosy in Italy: New Skeletal Evidence," *HOMO: Journal of Comparative Human Biology* 65 (2014): 13–32, but it is described under the label of *elephantiasis* in the medical texts of the Roman Empire. In Leviticus (13:45–46) sufferers from "scale-disease" are removed "from the camp."

81. Soranus, *Gynecology* 3.45 (Temkin, 168–9).

82. Vertue, "Enquiry into Venereal Disease," 271, 289–91.

83. The Roman partnership of prostitution and marriage is stressed particularly in Rebecca Flemming, "*Quae corpore quaestum facit*: The Sexual Economy of Female Prostitution in the Roman Empire," *Journal of Roman Studies* 89 (1999): 38–61; see more generally on Roman prostitution, Thomas McGinn, *Prostitution, Sexuality, and the Law in Ancient Rome* (Oxford: Oxford University Press, 1998); and McGinn, *The Economy of Roman Prostitution: A Study of Social History and the Brothel* (Ann Arbor: University of Michigan Press, 2004).

84. Horace, *Satire* 2.1.31–35.

85. This anecdote is in the marginal scholia on Horace's satires, collected together under the name of Pseudo-Acron. O. Keller, *Pseudoacronis scholia in Horatium vetustiora*, vol. 2 (Leipzig: Teubner, 1904), 20. For the general point see Flemming, "*Quae corpore quaestum facit*."

86. On the tax, see McGinn, *Prostitution*, 248–87; and Flemming, "*Quae corpore quaestum facit*," 50–56. The allegation that financial dependence prevented successive Christian emperors from ceasing tax prostitution is made by Evagrius,

Ecclesiastical History 3.39, on the occasion of the final repeal in AD 498, over a century and a half after the conversion of Constantine.

87. Details are debated, and figures vague, but there is a scholarly consensus that the population and economy of empire expanded over the period from the end of the civil wars in 31 BC to the first outbreak of the Antonine Plague in AD 165: see, for example, the range of population figures used by Myles Lavan, "The Spread of Roman Citizenship, 14–212 CE: Quantification in the Face of High Uncertainty," *Past and Present* 230 (2016): 3–46; and the relevant chapters in Walter Scheidel, Ian Morris, and Richard Saller, eds., *The Cambridge Economic History of the Greco-Roman World* (Cambridge: Cambridge University Press, 2007).

88. Leonor Sánchez-Busó et al., "Antimicrobial Exposure in Sexual Networks Drives Divergent Evolution in Modern Gonococci," preprint at *bioRxiv*, https://doi.org/10.1101/334847.

89. See, for example, Worboys, chap. 5, in this volume; these claims were in part about funding and politics.

Chapter Two

"Poxt and Clapt Together"

Sexual Misbehavior in Early Modern Cases of Venereal Disease

Olivia Weisser

The connection between infertility and venereal disease was probably widely understood in the early 1700s, though evidence of this is elusive, and it has received little historical attention.[1] The association is clearest in instances of healers who specialized in both curing venereal disease and treating infertility, and a few remedies for the disease doubled as fertility treatments.[2] Venereal scabs, ulcers, and scars were thought to hamper the physical processes involved in procreation. As one book put it quite brusquely, "the Seed does not squirt out with that Jirk as is necessary to keep up its conveyance to the Ovarium of the Woman." Likewise, the vaginas of infected women could become inflamed or fluxed, thereby inhibiting sexual activity. The disease was also thought to cause infertility in two other ways. First, it could weaken the seed. For instance, when a thirty-year-old man "much given to Venery" in his youth continued acting in lewd ways, "his Genital Parts became very much weakened, and at last Impotent." Second, venereal cures could lead to infertility by creating "lankness, softness, or withering" of the genitals.[3] A woman who contracted venereal disease from her husband told her doctor that she took treatments for years "by means of which, and the Disease, she believ'd she was rendred Sterill."[4]

This chapter approaches the link between sex and disease from a different angle, however. Rather than examining how the disease was thought to cause infertility, I analyze how ideas and anxieties about sex shaped clinical encounters. Using medical cases spanning 1675 to 1750, this chapter shows how beliefs and concerns about sexual misbehavior could inform interactions between venereal healers and patients. Such a focus highlights the moral nature of the disease and how sexual anxiety was key to treating and diagnosing it.

In their accounts of medical practice, venereal healers presented themselves as shrewd interpreters of patients' bodies and souls. They had to be such skilled observers, I suggest, because they did not trust their patients. In the early modern period, patients' verbal, subjective accounts of illness were crucial to medical practice.[5] Diseases were not viewed as tangible entities that manifested uniformly in all bodies. Rather, they were unique, continually transforming clusters of symptoms that patients and healers interpreted according to individual lifestyles and constitutions. Bodily signs were ambiguous, and diagnoses could be difficult to discern. Venereal disease was particularly vexing to diagnose because its symptoms were linked to a range of disorders, and the bodily marks associated with the disease could be difficult to read.[6] As a result, discerning whether a case was venereal was fairly dependent on patients' subjective expressions of their symptoms and sexual histories. Yet, I have found, several venereal healers viewed patients' words as unreliable. Healers described patients who were intentionally misleading or who denied shameful diagnoses of venereal disease. This chapter examines how healers exhibited diagnostic expertise by sagely navigating such constraints. They characterized themselves as medical detectives who gathered clues and made diagnoses in spite of patients' untrustworthy speech. This work entailed moral integrity, astute observations, and the ability to persuade patients to divulge their most shameful sexual secrets.

Methods and Sources

Before turning to the evidence, I want briefly to explain my approach within the context of this volume. Rather than a demographic or epidemiological study of the relationship between disease and fertility, this chapter offers a cultural history of disease. As many of the chapters in this volume demonstrate, epidemiological histories recover the changing occurrence of diseases and their impact on society. This approach to studying the past is valuable for helping us make sense of how epidemics occur and how to respond to them.

The premise of these studies is that modern-day understandings of diseases are "correct," and we can recover that truth in the historical record using the tools of modern science. Even diseases that evolve into new ones with different names and histories maintain traceable, epidemiological identities.

Rather than view diseases of the past as precursors to modern-day categories, a cultural approach attempts to understand diseases of the past in the terms of people living at the time.[7] Past explanatory frameworks do not always fit with our own modern views, of course. In the early modern period, for example, diseases were thought to roam around the body. They could even morph into entirely new disorders altogether. One woman endured a headache for years before the pain suddenly sunk into her pelvis. Another woman suffered from lifelong migraines that she ascribed to a fever contracted at the tender age of twelve.[8] Recovering how these women perceived and explained their ailments, rather than trying to make sense of them in modern terms, exposes the ever-shifting construction of biology and teaches us to question the contingency of our own convictions. Were the men and women in this chapter truly suffering from the diseases we know today as syphilis and gonorrhea? From a cultural historian's perspective, the question is beside the point. Diseases of the past are culturally incommensurable with our own.

In addition to taking an anthropological perspective, cultural historians have moved away from measuring responses to disease and have become increasingly invested in the assumptions, mind sets, and narratives that gave shape and meaning to experiences of health and illness. Scholars taking this approach have paid particularly close attention to language and writing practices—not only *what* texts say but *how* they say it.[9] The ways people wrote about disease, after all, expose the assumptions and preoccupations embedded within their explanations and experiences, not to mention medical knowledge itself. For many cultural historians, diseases are not clearly delineated entities plucked from the historical record so much as contested, negotiated, and produced through acts of writing and the medium of language.

The analysis that follows centers on a curious pattern I found in healers' cases of venereal disease: a tendency to characterize patients as unreliable and to end cases with patients' confessions of sexual misbehavior. Why were patients depicted as unreliable narrators? And why was confession such a persuasive literary frame for venereal cases? To answer these questions I approach cases as both carefully crafted narratives aimed at promoting practice and demonstrating authority and documents that can tell us something very real about past experiences of disease. Most of the cases I discuss were probably embellished; some may have been entirely fictional. Yet they had to be plausible to be effective promotional material and, as such, offer illuminating insights into medical practice. Rather than read these sources as unproblematic reflections of what actually transpired in the consulting room, I instead attempt to uncover the assumptions and preoccupations underlying healers' words—particularly the meanings of confession for early modern individuals and the implications of unreliable speech for healers' work.

My analysis is based on two types of sources: cases recorded in over sixty books on venereal disease, many of which were authored by nonlearned or unlicensed healers, and 206 nonrecurring printed advertisements for venereal cures spanning the late 1600s and early 1700s.[10] Who were the healers who produced these books and handbills? Only 94 of the 206 advertisements include a name. Some provide a mere initial—Dr. S., for example. Those possessing traditional credentials were certain to highlight them. Healers listed their affiliations with universities or licensing bodies or their previous roles as healthcare providers in royal courts.[11] Several noted the former patients or physicians—invariably "Gentlemen of Quality"—who referred patients to their practices.[12] John Marten apprenticed for a surgeon and worked for the Sick and Wounded Hospital in Ireland before striking out on his own. According to a competitor, however, he performed only simple procedures like cutting corns and letting blood.[13]

These men and women sold purges, injections, and balsams that purportedly cleansed the body of venereal poisons, though many kept their ingredients secret. John Marten claimed to possess prescriptions for a pill and diet drink passed down from his master's master, a surgeon named Samuel Smith who worked at Saint Thomas' Hospital for eighteen years. Marten shared the ingredients of the pills, but he kept the drink a secret, "being so particular and uncommon."[14] The rarity of the drink made it all the more alluring to customers. The two most common treatments for venereal disease were "salivations" and "frictions." Salivations contained mercury that caused excessive spitting. They ranged from pills and drinks to smoke that users inhaled, and they were composed of mercury in all its forms. While today we attribute extreme salivation to mercury poisoning, this response was desirable within the humoral framework of disease. Prolific spitting signified the release of pent-up matter, which was evidence of a potentially curative bodily transformation. Frictions were topical ointments that contained mercury but did not always result in salivation. Frictions were also known as the "French method" or "Montpellier method," references to the university that employed the treatment's alleged creator, Francois Chicoyneau. Although patients endured multiple courses of frictions, and some spent weeks recuperating, proponents of the method promoted it as gentler and more discreet than salivations.[15]

More than a few healers avoided mercury altogether. Of the advertisements analyzed here, thirty-nine characterized cures as mercury-free or as targeting venereal disease while also cleansing bodies "Damnified by Mercury."[16]

Early stages of the disease, known colloquially as a "clap," "running of the reins," or gonorrhea, entailed burning sensations while urinating, chancres, ulcers, inflammations, and excretions from the genitals. Improperly treated or neglected, these symptoms developed into a more serious disorder that corrupted the entire body, known as a "confirmed" or "true" pox. Healers tended to view this process as a slow spread of venereal venom from the genitals out to the body's extremities. Eventually the poison seeped into the nerves and bones, "a dismal Scene indeed."[17] At this stage the patient might develop paralysis, a fallen palate, or sunken nose.

"Venereal disease" was the catchall term that English men and women in the 1700s used to describe a group of related symptoms that we now associate with discrete disease categories, such as syphilis or gonorrhea. Yet the difference between venereal disease in early modern England and today is not just one of semantics. Disease was thought to look different in each individual, and symptoms, causes, and cures were understood within a humoral framework of health that associated illness with clogged or corrupted internal fluids.[18] Moreover, while many healers and patients in the period recognized a link between sex and venereal disease, they did not perceive that link the same way we do. It was not simply sexual contact that was presumed to produce infection, but the "wrong" kind of sex—illicit, frequent, fervent. Like any aspect of regimen, sex must be moderate and suited to one's constitution. In her work on sixteenth-century Germany, Claudia Stein has shown how some patients attributed the disease to events that had no apparent connection to sex, such as shifts in weather.[19] English cases from the early 1600s recorded by clergy healer and astrologer Richard Napier likewise linked venereal disease to nonsexual sources, such as spraining an ankle while jumping over a hedge or getting struck in the chest by a stone.[20] Early modern theories of disease are not the focus here, but they do provide important context for healers' accounts of medical practice. The connection between infection and improper sex, after all, made it plausible that patients might mislead their healers. And because disease was presumed to look different in everyone, interpreting and diagnosing it was fairly subjective. Symptoms varied by constitutions and lifestyle choices, and diagnoses were determined in part by listening to patients describe their conditions and health histories. This view of disease contextualizes venereal healers' self-characterizations as diagnostic experts. They claimed to root out the truth despite lacking information—reliable patient testimony—considered essential to that work.

Cases of Sexual Misbehavior

I have found thirty instances in which healers characterized venereal patients as unreliable narrators—that is, as deceptive, evasive, or otherwise untrustworthy. Such unreliability, I argue, served to highlight practitioners' diagnostic acumen, as they had to navigate the constraints of patients' lies and omissions to evaluate disease. Literary scholars have suggested that medical cases can resemble moral tales or stories driven by heroic action.[21] The most apt literary construct in early modern venereal cases is the rather anachronistic detective story. Healers characterized consultations as sleuth work that required shrewd observations and ended with confessions of sexual secrets. When a young maid sought out treatment for a sore throat, for example, John Marten claimed to detect signs of venereal disease. She initially denied this diagnosis but then confessed to sharing her bed with an apprentice. She conceded to contracting an infection from him but claimed to remain a virgin. According to Marten, her symptoms suggested otherwise: "she was both Poxt and Clapt together, and without doubt no Virgin."[22]

Alexander Morgan, a surgeon's apprentice from Bristol, recorded another typical case. A woman came to see him for sores on her arms and thighs. Morgan dressed the area "as I use to do others in like cases," but he grew wary when his remedies failed to work. When he uttered the word "pox" the patient grew angry "at such plain de[a]ling." She would have preferred a euphemism or perhaps even a false diagnosis that allowed Morgan to treat her symptoms without acknowledging the true nature of her infection. Despite her wrath, the patient "at last consented she had been salivated by Unction & for 2 years." She had spent two years rubbing mercurial ointments on her skin, which suggested a prior diagnosis of pox. His suspicions confirmed, Morgan claimed to have cured her with his own ointment in just five weeks.[23]

Some patients were portrayed as intentionally misleading. When questioned about his sore nose, a young servant denied having venereal disease and instead attributed his malady to the most wholesome of activities: playing with a kitten.[24] Daniel Turner likewise treated a man's swollen testicle as a "simple Contusion" based on his patient's assertion that the swelling developed from sleeping with his legs crossed. Turner let blood, applied a truss, and prescribed a topical mixture to keep the swelling ripe and soft. Like the case from Morgan, Turner was tipped off when his usual remedies proved ineffective. He suspected a venereal disorder but, given the man's "Habit and State of Life"—chaste in this instance—he also considered a malady rooting from "seminal Retention." The man's swelling improved the next morning, but his continual sighs, as Turner put it, "increased my Suspicion of the real Cause." Turner's hunch was later confirmed when he noticed stains on the bed linens and fluid issuing from the patient's penis, which he had concealed in previous examinations. The patient blushed and "fell a weeping," admitting that he suffered from a disease acquired through venery and begging Turner to protect his reputation.[25]

In other instances healers suggested that patients legitimately misdiagnosed themselves. A couple took their daughter to see John Sintelaer in 1705 because her legs were covered in painful ulcers. The couple had been poxed previously, but they neglected to mention their medical history. Rather than acting "stupid and thoughtless," Sintelaer believed that they simply failed to associate their daughter's ailment with their own past conditions: "they were so far from entertaining any such Thoughts," Sintelaer explained, "that without dreaming in the least of any thing like it, they consulted divers Physicians to cure this young Woman of the Consumption, without mentioning a Word of their own former Disaster." Sintelaer recalled having cured the couple for venereal disease some twelve years earlier and asked if perhaps the mother unknowingly infected her daughter while pregnant. The woman was "thunder-struck" upon hearing this theory, a reaction that affirmed Sintelaer's diagnostic insight, not to mention his impressive memory.[26]

Why was this couple deemed honest and forgetful, while the man with the swollen testicle was deceptive? Such characterizations may indeed have been accurate, but they also performed the work of exhibiting healers' diagnostic skills. Sintelaer was able to make a connection between two disparate episodes of illness that even those afflicted failed to see. And Turner displayed his expertise by overcoming the dual challenge of diagnosing a deceptive patient who also appeared chaste and therefore less likely to have venereal disease in Turner's mind. The ability to assess moral character presented practitioners as principled and capable. Such assessments were in fact common ways that venereal healers claimed to circumvent patients' untrustworthiness. By noting another patient's "Way of Living," Turner suspected there was more to his sore throat than the "common Catarrh, or Cold, that he pretended of late to have contracted."[27] And Marten suspected venereal disease in a man suffering from fever and headaches after inquiring about his symptoms, as well as "his Life, which I understood to be very dessolute."[28] Likewise, Richard Wiseman noted "the manner of life of the Patient" when treating an ulcer on the leg of a twenty-eight-year-old man. This information, in combination with the inefficacy of his standard remedies, led Wiseman to suspect the ulcer developed from a poorly cured clap. He treated it with mercury and an enema made of milk and egg yolks.[29] When dealing with such a moralizing disease, depravity could be just as significant a symptom as headaches, fevers, and sores.

These healers stressed their ability to detect disease in spite of sufferers' alleged omissions, deceptions, and denials. These cases suggest some of the ways they did so: by noting the inefficacy of their cures, by investigating prior treatments, and by evaluating patients' habits and lifestyles. A fourth approach was to use sensory observations to read patients' bodies. Patients' speech may have been viewed as suspect, but bodies did not lie. A servant suspected that he had a kidney stone, but John Douglas interpreted his malady as venereal by watching him urinate. The patient strained and only a few drops dripped out. Douglas asked if it hurt to ride in a coach or on horseback. The patient could endure both without a problem, which confirmed Douglas' suspicions: "I don't think you have the stone in the bladder, for I never knew one that had, who could bear either of them." When he asked about the pox, the man freely admitted to having the disease years ago. Douglas again looked to the body as validation: he inserted a probe toward the bladder but could get no further than the prostate gland on account of a large swelling. He suspected it developed from medicines prescribed for a venereal disorder. Some treatments provided only temporary relief, leaving behind scars and poisons that materialized years later.[30]

Daniel Turner had no need to interrogate a woman covered in ulcers. Nor could he, since her speech was garbled due to a damaged palate. Her husband's case was even more obvious. Turner noted how "without telling his Tale," his body communicated the nature of his affliction. While historians have emphasized the visual effects of venereal disease, these cases show that infections were also conspicuous by altering patients' voices. Venereal ulcers ate away at the throat and palate, creating a mode of speech that healers definitively identified with the disease. Turner referred to it as "snuffling." In several instances it was the sound of a patient's voice, rather than the words themselves, that led healers to a diagnosis.[31]

They also pushed, poked, and pressed. Such manipulations revealed the location and consistency of internal matter, as did the subsequent yelps of patients. One man complained when Thomas Garlick pressed down on his groin, but this allowed Garlick to link fluid seeping from his penis to ulcers.[32] Healers also observed the "intolerable Noysomness and Stench" emanating from mortified body parts.[33] John Sintelaer characterized the odor of one man's ulcer as so putrid "it was ready to strike me down," and Charles Peter ominously described a patient's smell as "cadaverous."[34] Others noted the smell of effluvia, such as urine and spit, and one healer even relied on taste. The fluid seeping from a woman's ulcerated breast tasted "sharp as Oyl of Vitriol."[35]

Finally, venereal healers made and confirmed their interpretations by garnering patients' trust and eliciting stories of sexual misbehavior. Trust was a key component of clinical relationships, particularly those between female patients and male practitioners.[36] Several of the healers here diagnosed disease by asserting authority and instilling confidence in their patients, ultimately convincing them to divulge sexual secrets. Such confessions are significant, I argue, because they verified healers' clinical interpretations and further established their expertise.

John Marten seemed to rely on these tactics more frequently than others. Again and again he refused to capitulate to patient demands for alternate treatments or to acknowledge interpretations of illness that contradicted his own. Given his notoriety for circulating medical material as provocative entertainment, perhaps Marten's need to establish his authority was more pressing than that of his contemporaries. In fact, he recorded seventeen of the thirty cases of unreliable patients.[37] In one instance he was called to treat a nursery maid who cared for two young children of an eminent London shopkeeper. Another servant in the house noticed that the maid owned a trunk of pills and powders. When asked about it, the maid explained that the medicines were for emergencies. Shortly following this interchange, the children developed fevers, stomachaches, and swellings. They also presented sores on their faces and bodies and "a violent hot, sharp Humour upon the lower Parts." Most suspiciously of all, they fell ill at precisely the same time. Marten began his investigation, like so many of these cases, by inquiring about the medicines the children had taken previously. This information could hint at a prior diagnosis or the possibility that they ingested a hazardous substance. He also asked the maid if she had any "Breakings out," suggesting that she may have transmitted an infection to the children by sharing a bed with them. The maid, in response, claimed to be "as well as ever she was in her Life." Marten wrote down instructions for the children's parents and promptly left.[38]

The parents remained uneasy, however. So too did the servant who initially spotted the trunk. She suspected her colleague of secretly administering medicine to the children, and she said as much to their parents. The nurse denied it. But when the parents looked inside the trunk, they found it filled with boxes of pills and pots of unguents, as well as directions for treating sores on the groin. Marten was called back again and, given the situation, "told them plainly I believ'd their Children had got the foul Disease." The maid continued to deny the diagnosis, even after Marten examined her body for signs of the pox: "she with a great deal of Confidence denied it, and not only so, but that she would make me prove my Words." Marten, in turn, continued to assert his authority by stating his view in increasingly strident tones: "the more she denied it, the more I asserted it." He not only urged her to concede but was "threatning her, and telling her I was sure what I said was true." She finally relented and admitted her guilt.[39]

When another patient rejected a diagnosis of venereal disease, instead insisting that he contracted King's Evil from his late wife, Marten threatened to withhold treatment altogether. According to Marten, the patient was concerned about his reputation and consistently denied engaging in any kind of activity that would lead to venereal disease. The healer explained, "I could not help, for that he must be Cured as such or not at all; he gave me my Fee, made me a Bow, and away he went." The gamble paid off. The man returned the next day and conceded that he had slept with a woman eight weeks earlier. The unmarried daughter of a local merchant similarly contested a diagnosis of pox. Venereal treatments were slow and conspicuous and would have exposed her malady. But any other treatment, Marten explained, "would be in vain" and would only make her ailment more difficult to cure down the road. He related, once again, how his insistence led to a confession. She admitted to having the pox but demanded an inconspicuous remedy for it lest her parents find out.[40]

In one case Marten had no need to dwell on a diagnosis. A woman came to see him after contracting pox from her husband, and she was well aware of what ailed her. Yet Marten still managed to brandish his interpretive skills by assessing her character, as well as that of her husband. She developed sores just one week after her wedding day. She consulted a midwife but began to suspect a venereal disorder when her symptoms persisted. Her parents confronted her new husband, who denied any wrongdoing and "fell a Cursing and Swearing, as if they had done him Wrong." Based on this story and "her Husband's Behavior during her telling it," Marten determined that she was a "discreet, modest Woman" and her husband was the source of her infirmity. Marten confronted the man one-on-one. After a few stubborn refusals, he admitted to having contracted a clap a few months before the wedding.[41] Pinpointing the cause of infection might seem irrelevant. The couple, after all, hired Marten to cure them, not root out the source of their sickness. But by correctly assigning blame, Marten exhibited his role as moral as well as medical authority.

Among the thirty cases of unreliable patients, eleven involved men like this one who secretly infected their unsuspecting wives. Another such case originates from Martin Lister. A woman came to him to treat a common reproductive ailment known as "the whites." She had taken spa water and astringents mixed with roasted rhubarb and opium, but she continued to suffer from diarrhea and "gripings" in her bowels. After observing her symptoms and hearing her story, Lister pulled her husband aside and admonished him for infecting his wife. The man responded to this accusation "very heinously" but then admitted to having contracted venereal disease years earlier.[42] The eleven cases that fit this pattern all involve innocent female patients and healers who claim to identify deceptive husbands.[43] They also tend to end with private confrontations between healer and husband and, ultimately, admissions of sexual misdeeds. Kevin Siena has valuably shown that venereal healers highlighted private conversations to demonstrate their discretion and appeal to potential clients.[44] These cases suggest that discretion was also a tool that enabled healers to exhibit expertise. It was the guarantee of confidentiality, after all, that convinced patients to divulge their sexual histories. And it was those histories that validated healers' diagnoses of disease. Of course, healers ultimately violated patients' confidence by putting those sexual histories and diagnoses in print.

Two-thirds of the cases of unreliable patients (twenty-one out of thirty) end with confessions of sexual misbehavior. These cases took this form, I suggest, because of the persuasive power of confessions as validation of healers' diagnostic ability. As proof of clinical evaluations, confessions functioned much the same as patient testimonials and certificates of cures in handbills and advertisements. While these other modes of validating expertise or the efficacy of cures were derided as instruments of quacks, confessions in medical cases were couched within a sanctioned genre of medical writing.[45] The prevalence of confessions also reflects the presumption that venereal infection resulted from illicit sex. A diagnosis of venereal disease, in other words, would be difficult to prove if patients only ever slept with their spouses. Confessions confirmed that forbidden liaisons took place.

Confessions held a range of meanings in the period that further suggest why so many of these cases end with one. While the days of confessing to priests in England were long past, confession in the early eighteenth century retained its associations with penance. For Protestants confession took new forms within the private realm of account keeping and routine self-examination.[46] Confession too continued to be linked to divulgence of sin and expressions of remorse in more secular dimensions of early modern life. For many English men and women, the most familiar form of confession was the last-minute admission of guilt typically included in gallows speeches. Historians have interpreted the "last dying speeches" of those condemned to public execution as warnings, a form of repentance, and even a last-ditch attempt at redemption.[47] The early modern stage provided a venue for another type of confessional performance. According to literary scholar John Parker, confessions onstage exposed the duplicity of villains and enabled theatergoers to witness characters' transgressions guiltlessly.[48] Like these various types of confession from the period, the disclosure of sexual misconduct in venereal cases provided warnings, exposed deceit, and invited readers to delight in others' misdeeds. The men and women who read books on venereal disease were voyeurs, observing the sins of others from the safety and privacy of their homes.

There was perhaps a healing component to confession too. Venting clogged matter was deemed healthful in this period, as illness was thought to result largely from obstructions and corruptions within the body. As a result, common medical treatments, including vomits, bloodletting, emetics, and even mercury that caused excessive salivation, were thought to work by releasing pent-up fluid. Confessing secrets to a confidante could be similarly cleansing. Francis Bacon compared unburdening the heart by means of a "kind of civil shrift or confession" to the wholesome release provoked by medical therapies.[49] Confession incited a therapeutic opening of the heart much like the purgative effects of many medicinal cures.

Associations between confession and health are perhaps most prevalent in religious writing from the period. Scripture explicitly characterized confession as a nourishing act: "Confess your faults one to another, and pray one for another, that ye may be healed."[50] If sinful behavior caused infection then repenting sins cured it. Early modern sermons and devotional literature further suggested a link between confession and health by characterizing repentance in medical terms. Moral transgressions were likened to disease and purging the soul of impurities to a beneficial dose of physic.[51] A Lancashire shopkeeper copied out lengthy instructions for repentance using the structure and vocabulary of one of the most familiar forms of medical writing from the period—a medical recipe:

> Take a quart of repentance of Ninivah, and [pu]t nine handfulls of faith in the bloud of Christ with as much hope and charitee as you can gett, and put into a vessell of a clean consciance. Then boile it on the fire of love. . . . Then scum it of cleane with the spoone of faithfull prayers. When this is done, put in the pouder of patiance; then straine altogather in the cupp of a humble hart; then drinke it burneing hott next thy heart, and cover thee warme with as many clothes of amendment of life as God shall enable thee to beare.[52]

Overlaps between health and confession were even apparent in the act of repentance itself. While Protestants took stock of their sins through prayer, reading, and private writing, repentance could also take the form of weeping. Devotional tears were thought to demonstrate contrition and aid spiritual health, an outflow that mirrored the purgative effects of medicinal pills and potions.[53] Patients and healers did not make an explicit link between confession and physical recovery. Yet they surely viewed confessions of sexual misbehavior as cleansing, and prevailing understandings of penance, health, and recovery imbued those confessions with meaning. Divulging sexual secrets provided relief much the way a spiritual confession cleared sin from the soul and a medical remedy purged the body of corruption.

If patients were confessors, then practitioners were the priests who arbitrated the moral status of their flocks and doled out penance in the form of medicines. There was a widely held belief that the punitive nature of venereal cures was justified, and even necessary. Punishing remedies were acts of atonement: infected men and women suffered for their sinful ways by enduring the physical toll of mercury ointments, fumigations, and pills. These remedies caused sweats, fevers, shaking, and rotten palates. Patients' teeth fell out from a combination of decayed gums and trembling fits. Others lost their hearing and vision.[54] "It is an old saying, that Mercury cures the Pox, but what cures Mercury?" posed one practitioner.[55] John Sintelaer used the term "martyr" to describe patients undergoing such treatments, a term that overtly likened mercurial remedies to redemptive torture.[56] Advertisements for venereal cures further suggested that poxed patients should ingest medicine to cleanse the soul as well as the body. Rose's Balsamick Elixir purportedly made "any Man tho' as rotten as a Pear, to be as sound as a Sucking Lamb." "Rotten" could define the physical state of the body but was also a term that connoted the moral fitness of the soul. "Sound as a Sucking Lamb," on the other hand, implied purity. One healer invited patients who had "slipp'd in between the Thighs of Venus" to sample his cures. "I will cleanse them from all Defilement and make them as white as Snow," he wrote.[57] These remedies promised to both cure disease and absolve sin.

Assumptions about gender and status framed portrayals of patients as confessors. In early modern England women were presumed to be duplicitous, and blame for the spread of venereal disease was typically pinned on them.[58] Prostitutes were linked to contagion, while some medical authorities posited that all women bred infection on account of their physiology. Pioneering studies have shown how these assumptions reflected anxieties about women's sexuality, most especially outside the confines of marriage.[59] A case by Daniel Turner typifies these views. A man went out "drinking harder than usual," but, despite his gluttony, Turner pinned responsibility for his infection on one of the "Night-walkers in Cheapside." She picked up the man, "carry'd him to the Tavern," and "clap'd him also." Turner assigned the man no agency in the matter, characterizing him instead as "prey."[60] Despite such stereotypes, it was men rather than women who were depicted as dishonest and lascivious most often in cases of unreliable venereal patients. Of the thirty cases twenty-two entailed male patients who contracted the disease or spread it knowingly to innocent women. Eleven of those men were married and brought infections home to their unsuspecting spouses. Although this sample is very small, it shows that gender informed thinking and writing about venereal disease in ways that extended beyond typical associations between devious women and infection. The disgraceful behavior of married men suggests anxieties about preserving domesticity rather than restraining women's promiscuity.

Two of John Marten's cases—one involving the virgin servant girl and the other the nursery maid with the trunk of pills—demonstrate how gender worked together with age and status to shape these accounts.[61] As the son of a tailor who purportedly shared a house with his brother to make ends meet, Marten was especially sensitive to issues of status. There were instances when he convinced gentlewomen to confess to sexual misdeeds, but he seemed to assert his moral and diagnostic authority most forcefully in cases involving young girls at a particularly vulnerable stage of the early modern life cycle. It was common for women between the ages of fourteen and twenty-four to work as domestic servants in other people's homes. These young, unwed women occupied tenuous positions in early modern English society. They were more commonly associated with depravity and deception than their older, married, or genteel counterparts, and they enabled healers like Marten to flaunt their intellectual and moral authority most effectively. Of the thirty cases of unreliable patients, only eight women were blamed for their infections, but most of those women were relatively disempowered on account of their youth, economic status, or singlehood: one was a wet nurse, three were servant maids, one was a young girl, and one was an unmarried daughter of a merchant.[62] The remaining two female patients included a gentlewoman and a woman characterized only by her age of forty years. Venereal practitioners did not characterize solely workers and youths as unreliable. Over half of the male patients in my sample (twelve out of twenty-two) were defined as gentleman or "of great repute." The remaining ten cases involving men did not include information about age or status, save for one "country lad." The fact that so many unreliable patients were characterized as low-status single women or high-status married men again reflects contemporary anxieties about the fragility of the bourgeois family. The deceptions of gentlemen belied the security of domesticity, while wet nurses and maids posed further threats. These women were commonly targeted as potential sources of disruption for engaging in extramarital affairs or infecting their nurslings.[63]

The Ramifications of This Study

Although contemporaries probably believed that venereal diseases could imperil fertility, other considerations concerning the cultural understandings of sexual behavior and the meanings of venereal infection appear to have taken precedence in shaping the accounts of encounters that have survived. Not all venereal healers convinced patients to divulge shameful acts, of course. Some practitioners conceded to demands for alternate diagnoses or chose not to contradict sufferers' views. If a patient disagreed with his assessment, John Douglas diagnosed the patient's disease of choice. "I never differ with patients about names," Douglas explained, "but leave them always to call their disease what they please." This attitude resulted in innocuous diagnoses like strains and scurvy.[64] Yet even these concessions presumed patients to be untrustworthy. I have shown how such characterizations of unreliability comprised a common tactic that venereal healers employed to highlight their diagnostic know-how.

Such portrayals are significant for illuminating two key aspects of early modern medicine. First, they expose how one group of healers represented themselves and their work. While there is an abundance of literature on the promotional strategies of quacks, switching the focus to the consultation room recovers how healers specializing in venereal disease framed their expertise in terms of diagnostic skill and moral superiority. They claimed to detect patients' reluctance to speak and to diagnose in spite of it. This work involved evaluating bodies and characters and also displaying authority in ways that won clients' trust and convinced them to divulge sexual secrets. These findings resonate with Lauren Kassell's study of astrological healer Simon Forman. Although Forman did not specialize in treating venereal disease, he too distrusted patients' words and exposed patients' sexual secrets. When patients refused to respect Forman's authority, he chose not to treat them, much like John Marten. Perhaps this power dynamic between patient and healer, especially in cases involving sexual misbehavior, was more common in the period than historians supposed.[65]

Second, the cases here deepen our view of medical practice by allowing us to peek inside the consultation room. Diagnosing venereal disease entailed instilling trust, eliciting confessions, and closely scrutinizing patients' characters, behaviors, and bodies. These details of medical practice—a balance of words and bodies—reflect both older seventeenth-century cases that privileged patients' narratives and newer eighteenth-century ones that centered on observed signs. The majority of the cases, after all, end with patients' verbal confessions that served largely to confirm healers' assessments. The validation of healers' knowledge ultimately lay in patients' words, as well as the healers' ability to elicit them. Yet the cases also point to a later emphasis by physicians on expertise and observation over university credentials and reason.[66] Because venereal healers did not trust patient reports, they looked to empirical modes of evaluation. They analyzed mannerisms, deduced prior treatments, and evaluated characters. They also watched, listened, smelled, and tasted. The shift from patient narrative to observed sign, these cases suggest, was more complex than the one simply replacing the other. Cases here show that both could coexist in medical practice.[67] Perhaps the moral nature of venereal disease resisted new definitions of diseases as entities that affected all bodies the same way.

Despite their authorship and potential exaggerations, the sources here provide a sense of what it meant to receive a diagnosis of venereal disease in early modern England. The disgrace and guilt that may have driven patients to deception are echoed, for instance, in some personal writing. Upon learning of his brother Tom's venereal diagnosis in 1664, the famous diarist Samuel Pepys enumerated Tom's many transgressions as if to couch his alleged infection in a greater web of moral decay. Tom was in debt to a number of people, including doctors and family members, and, according to his maid, "hath been a very bad husband as to spending his time." In the hope of obtaining a more dignified diagnosis, family and friends hired a new doctor to evaluate him as he lay on his deathbed. After his death a group of women stripped him bare to prepare him for burial, reporting afterward to Pepys that he was "as clear as any they ever saw."[68] Such accounts expose the moral assumptions, fear, and shame that could accompany a diagnosis of pox.

The cases here functioned in multiple ways. They were structured to highlight healers' abilities to see through patients' unreliable words and recover the "truth." Yet they also functioned as didactic texts that taught potential patients how to view clinical encounters and perhaps even how to deceive. We will never know whether patients were truly as untrustworthy as their healers claimed. But historians who have studied diseases that entailed similar assumptions about the moral fiber and behaviors of particular populations suggest that deception and incredulity are fairly standard reactions to stigmatizing diagnoses.[69] In cases of venereal disease in early modern England, the moralizing nature of the disease structured patients' alleged behaviors and choices, as well as healers' work as interpreters of patients' bodies and souls. Such findings demonstrate how the values and meanings that we, as patients and as healers, attribute to a disease are crucial to representations of expertise and the negotiation of care.

Notes

1. I am not aware of secondary literature that has examined the link between venereal disease and infertility in the early modern period. Mary Fissell (email message to Simon Szreter, September 4, 2018) has advised that she has found no such link mentioned in the various editions of *Aristotle's Masterpiece* between 1684 and the early nineteenth century. But see Kevin Siena, who has written of the eighteenth century in London that "venereal disease hospitals were part of a larger pronatalist concern," reflecting the perception that widespread venereal disease produced "low birth rates and the sickly children that accompanied it." "'The Venereal Disease,' 1500–1800," in *The Routledge History of Sex and the Body 1500 to the Present*, ed. Sarah Toulalan and Kate Fisher (New York: Routledge, 2013), 463–78, 473.

2. For example, see British Library (hereafter cited as BL), 551.a.32(31). On early modern infertility more generally, see Jennifer Evans, *Aphrodisiacs, Fertility and Medicine in Early Modern England* (London: Boydell, 2014); Lisa Smith, "Imagining Women's Fertility before Technology," *Journal of Medical Humanities* 31 (2010): 69–79; and Daphna Oren-Magidor, *Infertility in Early Modern England* (London: Palgrave Macmillan, 2017).

3. John Marten, *A Treatise of the Venereal Disease* (London, 1711), 826, 827, 822.

4. Joannes Groeneveld, *A Treatise of the Safe, Internal Use of Cantharides* (London, 1706), 219.

5. Mary E. Fissell, *Patients, Power, and the Poor in Eighteenth-Century Bristol* (Cambridge: Cambridge University Press, 1991); Roy Porter and Dorothy Porter, *In Sickness and in Health: The British Experience, 1650–1850* (New York: Blackwell, 1988); Gianna Pomata, *Contracting a Cure: Patients, Healers, and the Law in Early Modern Bologna* (Baltimore: Johns Hopkins University Press, 1998). On the ways patients' narratives structured the diagnosis of venereal disease in particular, see Claudia Stein, "The Meaning of Signs: Diagnosing the French Pox in Early Modern Augsburg," *Bulletin of the History of Medicine* 80 (2006): 617–48.

6. See Cristian Berco, "The Great Pox, Symptoms, and Social Bodies in Early Modern Spain," *Social History of Medicine* 28 (2015): 225–44; Susan Staves, "The Puzzle of the Pox-Marked Body," in *A Cultural History of the Human Body: The Age of Enlightenment*, ed. Carole Reeves, vol. 4 (Oxford: Berg, 2010), 155–74.

7. For examples, see Claudia Stein, *Negotiating the French Pox in Early Modern Germany* (Farnham: Ashgate, 2009); Andrew Wear, *Knowledge and Practice in English Medicine, 1550–1680* (Cambridge: Cambridge University Press, 2000), 104–53;

and Jon Arrizabalaga, John Henderson, and Roger French, *The Great Pox: The French Disease in Renaissance Europe* (New Haven: Yale University Press, 1997). For a helpful discussion of what newer cultural histories of disease entail, see Mary E. Fissell, "Making Meaning from the Margins: The New Cultural History of Medicine," in *Locating Medical History: The Stories and Their Meanings*, ed. Frank Huisman and John Harley Warner (Baltimore: Johns Hopkins University Press, 2004), 364–89.

8. Royal College of Physicians, London, MS 206/4, George Colebrook, "Letters on Medical Cases" (ca. 1690), 95; Marjorie Hope Nicolson and Sarah Hutton, eds., *Conway Letters: The Correspondence of Anne, Viscountess Conway, Henry More, and Their Friends, 1642–1684*, rev. ed. (Oxford: Clarendon, 1992).

9. Much of this scholarship is literary. For a few examples, see Sabine Arnaud, *On Hysteria: The Invention of a Medical Category between 1670 and 1820* (Chicago: University of Chicago Press, 2015); Deborah N. Losse, *Syphilis: Medicine, Metaphor, and Religious Conflict in Early Modern France* (Columbus: Ohio State University Press, 2014); David Shuttleton, "A Culture of Disfigurement: Imagining Smallpox in the Long Eighteenth-Century," in *Framing and Imagining Disease in Cultural History*, ed. George Sebastian Rousseau et al. (Houndmills: Palgrave Macmillan, 2003), 68–91; and Jennifer C. Vaught, *Rhetorics of Bodily Disease and Health in Medieval and Early Modern England* (Farnham: Ashgate, 2010).

10. These advertisements are from four collections: BL, 551.a.32 (1675–1715); BL, C.112.f.9 (1660–1716); BL, Harley 5931 (n.d.); and "17–18th Century Burney Collection Newspapers," (1650–1750), Gale news vault.

11. For example, see BL, 551.a.32(121); BL, 551.a.32(9); and BL, 551.a.32(169); John Douglas, *A Dissertation on the Venereal Disease* (London, 1737), 6.

12. John Sintelaer, *The Scourge of Venus and Mercury* (London, 1709), 281. See also John Marten, *Gonosologium Novum* (London, 1709), A7r; *Country Journal, or The Craftsman* 21 December 1734, April 3, 1736, in "Burney Collection Newspapers."

13. Marten, *Treatise* (1711), xxvii, xxvi; John Spinke, *Quackery Unmask'd* (London, 1711), 27. On Marten, see Roy Porter, "'Laying Aside Any Private Advantage': John Marten and Venereal Disease," in *The Secret Malady: Venereal Disease in Eighteenth-Century Britain and France*, ed. Linda Merians (Lexington: University Press of Kentucky, 1996), 51–67; and Michael Stolberg, "Self-Pollution, Moral Reform, and the Venereal Trade: Notes on the Sources and Historical Context of *Onania* (1716)," *Journal of the History of Sexuality* 9 (2000): 37–61.

14. John Marten, *A Treatise of All the Degrees and Symptoms of the Venereal Disease* (London, 1707), 144–45, at 145. There are too many additional examples of secret remedies to cite. For a few, see BL, 551.a.32(153); BL, 551.a.32(156); and BL, 551.a.32(114).

15. George Key, *A Dissertation on the Effects of Mercury on Human Bodies* (London, 1747), 25; *A Collection of Recipe's* [*sic*] *and Letters Lately Inserted in the Daily Journal* (London, 1730), esp. 7–8. On mercury, see Philip K. Wilson, *Surgery,*

Skin and Syphilis: Daniel Turner's London (1667–1741) (Amsterdam: Rodopi, 1999), 161–67, 172–76; and Arrizabalaga, Henderson, and French, *Great Pox*, 139–42.

16. BL, 551.a.32(88).

17. Joseph Cam, *A Short Account of the Venereal Disease* (London, 1719), 9, 10.

18. For a valuable study of pox in early modern Germany that situates the disease within contemporary medical theories, see Stein, *Negotiating the French Pox*.

19. Stein, *Negotiating the French Pox*, esp. 140; Claudia Stein, "'Getting' the Pox: Reflections by an Historian on How to Write the History of Early Modern Disease," *Nordic Journal* 2 (2014): 53–60. On the link between improper sex and venereal disease, see, for example, Mary Hewlett, "The French Connection: Syphilis and Sodomy in Late Renaissance Lucca," in *Sins of the Flesh: Responding to Sexual Disease in Early Modern Europe*, ed. Kevin Siena (Toronto: Centre for Reformation and Renaissance Studies, 2005), 239–60.

20. Lauren Kassell, ed., "CASE14392 (Normalised Version)" and "CASE29160 (Normalised Version)," with Michael Hawkins, Robert Ralley, and John Young, *Casebooks Project*, accessed October 9, 2015, https://casebooks.lib.cam.ac.uk/.

21. Rita Charon, "To Build a Case: Medical Histories as Traditions in Conflict," *Literature and Medicine* 11 (1992): 115–32; Howard Brody, "'My Story Is Broken: Can You Help Me Fix It?' Medical Ethics and the Joint Construction of Narrative," *Literature and Medicine* 13 (1994): 79–92; Arnaud, *On Hysteria*, esp. 195–202.

22. Marten, *Treatise* (1707), 38–39. Much of the research discussed in this chapter has been published in Olivia Weisser, "Treating the Secret Disease: Sex, Sin, and Authority in 18th-Century Venereal Cases," *Bulletin of the History of Medicine* 91 (2017): 685–712.

23. Wellcome Library, MS.3631, Alexander Morgan, medical casebook (1714–47), 17. In another instance, Morgan diagnosed the pox by talking to a neighbor: 48–49.

24. Richard Wiseman, *Severall Chirurgicall Treatises* (London, 1676), 32.

25. Daniel Turner, *Syphilis: A Practical Dissertation on the Venereal Disease* (London, 1717), 159, 160.

26. Sintelaer, *Scourge*, 308–9. See also Marten, *Treatise* (1711), 563.

27. Daniel Turner, *Syphilis: A Practical Dissertation on the Venereal Disease* (London, 1724), 247–48.

28. Marten, *Treatise* (1711), 520.

29. Wiseman, *Severall Chirurgicall Treatises*, 37.

30. John Douglas, *A Dissertation on the Venereal Disease* (London, 1739), 56–57. For similar examples, see Douglas, *Dissertation* (1737), 68; and Sintelaer, *Scourge*, 327. On physical examination, see Stein, *Negotiating the French Pox*, 136–38; Luke E. Demaitre, *Leprosy in Premodern Medicine: A Malady of the Whole Body* (Baltimore: Johns Hopkins University Press, 2007), 200–205; and Olivia Weisser, "Boils, Pushes, and Wheals: Reading Bumps on the Body in Early Modern England," *Social History of Medicine* 22 (2009): 321–39.

31. Turner, *Syphilis* (1717), 224, 209. On diagnosing venereal disease by the sound of patients' voices, see Marten, *Treatise* (1707), 108; Marten, *Treatise* (1711), 586; Turner, *Syphilis* (1717), 223; Turner, *Syphilis* (1724), 304; and Wiseman, *Severall Chirurgicall Treatises*, 32.

32. Thomas Garlick, *A Mechanical Account of the Cause and Cure of a Virulent Gonorrhaea* (London, 1727), 44. On touch, see also Marten, *Treatise* (1707), 185, 277; Douglas, *Dissertation* (1739), 57; Garlick, *Mechanical Account*, 6; and Turner, *Syphilis* (1717), 74, 220, 229.

33. Marten, *Treatise* (1707), 171.

34. Sintelaer, *Scourge*, 154; Charles Peter, *New Observations on the Venereal Disease* (London, 1704), 25. For additional examples of smell, see Marten *Gonosologium novum*, 122; Marten, *Treatise* (1707), 124; Marten, *Treatise* (1711), 435–36; and Sintelaer, *Scourge*, 319.

35. Marten, *Treatise* (1707), 261; see also Marten, *Treatise* (1711), 575, 820.

36. Wendy D. Churchill, *Female Patients in Early Modern Britain: Gender, Diagnosis, and Treatment* (Burlington: Ashgate, 2012), 70, 82–89; Hannah Barker, "Medical Advertising and Trust in Late Georgian England," *Urban History* 36 (2009): 379–98; Steven Shapin, "Trusting George Cheyne: Scientific Expertise, Common Sense, and Moral Authority in Early Eighteenth-Century Dietetic Medicine," *Bulletin of the History of Medicine* 77 (2003): 263–97.

37. For Marten's seventeen cases of unreliable patients, see *Treatise* (1707), 13–14, 17, 20, 24–25, 38–39, 100, 102, 103, 106, 269, 323; and Marten, *Treatise* (1711), 144, 305–6, 306–7, 307–8, 522, 588.

38. Marten, *Treatise* (1707), 17–18.

39. Marten, *Treatise* (1707), 18–19.

40. Marten, *Treatise* (1711), 307–8, 523.

41. Marten, *Treatise* (1711), 590, 591, 589.

42. This case is recorded in Marten, *Treatise* (1707), 103–4.

43. For the eleven cases, see Marten, *Treatise* (1707), 24–25, 102–3, 103–4, 106; Marten, *Treatise* (1711), 306–7, 588–91; Sintelaer, *Scourge*, 327; Turner, *Syphilis* (1717), 180; Turner, *Syphilis* (1724), 304, 316; and Wiseman, *Severall Chirurgicall Treatises*, 63.

44. Kevin Patrick Siena, "The 'Foul Disease' and Privacy: The Effects of Venereal Disease and Patient Demand on the Medical Marketplace in Early Modern London," *Bulletin of the History of Medicine* 75 (2001): 199–224, esp. 215.

45. On cure testimonials, see Pomata, *Contracting a Cure*, 50–52.

46. Effie Botonaki, "Seventeenth-Century Englishwomen's Spiritual Diaries: Self-Examination, Covenanting, and Account Keeping," *Sixteenth Century Journal* 30 (1999): 3–21; Margo Todd, "Puritan Self-Fashioning: The Diary of Samuel Ward," *Journal of British Studies* 31 (1992): 236–64, esp. 257. On the continued importance of confession for English Protestants, see Christopher Tilmouth, *Passion's Triumph over Reason: A History of the Moral Imagination from Spenser to Rochester* (Oxford: Oxford University Press, 2007), 103–4; for English Catholics, see Lisa McClain,

"Troubled Consciences: New Understandings and Performances of Penance among Catholics in Protestant England," *Church History* 82 (2013): 90–124.

47. J. A. Sharpe, "'Last Dying Speeches': Religion, Ideology and Public Execution in Seventeenth-Century England," *Past and Present* 107 (1985): 144–67; Richard Wunderli and Gerald Broce, "The Final Moment before Death in Early Modern England," *Sixteenth Century Journal* 20 (1989): 259–75, esp. 272–74.

48. John Parker, "Faustus, Confession, and the Sins of Omission," *ELH* 80 (2013): 29–59, esp. 29, 47.

49. This point builds on Michael Schoenfeldt's discussion of the physiological benefits of speaking about—or "verbally ventilating"—grief in literature: "'Give Sorrow Words': Emotional Loss and the Articulation of Temperament in Early Modern England," in *Dead Lovers: Erotic Bonds and the Study of Premodern Europe*, ed. Basil Dufallo and Peggy McCracken (Ann Arbor: University of Michigan Press, 2007), 143–64. The quotation is from Francis Bacon, *The Essays or Counsels, Civill and Morall*, ed. Michael Kiernan (Cambridge: Harvard University Press, 1985), 81, cited in Schoenfeldt, "Give Sorrow Words," 155.

50. King James Bible 5:16, cited in Anne Harrington, *The Cure Within: A History of Mind-Body Medicine* (New York: Norton, 2008), 69.

51. See David Harley, "Medical Metaphors in English Moral Theology, 1560–1660," *Journal of the History of Medicine and Allied Sciences* 48 (1993): 396–435; and Tilmouth, *Passion's Triumph*, 108.

52. Roger Lowe, *Diary of Roger Lowe, of Ashton-in-Makerfield, Lancashire, 1663–74*, ed. William L. Sachse (New Haven: Yale University Press, 1938), 17. The excerpt is taken from Michael Sparke, *Crumms of Comfort* (London, 1627).

53. On repentant sorrow, see Raymond A. Anselment, "Mary Rich, Countess of Warwick, and the Gift of Tears," *Seventeenth Century* 22 (2007): 336–57.

54. See Sintelaer, *Scourge*, 153; Turner, *Syphilis* (1724), 246; and Douglas, *Dissertation* (1739), 59.

55. Nathaniel Lomax, *Launaeus Redivivus, or A True Narrative of the Admirable Effects of Delaun's Pill* ([London], 1675), 12.

56. Throughout his book *Scourge*, Sintelaer refers to mercury treatment as the "mercurial rack" and to venereal patients as "martyrs of Venus."

57. BL, C.112.f.9(11); BL, 551.a.32(182).

58. On assumptions about women's duplicity, see Lauren Kassell, "How to Read Simon Forman's Casebooks: Medicine, Astrology, and Gender in Elizabethan London," *Social History of Medicine* 12 (1999): 3–18; and Cathy McClive, "Blood and Expertise: The Trials of the Female Medical Expert in the Ancien-Regime Courtroom," *Bulletin of the History of Medicine* 82 (2008): 86–108.

59. Kevin Siena, "Pollution, Promiscuity, and the Pox: English Venereology and the Early Modern Medical Discourse on Social and Sexual Danger," *Journal of the History of Sexuality* 8 (1998): 553–74; Winfried Schliener, "Infection and Cure through Women: Renaissance Constructions of Syphilis," *Journal of Medieval and Renaissance Studies* 24 (1994): 499–517; Louis F. Qualtiere and William W. E.

Slights, "Contagion and Blame in Early Modern England: The Case of the French Pox," *Literature and Medicine* 22 (2003): 1–24, at 12; Laura J. McGough, *Gender, Sexuality, and Syphilis in Early Modern Venice* (New York: Palgrave Macmillan, 2011).

60. Turner, *Syphilis* (1724), 209; Turner, *Syphilis* (1717), 162.

61. On some of the ways that gender, status, and anxiety about authority informed early modern healers' writing, see Olivia Weisser, *Ill Composed: Sickness, Gender, and Belief in Early Modern England* (New Haven, Yale University Press, 2015), 33–45.

62. Marten, *Treatise* (1707), 13, 17, 20, 38; Marten, *Treatise* (1711), 305, 522–23.

63. For example, see Marissa C. Rhodes, "Domestic Vulnerabilities: Reading Families and Bodies into Eighteenth-Century Anglo-Atlantic Wet Nurse Advertisements," *Journal of Family History* 40 (2015): 39–63.

64. Douglas, *Dissertation* (1739), 42; see also 77. For examples of altering venereal treatments or diagnoses to suit patient demands, see Douglas, *Dissertation* (1737), 66; Garlick, *Mechanical Account*, 49; Turner, *Syphilis* (1717), 154, 180; and Turner, *Syphilis* (1724), 211, 74.

65. Kassell, "Simon Forman's Casebooks"; Lauren Kassell, *Medicine and Magic in Elizabethan London: Simon Forman: Astrologer, Alchemist, and Physician* (Oxford: Clarendon, 2005), 131, 150, 160–70.

66. Harold J. Cook, "Bernard Mandeville and the Therapy of 'The Clever Politician,'" *Journal of the History of Ideas* 60 (1999): 101–23.

67. Michael Stolberg makes this same point in *Uroscopy in Early Modern Europe* (Farnham: Ashgate, 2015).

68. Robert Latham and William Matthews, eds. *The Diary of Samuel Pepys: A New and Complete Transcription*, vol. 5 (Berkeley: University of California Press, 1971), 82, 84–85, 86.

69. Examinations for leprosy from the Middle Ages, for example, included oaths of honesty: Demaitre, *Leprosy in Premodern Medicine*, 198. See also Judith Walzer Leavitt, *Typhoid Mary: Captive to the Public's Health* (Boston: Beacon, 1996); and Laura McGough, "HIV/AIDS Stigma: Historical Perspectives on Sexually Transmitted Diseases," *Virtual Mentor* 2005 (10): 710–15.

Part Two

The Biomedical Sciences and the History of the STI Microorganisms

Chapter Three

Bioarchaeological Contributions to Understanding the History of Treponemal Disease

Charlotte Roberts and Rebecca Redfern

Introduction and Aims

Sexually transmitted infections (STIs) remain common today, both in developed and developing countries, and they can have serious consequences for fertility and pregnancy. There are over thirty bacterial, parasitic, and viral STIs. The World Health Organization states that more than 1 million people contract one of eight STIs on a daily basis and that each year, independently of the four incurable STI viruses (hepatitis B, herpes simplex virus, the human immunodeficiency virus, and the human papillomavirus), an estimated 357 million new infections are caused by one of the four frequently occurring and treatable bacterial STIs (chlamydia, gonorrhea, syphilis, and trichomoniasis).[1] The US Centers for Disease Control and Prevention also list pelvic inflammatory disease as a complication of chlamydia and gonorrhea.[2] Clearly, it is possible to have more than one STI. In England, during 2014, almost half a million diagnoses of STIs were made, mostly in heterosexuals less than twenty-five years old and in men who have sex with men. Chlamydia was the most common, and between 2013 and 2014 the highest proportional increases were for venereal syphilis (VS) (33 percent) and gonorrhea (19 percent). A number of factors have been linked to STIs, including travel and migration, a high rate of partner exchange, poor access to health care, social marginalization, and a low socioeconomic status.[3]

Detecting these STIs in the past can be challenging both for scholars who focus on historical documents and for those who work on the evidence for disease gleaned from human remains, either skeletons or preserved bodies.[4] Bioarchaeology describes the contextualized study of archaeological human remains, with paleopathology focusing specifically on health and well-being, as seen in the results of encounters of once-living people with health risks in their environment, including exposure to pathogens.[5]

One of the more popular areas of interest in paleopathology is infectious disease and, within that category, specific infections rate highly as of particular interest—that is, those where the disease-causing organism is known. While it is possible to identify infectious disease changes to body tissues, actually diagnosing what specific infection affected a person in life can be very challenging when studying skeletons, in particular.[6] Nevertheless, of the specific infectious diseases that have been recognized in the bioarchaeological record, leprosy, tuberculosis, and the treponemal diseases are perhaps the most commonly reported.[7] Within the category of treponemal diseases, VS and congenital syphilis (CS) are the infections of particular relevance to this chapter.

This chapter takes a paleopathological approach to focus primarily on VS and considers the long-running debate about its relationship with Christopher Columbus and his crew in both Europe and the Americas. In doing so it provides a short introduction to paleopathology and its challenges and the extant evidence for VS in human remains, focusing on Eurasia, and then considers approaches that might be used to assess its impact on fertility and mortality in the past.

Paleopathology

Paleopathology considers the origin, evolution, and history of disease as seen in archaeological human remains. It is a contextually and question-driven multi-methodological and multidisciplinary field of study that benefits from a global resource for study (human remains) that has longtime depths. Its research is not limited to the macroscopic examination of human remains, as it regularly employs imaging (for example, computed tomography and plain film radiography) and biomolecular (most commonly aDNA, or ancient DNA) and histological techniques to identify, diagnose, and interpret health changes. In essence, it complements the emerging field of evolutionary medicine.[8]

In Britain most human remains are excavated in advance of new construction or infrastructure projects, and they are studied by bioarchaeologists. The majority of human remains are skeletons (inhumations), and thus most of the evidence used to reconstruct the origin, evolution, and history of disease derives from skeletons rather than preserved bodies. However, in some parts of the world environmental conditions, such as extremes of heat and cold, can be conducive to the preservation of whole bodies. A bioarchaeologist records data from skeletons to estimate biological sex and age at death and documents normal and abnormal variations. Normal variation recording includes measuring the teeth and bones of skeletons, such as female (top) and male (below) pelves (figs. 3.1–3.2), as well as using specific bone dimensions to estimate stature (fig 3.3), and observing nonmetric traits, which can be inherited. Specific types of traits can even illustrate geographic groupings; for example, the Inca bone in the skull shown in figure 3.2 has a higher frequency in Latin America.[9] Abnormal variation encompasses pathological changes caused by disease or trauma. In the case of skeletons, the basic premise on which to attempt disease diagnosis initially rests on the detailed (macroscopic) recording of preserved bones and teeth. If a disease affects bones, it can precipitate bone formation (e.g., in infection) or bone destruction

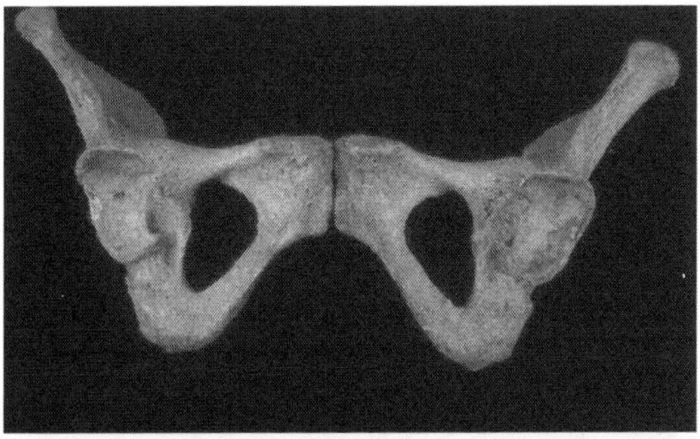

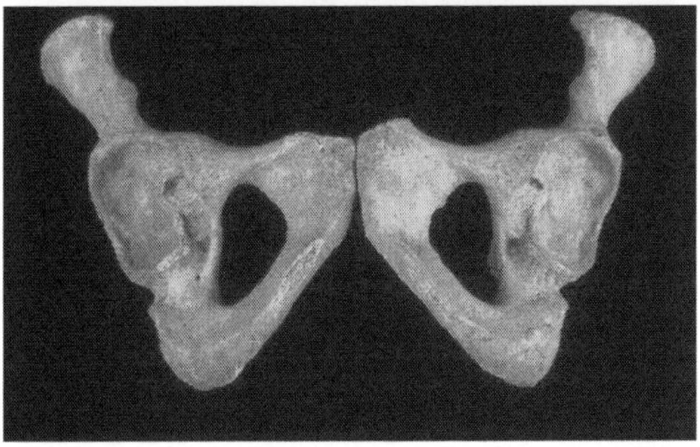

Figures 3.1a. and 3.1b. Pelves.

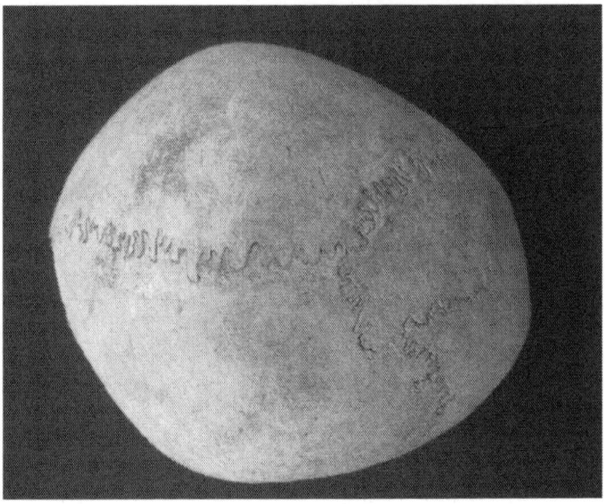

Figure 3.2. Skull with Inca bone (the roughly oval plate on the right, middle).

(e.g., in cancer), or both (figs. 3.4 and 3.5). It is also possible to observe destruction of the teeth (e.g., carious lesions) and their supporting jaws (e.g., periodontal disease or dental abscess) (fig. 3.6). Only a small number of diseases affect the skeleton, and, of those, only a small proportion will affect an untreated person; for example, only 3 to 5 percent of those experiencing leprosy and tuberculosis will show evidence of the disease.[10]

These abnormal changes are documented in a detailed description and in their distribution pattern in the bones and teeth of the skeleton studied (fig. 3.7). In particular, different diseases make their mark on and within specific bones (e.g., the vertebral bodies of the spine in tuberculosis) and parts of bones (e.g., the different joint diseases). It is therefore important when attempting disease diagnosis that complete, well-preserved skeletons are available.

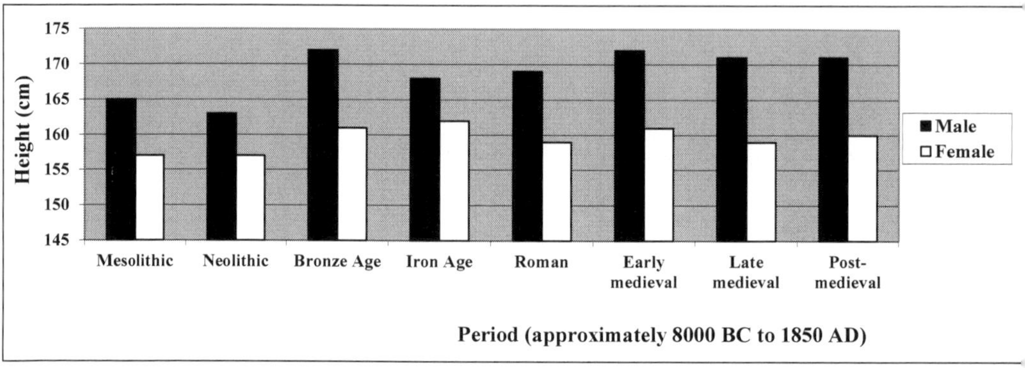

Figure 3.3. Variation in stature through time in Britain.

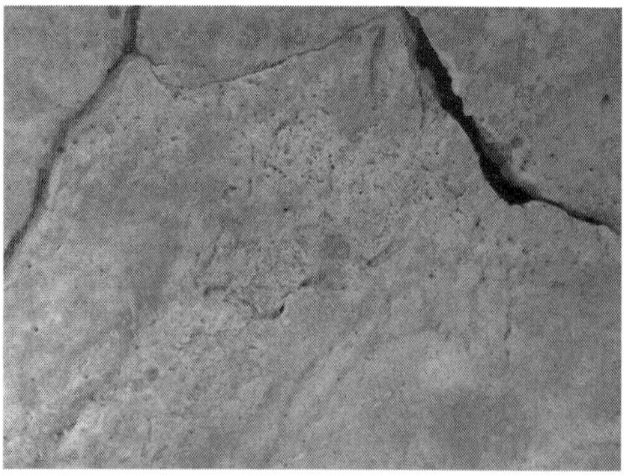

Figure 3.4. Example of bone formation on the inner surface of a cranium.

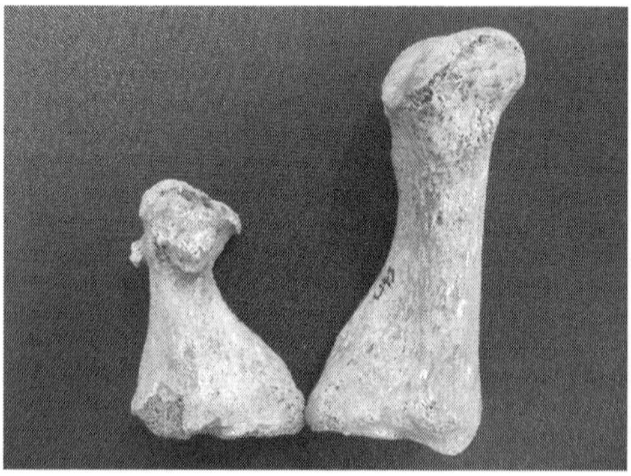

Figure 3.5. Example of bone destruction, to a 1st metatarsal bone in the foot (left)—normal on the right.

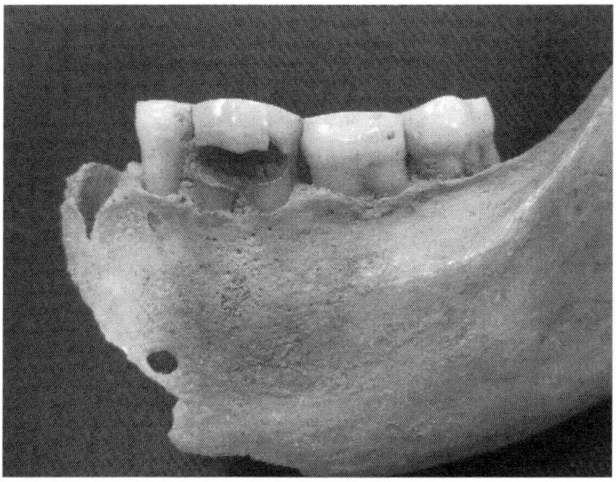

Figure 3.6. Example of destruction of tooth and, below, bone formation due to inflammation from an underlying dental abscess due to caries.

However, it is unusual to recover a totally complete and well-preserved archaeological skeleton, because the environment of burial is often detrimental to the preservation of the skeleton. Therefore, it is often the case that incomplete, poorly preserved skeletons may be encountered. Once the characteristics and distribution pattern of the pathological lesions have been recorded, differential diagnostic options are considered because bones can react only in two limited ways—that is, bone formation and destruction—and therefore some diseases may produce very similar bone changes. For example, leprosy, VS, and tuberculosis can damage the facial bones, and so accompanying bone lesions in other parts of the skeleton may help refine a diagnosis. Skeletons showing pathological lesions usually exhibit chronic healed lesions, suggesting that the person had a strong immune system to withstand death in the acute stages of the disease and survived long enough for the bone changes to occur and become healed—these people were, in effect, the healthy "survivors," even though they of course subsequently died. Those skeletons without bone changes reflect the people who likely died in the acute stages of the disease or of a disease that did not affect the bones, or they died before bone changes could develop. This is termed the "osteological paradox" when inferring health from the skeleton: those with lesions are in fact the survivors of the disease that caused them, not its fatal victims.[11]

Treponemal Disease

The focus of this chapter is venereal (and congenital) syphilis, but to understand the context of this infection, it is necessary to be aware of the spectrum of treponematoses. The treponemal diseases (or treponematoses) are caused by bacteria of the genus *Treponema* (a spirochete). There are four "syndromes," and they appear to have different global distribution patterns

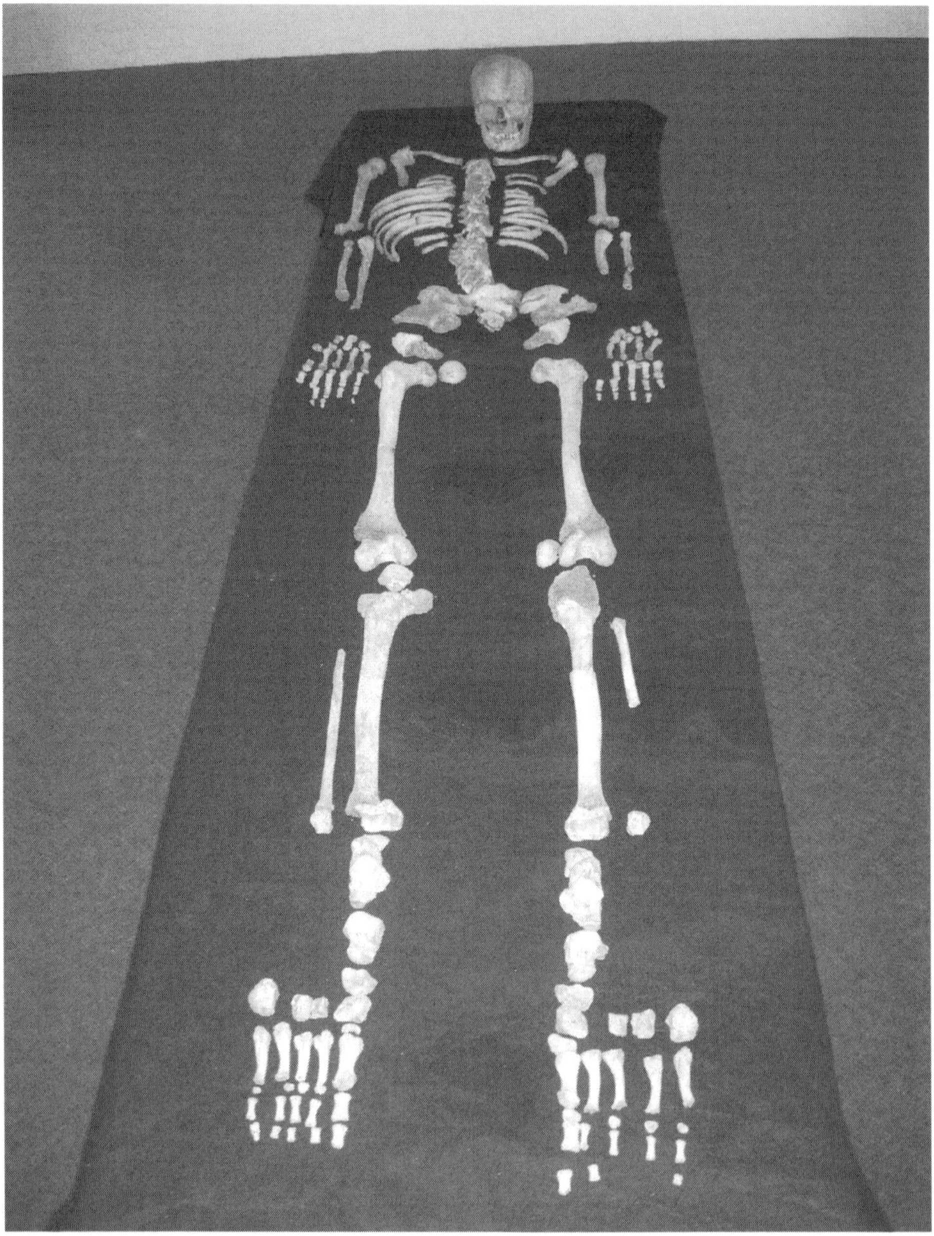

Figure 3.7. Skeleton laid out to record the distribution of lesions for a diagnosis.

today.[12] There has been some debate about whether they are caused by different species of the bacterial genus, *Treponema*, or reflect different clinical manifestations of one species, *Treponema pallidum*. Ellis Herndon Hudson was of the opinion that the organisms were identical and that the environment and climate led to different clinical manifestations.[13] However, Cecil Hackett believed that these organisms were genetically distinct, although very closely related, something that was more recently supported in 2006 using biomolecular techniques applied to an animal model (New Zealand white rabbits).[14] It was suggested that the basis for this research may be used for subspecies differentiation in ancient DNA research.

Causes and Characteristics of the Syndromes

Pinta is caused by *Treponema carateum* and today is seen in tropical Central and South America. It produces skin lesions and affects the lymph nodes. It is likely transmitted via contact with skin lesions. Late childhood and young adulthood are the key age categories at risk. There is no bone damage in this syndrome, and because most bioarchaeologists analyze mainly skeletons and not the soft tissues, it is not discussed further.[15]

The three other syndromes are yaws, endemic syphilis, and VS, the latter also being responsible for congenital syphilis. Endemic syphilis might also be called bejel and treponarid in the published literature. Therefore, when "syphilis" is mentioned, it should be differentiated as to whether endemic, venereal, or congenital syphilis is being described. These three syndromes (along with CS) can potentially affect the bones of the skeleton, but only CS may affect the dentition. Bone changes occur in the tertiary phases of these syndromes in varying percentages of untreated people but may be present in 8–20 percent of those affected with VS.[16]

Yaws is caused by *Treponema pallidum*, subspecies *pertenue*, and today is found in people living in the warm humid areas of equatorial Africa and southeast Asia, but larger parts of Africa and many areas of South America have previously been endemic for this disease.[17] The skin, lymph nodes, and bones may be affected, the latter comprising the upper jaw (maxillary and palatal bones), and the large lower-leg bones (tibiae).[18] Dactylitis of the hand bones may occur, due to inflammation of the fingers. Yaws is believed to be transmitted by skin-to-skin contact and exacerbated by poor hygiene, sanitation, and overcrowding. This syndrome affects young people and is acquired before puberty.[19] Endemic syphilis is caused by *Treponema pallidum*, subspecies *endemicum*, and is found in people today living in some areas of Africa and the Middle East.[20] Contact with skin lesions and infected mucous membranes are the most likely routes of transmission, and children are most affected.[21] The skin, bones, and mucous membranes are involved, and the tibiae and nasal bones are affected. Yaws and endemic syphilis are classified as non-venereal treponemal diseases, and factors that may be relevant are the lack of clothing, thereby permitting greater likelihood of skin-to-skin contact; sharing contaminated eating and drinking utensils, clothing, and bedding; and poor personal hygiene.[22]

The final syndrome is VS caused by *Treponema pallidum*, subspecies *pallidum*. It affects the skin, bones, and cardiovascular and central nervous systems, with the bone changes occurring in the tertiary phase. The key bones affected are the cranial vault, nasal and palatal bones, and those of the lower leg.[23] Damage to the joints (Charcot joints) and bone changes in the spine due to aortic aneurysm (weakened blood vessel walls) may also be associated with the tertiary phase, when the central nervous and cardiovascular systems are involved.[24] It is spread via sexual intercourse, and infected mothers can transmit the infection to their unborn babies to cause CS.[25]

VS has three stages to its course. The primary stage generates a painless skin lesion (chancre) at the site of infection and involvement of the lymphatic system. Healing occurs in two to three weeks. The secondary stage occurs after four to ten weeks of the primary lesions and consists of a generalized infection, with a fever, sore throat, skin rash, mucosal ulcers (mouth and genitalia), lymphatic involvement (in 50 percent of people), kidney involvement (in 10 percent), and bone pain; this disappears in up to twelve weeks but may recur.[26] The third stage appears two to thirty years later, with necrotic swellings called gummata in the skin, liver, testes, bones, and meninges; gummata in the skin can cause underlying bone-forming and destructive changes.[27] Congenital syphilis occurs as a result of the infection of the mother with VS and is apparent between the second and sixth weeks after birth.[28] Periostitis, osteitis, and osteomyelitis of the femora and tibiae can be seen, along with metaphyseal irregularities, dactylitis, and dental defects.[29] Dactylitis can also be caused by other conditions (e.g., sickle cell anemia). However, the dental changes are quite specific to this disease and include Hutchinson's incisors and Moon's molars, which are suggested to be pathognomonic; "Mulberry" molars may also be present.[30]

Differentiating the Bone Changes for Diagnosis

Differentiating the three syndromes that affect the adult skeleton is challenging in paleopathology, especially if the skeleton is not well preserved, because differential diagnostic options need to be considered. Hackett, has described the bone changes used to diagnose the treponemal diseases, based on clinical data.[31] They include porosity and bone formation and destruction represented by periostitis, osteitis, and osteomyelitis, particularly on the lower-leg (long) bones. People with any of these three syndromes can have this bone change, but a person with yaws may also have involvement of the ends of the thigh bones (femurs). However, the bone changes of the lower legs can also be caused by many other diseases (e.g., leprosy), as highlighted by Darlene Weston.[32]

In VS gummas are further observed on the long bones (fig. 3.8), as is destruction of the cranial vault bones of the skull, especially of the frontal bone (fig. 3.9). Here the lesions (*caries sicca*) are destructive and focal in nature and may appear as active (unhealed) or chronic healed lesions, the latter also referred to as stellate, because of the starlike scarring. This is very characteristic of VS. The destruction and remodeling (healing) of the nasal bones and upper jawbone (maxilla) and perforation of the palate may occur. Other causes producing facial bone damage of this type may be cancer, tuberculosis, and leprosy, and even endemic syphilis.[33] It is therefore important to have a skeleton that has both the skull and long bones preserved, at the very least, for a realistic attempt at a positive diagnosis of VS, since its unique signature is the combination of both *caries sicca* in the skull and lower-leg bone changes. However, the presence of this latter bone change on other long bones, such as those of the arms, alongside gummas, is also diagnostic.

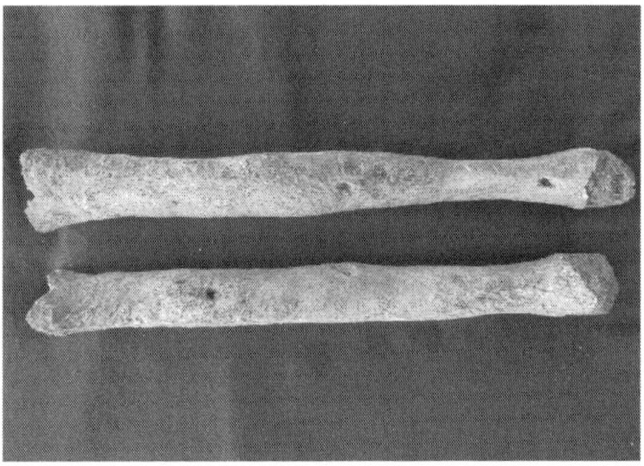

Figure 3.8. Syphilitic lesions (gummas) in long bones (black "holes," *top right*; *bottom left*).

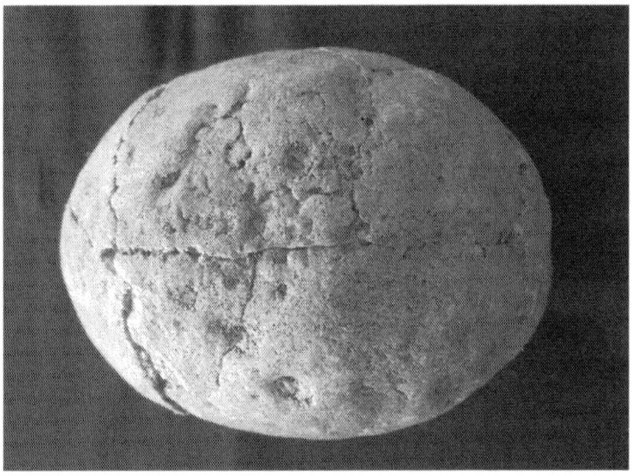

Figure 3.9. Skull showing destructive lesions (*caries sicca*) from venereal syphilis.

There have also been rare diagnoses of VS in mummified remains, based on skin lesions. The study of a female mummy from sixteenth-century Italy identified an oval ulcer, which was covered with a linen dressing containing ivy leaves and sulfur (both have healing properties). Indirect immunofluorescence identified filaments that had the appearance of fluorescent treponemes, and spirochetes were observed using electron microscopy. These findings suggest a treponemal, probably venereal, infection.[34]

At present the macroscopic approach to the diagnosis of VS is the only viable method. Histological analysis has been attempted, but this has shown that the characteristic, changed appearance of the bone microstructure could be seen in other infections too, such as leprosy.[35] To date diagnosis using ancient DNA (aDNA) analysis has only had limited success in adult human remains with specific bony changes (i.e., no treponemal aDNA seems to survive in adult skeletons with tertiary bone changes).[36] The latter outcome has been supported by experimental work that has indicated that by the tertiary phase of the infection, no bacteria are present in the bones, which explains why the aDNA has been identified only in neonatal and infant remains with nonspecific infectious disease changes—that is, they were infected in utero and died while the disease was still active.[37] Because of the vagaries of preservation of skeletal remains, the lack of success with aDNA research is unfortunate, particularly when all the relevant bones for diagnosis of the different syndromes of treponemal disease are not preserved for observation. However, a number of bioarchaeologists are actually more comfortable with diagnosing "treponematosis" rather than a specific treponemal disease, a pattern of analysis observed more generally in paleopathological practice (e.g., joint disease rather than a specific type of joint disease).[38]

The Debated Hypotheses about VS

Accurately diagnosing VS is the first step toward testing hypotheses about the origin and transmission of VS around the world, as is having an accurate date, e.g., from radiocarbon or securely dated grave goods. The three key hypotheses that continue to be debated rely on the undisputed presence of VS of pre- or post-Columbian dates—that is, before or after 1493, when Christopher Columbus and his crew returned to Europe from the Americas. The hypotheses are as follows:

1. Columbian: treponemal disease, including VS, existed in the Americas prior to 1492 and returned with Columbus to Europe in 1493.[39]
2. Pre-Columbian: one or more forms of treponemal disease, including VS, existed in Europe, and Columbus took it to the Americas in 1492, but it was not previously recognized in Europe because it had been confused with leprosy.[40]

3. Unitarian: the four syndromes were environmentally determined expressions of treponemal disease present in both Europe and the Americas pre-Columbus.[41] This hypothesis is now discredited, as the three treponemal subspecies are genetically distinct.[42]

There are two more hypotheses that are also important to consider:

4. Evolutionary: pinta is considered to be the earliest syndrome and VS the most recent representation of the pathogen's "successful adaptation to a decrease in endemic transmission due to specific cultural changes, such as urbanisation."[43]
5. Evolutionary theory variation: The treponemal disease in the Americas was the nonvenereal form (yaws and endemic syphilis) endemic before 1492, and it was this, rather than the venereal form of treponematosis, that was taken from the Americas to Europe by Columbus, which then evolved rapidly (i.e., mutated) post-1492 into the venereal form in the different European environment.[44]

The Skeletal Evidence for Treponematosis in Europe

The skeletal evidence for the treponematoses, including VS, has been documented in monographs, books, and journal papers and has also been the subject of a meta-analysis.[45] Here we focus on Europe, especially Britain and Ireland. To a large extent many studies have placed reliance on published data without having the opportunity to access the actual skeletons with the bone changes to verify diagnoses. Therefore, the data are usually taken at face value. In addition, paleopathology is less developed in some parts of the world, and therefore training in recognizing treponematosis may not always be available, even though diagnoses are made and the environment or methods of disposal of the dead (e.g., cremation) may not preserve remains in a condition conducive to diagnosis.[46] Furthermore, absence of evidence anywhere in the world is not evidence of absence. As more excavations of human remains occur and those remains are analyzed, more data will become available.

It is safe to say that most data on treponemal disease as seen in skeletal remains derives from North America with both pre- and post-Columbian dates attributed.[47] There is much less evidence in South America. This perhaps reflects a longer history of work and research on identifying the disease, and available training, in North America. In Europe there is less evidence and less that is pre-Columbian in date, although in Britain and Ireland the majority appears to be from the late medieval period (twelfth to sixteenth centuries).[48] The skeletons listed in table 3.1 were generally well preserved, with the bones affected by treponemal disease available for study, thus legitimately supporting the diagnoses provided. However, for the London Road, Gloucester, and East Smithfield sites, preservation of the affected skeletons was not as good as for the other sites, and for three individuals only the skulls were preserved (St. Mary Spittle, London; St. Helen-on-the-Walls, York; Whithorn Priory). Suffice it to say, however, that pre-Columbian dated evidence is increasing in the Old World, for example, in England, France, Israel, Iraq, South Africa, and Turkey.[49] However, Olivier Dutour and colleagues have also documented other evidence in various chapters in their volume, and a summary also appears in the work by Kristin Harper and colleagues.[50] Thus, data have been reported from Africa, Asia and Australia, and Europe.[51]

In the present state of scholarship it can be asserted only that there is clear pre-Columbian treponemal disease evident in human remains in both the Americas and in Europe if the following issues are disregarded: the problem of older carbon 14 dates not taking into account the marine reservoir effect; an incorrect diagnosis of either yaws, endemic, VS, or CS; and the location the skeleton was buried.[52] The accuracy of dating and diagnosis are naturally the key to any discussions about the origin and history of the treponemal diseases, including VS. This has been the subject of a 2011 paper by Harper and colleagues, which reappraised the European skeletal evidence published between 1949 and 2001, including dating evidence; their reevaluation considered fifty-four papers based on fifty archaeological sites.[53]

Harper and colleagues considered data from the continents of Africa (four countries), Asia (five countries), Australia (two countries), and Europe (eleven countries). The later stages of *caries sicca* and the enlargement of long bones due to new bone formation along with gummata seen in adult skeletal remains were considered to be specific to treponemal disease in these publications, but two other categories were included for scoring the infection, with different definitions: "consistent with" and "suggestive of." Evidence for CS was considered as consistent, suggestive, or highly suggestive, the latter being identified if destruction of the edge of the metaphysis of a tibia (Wimberger's sign), Hutchinson's incisors, or Moon's molars were present. Harper and colleagues found that nondiagnostic lesions had been used in 22 percent of publications (eleven papers), that the dating methods were not described in 39 percent (twenty papers), and only 6 percent (three papers) had offered securely dated pre-Columbian evidence. The authors claimed that there "is not a single published case from the Old World than can be confidently diagnosed as [both] treponemal and that has a radiocarbon date that places it firmly in the pre-Columbian period."[54] However, we would argue that similar claims could be made about the published American

Table 3.1. Potential pre-Columbian skeletons with treponemal disease, from sites in Britain and Ireland.

Site name and location	Skeleton number and date	Description of skeleton (skeleton number given when multiple skeletons were diagnosed)	Reference
120–22 London Road, Gloucester, Gloucestershire (not considered by Harper et al. 2011)	1277: **50–220** 1672: Second century (archaeological date)	2–5 years old 15–18 years old	Simmonds et al. 2008
Apple Down, near Compton, Sussex	152: **427–634** (date not available when considered by Harper et al. 2011)	Young adult male	Cole and Waldron 2011, 2015
East Smithfield, London (not considered by Harper et al. 2011)	5279: 1348–50 (secure archaeological date)	Subadult	Grainger et al. 2008
Blackfriars, Gloucester, Gloucestershire	77: 1239–mid-fifteenth century (archaeological date) **1438–1635**b	Young adult female	Roberts 1994
Blackfriars, Ipswich, Suffolk	1965: **1440–1520** (73% probability of a pre-1493 date) **1518–1647** (Harper et al. 2011)	Female, older than 50	Mays et al. 2003
Castle Mound, Huntingdon, Cambridgeshire	HC017: **1050–1250** **1046–1217**c	Adult female	Mays et al. 2012
St. Mary Spittle, Londona (not considered by Harper et al. 2011)		Adult female	Brothwell 1961
Hull Magistrates Court, Kingston-upon-Hull, Humberside	1316–1539 (archaeological date) 932: **1492–1657** (Harper et al. 2011) 1121: **1497–1671** (Harper et al. 2011) 1216: **1492–1657** (Harper et al. 2011)	932: male, 34–36 years old 1121: female, 26–35 years old 1216: male, 17–25 years old	Boylston et al. 2001 Roberts et al 2013
Rivenhall, Essex	204: **1295–1445** (99% probability of a pre-1493 date) **1303–1618** (Harper et al. 2011)	Female, 25–50 years old	Mays et al. 2003

Table 3.1 (*continued*)

Site name and location	Skeleton number and date	Description of skeleton (skeleton number given when multiple skeletons were diagnosed)	Reference
St. Margaret's, Fyebridgegate, Norwich, Norfolk	1100–1468 (archaeological date) 68: **1451–1641** (Harper et al. 2011) 129: **1411–1633** (Harper et al. 2011) 227: **1434–1640** (Harper et al. 2011) 412: **1052–1270**c	68: mature adult female 129: mature adult male 227: mature adult male 412: young adult male	Stirland 1991, 1994
St. Mary Spital, London	**1200–1539** (archaeological dates) 28460: **1285–1390**c (Harper et al. 2011). This skeleton *did not have treponemal disease* but was buried directly above or below skeleton 6974, which showed signs of congenital syphilis (Connell et al. 2012). Siddell et al. (2007) dated 28460 to **1265–1295**. This date helped create the overall date for the phase (1285–1390). Twenty-five skeletons were affected by treponemal disease (from the largest late medieval cemetery excavated in Europe; 5,387 skeletons studied): 6482, 6910, 6974, *10566*, 10765, 10874, 10933, 11671, 11935, 12240, 12374, 13232, 13467, 13602, *13635*, 13715, 19485, *20360*, 20634, 20912, 21653, *22466*, *22251*, *23887*, *25749* (italics = skeletons 1200–1400; roman = skeletons 1400–1539)	3 subadults: 1 of unknown sex, 6–11 years old 2 of unknown sex, 12–17 years old 22 adults: 2 females, 18–25 years old 2 males, 18–25 years old 4 females, 26–35 years old 6 males, 26–35 years old 2 females, 36–45 years old 3 males, 36–45 years old 3 of unknown sex and age	Connell et al. 2012 Sidell et al. 2007 Walker 2012 Walker et al. 2015

Whithorn Priory, Dumfries and Galloway, Scotland	1300–1450 (archaeological date) **1459–1635**b	Young adult female	Cardy 1997
Waterford, Ireland	B253: Pre-late fifteenth century (archaeological date) **1440–1635** (Harper et al. 2011)	Subadult	Power 1992
St. Helen-on-the-Walls, York, Yorkshire	5556: 1197–1419 (archaeological date) **1197–1419**b **1457–1633** (Harper et al. 2011)	Male, 25–35 years old	Dawes and Magilton 1980
All Saints, York, Yorkshire (not considered by Harper et al. 2011)	3870: **1432–88** (95.4% probability)	Older adult female	McIntyre and Bruce 2010

Notes:
Bold in date column = radiocarbon dated
[a] This is the same cemetery as St. Mary Spital, but from a much earlier excavation.
[b] Uncorrected for marine signature (Harper et al. 2011); radiocarbon date corrected for marine component of diet (95% confidence interval).
[c] Accepted as pre-Columbian in date by Harper et al 2011.

References:
Boylston, Anthea., Malin Holst, and Charlotte A. Roberts. 2001. "The Human Skeletal Remains from Hull Magistrates Court." Unpublished skeletal report, Hull County Council.

Brothwell, Donald. 1961. "The Palaeopathology of Early British Man: An Essay on the Problems of Diagnosis and Analysis." *Man* 91: 318–44.

Cardy, A. 1997. "The Environmental Material: The Human Bones." In *Whithorn and St. Ninian: The Excavation of a Monastic Town, 1984–1991*, edited by P. Hill, 519–62. Stroud: Sutton Publishing.

Cole, G., and Tony Waldron. 2011. "Apple Down 152: A Putative Case of Syphilis from the Sixth Century AD, Anglo-Saxon England." *American Journal of Physical Anthropology* 144: 72–79.

Cole, G., and T. Waldron, T. 2015. Letter to the editor, "Apple Down 152 Putative Syphilis: Pre-Columbian Date Confirmed." *American Journal of Physical Anthropology* 156: 489.

Connell, Brian., Amy Gray Jones, Rebecca Redfern, Donald Walker. 2012. *A Bioarchaeological Study of Medieval Burials on the Site of St Mary Spital: Excavations at Spitalfields Market, London E1, 1991-2007*. Museum of London Archaeology Monograph Series 60. London: Museum of London.

Table 3.1 (*continued*)

Dawes, J. D. and J. R. Magilton. 1980. *The Cemetery of St Helen-on-the-Walls, Aldwark. The Archaeology of York.* The Medieval Cemeteries, vol. 12, no. 1. York: York Archaeological Trust, Council for British Archaeology.

Grainger, Ian., Duncan Hawkins, Lynne Cowal, and Richard Mikulski. 2008. *The Black Death Cemetery, East Smithfield, London.* Museum of London Archaeology Monograph Series 43. London: Museum of London.

Mays, Simon., Gillian Crane-Kramer, and Alexandra Bayliss. 2003 "Two Probable Cases of Treponemal Disease of Medieval Date from England." *American Journal of Physical Anthropology* 120: 133–43.

Mays, S., S. Vincent, and J. Meadows. 2012 "A Possible Case of Treponemal Disease from England Dating to the 11th–12th Century AD." *International Journal of Osteoarchaeology* 22: 366–72.

McIntyre, Lauren, and Graham Bruce. 2010. "Excavating All Saint's: A Medieval Church Rediscovered." *Current Archaeology* 245: 30–37.

Power, C. 1992. "Medieval Waterford—A Possible Case of Syphilis." *Archaeology Ireland* 6, no. 4: 20–21.

Roberts, Charlotte A. 1994. "Treponematosis in Gloucester, England: A Theoretical and Practical Approach to the Pre-Columbian Theory." In *L'origine de la syphilis en Europe avant ou après 1493? Actes du colloque international de Toulon, 25-28 Novembre 1993*, edited by Olivier Dutour, Györgi Palfi, Jacques Berato, and Jean-Pierre Brun, 101–8. Toulon, France: Centre Archeologique du Var, Editions Errance.

Roberts, C. A., A. R. Millard, G. M. Nowell, D. R. Gröcke, C. G. MacPherson. 2013. "Isotopic Tracing of the Impact of Mobility on Infectious Disease: The Origin of People with Treponematosis Buried in Hull, England, in the Late Medieval Period." *American Journal of Physical Anthropology* 150: 273–85.

Sidell, Jane, Christopher Thomas, and Alexandra Bayliss. 2007. "Validating and Improving Archaeological Phasing at St. Mary Spital, London," *Radiocarbon* 49, no. 2: 593–610.

Simmonds, Andrew, Nicholas Márquez-Grant, and Louise Loe, eds. 2008. *Life and Death in a Roman City: Excavation of a Roman Cemetery with a Mass Grave at 120–122 London Road, Gloucester.* Oxford Archaeology Monograph No 6. Oxford: Oxford Archaeological Unit.

Stirland, Ann. 1991. "Pre-Columbian Treponematosis in Medieval Britain." *International Journal of Osteoarchaeology* 1, no. 1: 39–47.

Stirland, Ann. 1994. "Evidence for Pre-Columbian Treponematosis in Medieval Europe." In *L'origine de la syphilis en Europe avant ou après 1493? Actes du colloque international de Toulon, 25-28 Novembre 1993*, edited by Olivier Dutour, Györgi Palfi, Jacques Berato, and Jean-Pierre Brun, 109–15. Toulon, France: Centre Archeologique du Var, Editions Errance.

Walker, D. 2012. *Disease in London, 1st–19th Centuries: An Illustrated Guide to Diagnosis.* Museum of London Archaeology Monograph Series 56. London: Museum of London.

Walker, Donald., Natasha Powers, Brian Connell, and Rebecca Redfern. "Evidence of Skeletal Treponematosis from the Medieval Burial Ground of St Mary Spital, London, and Implications for the Origins of the Disease in Europe." *American Journal of Physical Anthropology* 156 (2015): 90–101.

evidence, particularly regarding accurate diagnosis. Note that such a set of conclusions about both European and American skeletal remains, if correct, would be conducive to supporting the fifth alternative hypothesis considered earlier.

While a specific selection of the extant English skeletons that have been reported as supporting the pre-Columbian treponemal hypothesis were directly observed and reevaluated by some of the authors of the paper by Harper and colleagues, the vast majority of the English sites have not received the same detailed critical attention. Suffice it to say, reevaluation of the totality of the skeletal evidence for treponemal disease in both Europe and the Americas is badly needed for the debate to move forward. There is a particular need for direct observation and careful reevaluation of the human remains, rather than relying solely on reading published papers. In addition, there is a need for standardized accurate descriptions and diagnoses (including differential diagnoses) and AMS radiocarbon dating, as appropriate.[55] In terms of postmedieval evidence many reports are noted, but this period is not the focus of this chapter.[56] We now turn to focus on one site in England to illustrate how new data can change the way we view the history of treponemal disease.

Case Study from Medieval England

The Augustinian priory and hospital of St. Mary Spital was founded in 1197 by a group of wealthy London merchants with a charter to care for travelers, pilgrims, the sick and infirm, pregnant women, and children up to the age of seven. In 1235 it was refounded, and it is the cemetery associated with that phase of its history that is discussed here. It was the largest hospital in medieval England, and for many years in northern Europe. At the present time it is the largest late medieval cemetery excavated in Europe (containing the remains of more than 10,000 individuals) and the only cemetery in London subject to Bayesian carbon 14 dating, which has created four phases of cemetery use: period 1 (1120–1200), 2 (1200–1250), 3 (1250–1400) and 4 (1400–1539).[57] It has also enabled the differentiation of attritional and catastrophic (famine) burials.[58] A total of 5,387 individuals were recorded; twenty-five individuals with treponemal changes dating from 1200 to 1539 were recovered from the attritional burials (periods 2, 3, and 4). This is a "crude prevalence rate" and does not account for the fact that not every skeleton of the 5,387 individuals excavated and analyzed had the relevant bones preserved for a diagnosis of treponemal disease. The twenty-five skeletons affected by treponemal disease were the following: 6482, 6910, 6974, **10566**, 10765, 10874, 10933,

11671, 11935, 12240, 12374, 13232, 13467, 13602, **13635**, 13715, 19485, **20360**, 20634, 20912, 21653, **22466**, **22251**, **23887**, **25749** (**bold** = skeletons 1200–1400 CE; roman = skeletons 1400–1539).

The two earliest burials with treponemal disease were identified, first, in an indeterminate sex adult skeleton buried in the cemetery between 1200 and 1250. The skull had been truncated, but the long bones and hand and foot bones all had evidence of extensive new bone formation, and gummatous lesions were found in the left tibia (lower-leg bone), left humerus (upper-arm bone), and right scapula (shoulder-blade) bones. The second individual from the first period of the cemetery was a twenty-six- to thirty-five-year-old male, who appears to have died during the early stages of the disease, as there is evidence for multiple episodes of infection, much of which was active at the time of death. His facial bones, mandible, sternum, manubrium, and arm and leg bones were affected; although gummatous lesions are not present, the changes conform to the treponemal changes described by Donald Ortner.[59]

Classic treponemal and tertiary-stage gummatous lesions were observed in many other individuals from periods 3 and 4 of the cemetery, the latter period containing the majority (eighteen), suggesting that they had experienced the venereal form of this disease. The most poignant case, from period 4, is of a child around eleven years old at the time of death, whose entire skeleton is affected by late-onset CS (fig. 3.10). This child had extensive *caries sicca* lesions to the bones of the cranial vault, which had penetrated through the bone, and those of the palate and nasal cavity, producing extensive destruction; this indicates that the areas had developed and fused prior to the disease's onset. The arm and leg bones displayed multiple gummatous lesions, many of which had penetrated into the center of the bones (medullary cavity).[60] This child would have likely required extensive care, as the changes to the nose and mouth would have meant he/she lacked the ability to eat and drink without assistance, and the open gumma and *caries sicca* lesions would have necessitated dressing. It is also likely that these would have caused neurosyphilitic changes, such as hearing and sight loss and mental impairment.[61] From all the extant cemetery populations from medieval London, only at St. Mary Spital have subadults with skeletal changes associated with this disease been identified, and only this child, who seems to have needed such intensive care, has been found.[62] Donald Walker and colleagues propose that this hospital reflects the foundation charter of St. Mary Spital, which was the only hospital in London to care for children during this period.[63]

As the individuals were recovered from all periods of the cemetery, it was possible to establish that the levels of treponematosis were similar between

1200 to 1400, but there was a statistically significant increase from 1400 to 1539. More men than women were affected between 1200 to 1400 (five to one), but in the final period (1400 to 1539) women apparently had a higher rate of the disease. Interestingly, no individuals were over thirty-five years old at death, and the age distribution of this medieval sample conforms to that observed in clinical studies. The temporal span also afforded Walker and colleagues the opportunity to determine whether the appearance and distribution of the disease showed changes over time. The most frequently affected bones were the tibia (lower-leg bone) and ulna (one of the forearm bones), and there were temporal changes, with the skull bones being more affected from 1400 to 1539 (and particularly the frontal and parietal bones, known to be commonly affected by VS) (fig. 3.11). The disease affected both left and right sides of the skeleton in the majority of cases, but there were differences between the sexes in the number of bones affected, with males having more bones affected.[64] The majority of the skeletons with treponemal bone changes were buried in the later period of the site (i.e., 1400–1539), and they overall had the required combination of changes necessary for a secure diagnosis. However, no skeleton with treponemal disease was directly dated at this site, and thus it is not possible to say whether a majority—or indeed any—within the dating range of 1400–1539 were buried pre-1492.

Mortality, Fertility, and Venereal Syphilis

The question of whether and how much venereal syphilis (VS) contributed to early mortality and infertility in the past is not an area that has been considered in paleopathology, as far as the authors are aware. Estimating fertility, or the ability to conceive and produce children (which might be due to male or female infertility), is challenging in bioarchaeology, and fertility is heavily influenced by reproductive behavior. Work by Gwen Robbins has suggested that the gross reproduction rate for a population can be calculated using the proportion of infants to subadults in a skeletal population; this approach has not been attempted on medieval populations but may hold promise, despite issues associated with paleodemography.[65]

To complicate matters further, today there are many possible factors that can lead to infertility in men and women, apart from VS, most of which would be impossible to directly assess in skeletal remains, because they are restricted to the soft tissues. In women these include ovulation disorders, uterine and fallopian tube disorders, sterilization, and alcohol, medicine, and drugs, as well as increasing age. Male fertility is also affected by alcohol,

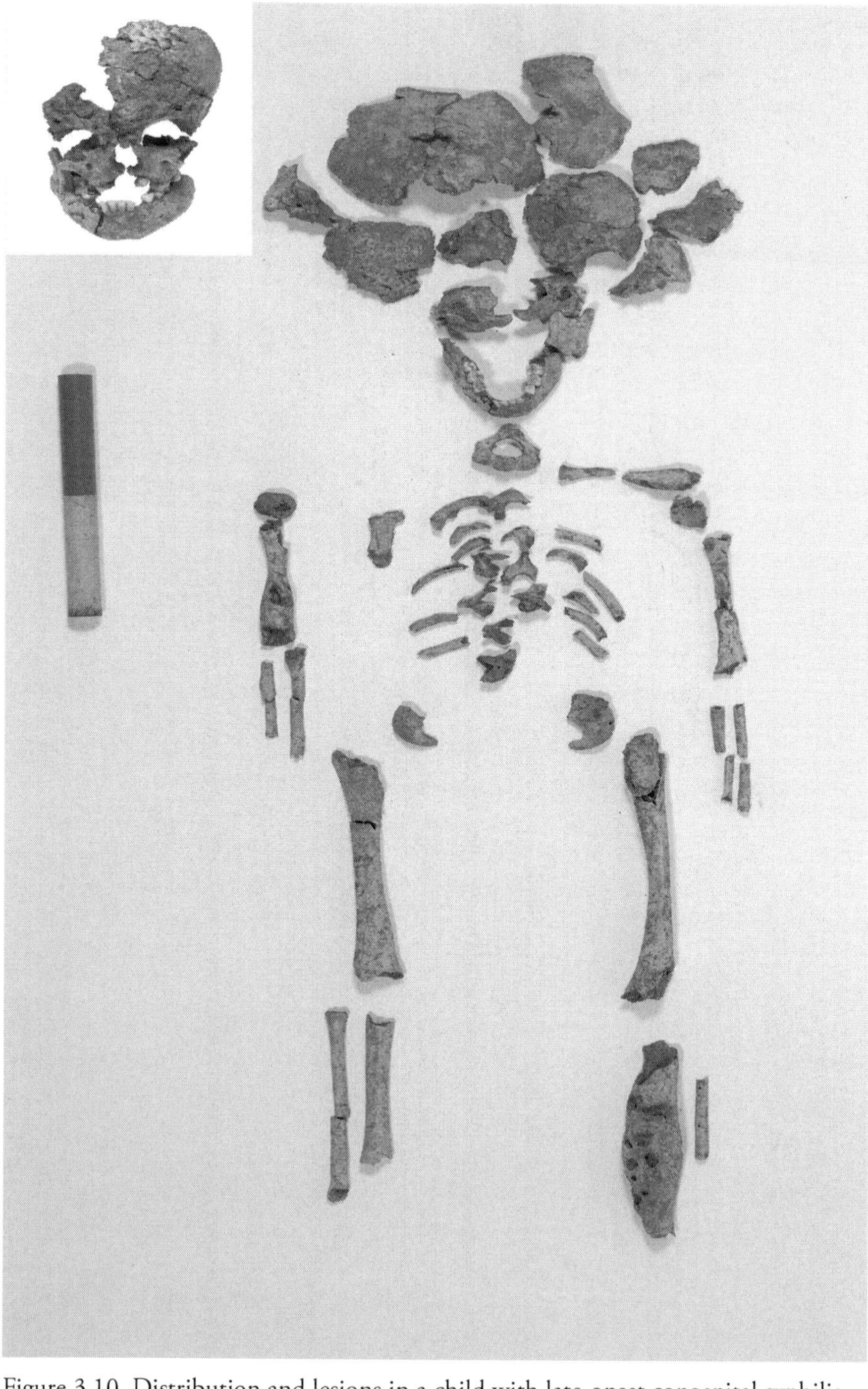

Figure 3.10. Distribution and lesions in a child with late-onset congenital syphilis. © Museum of London Archaeology, SRP98 sk 6974.

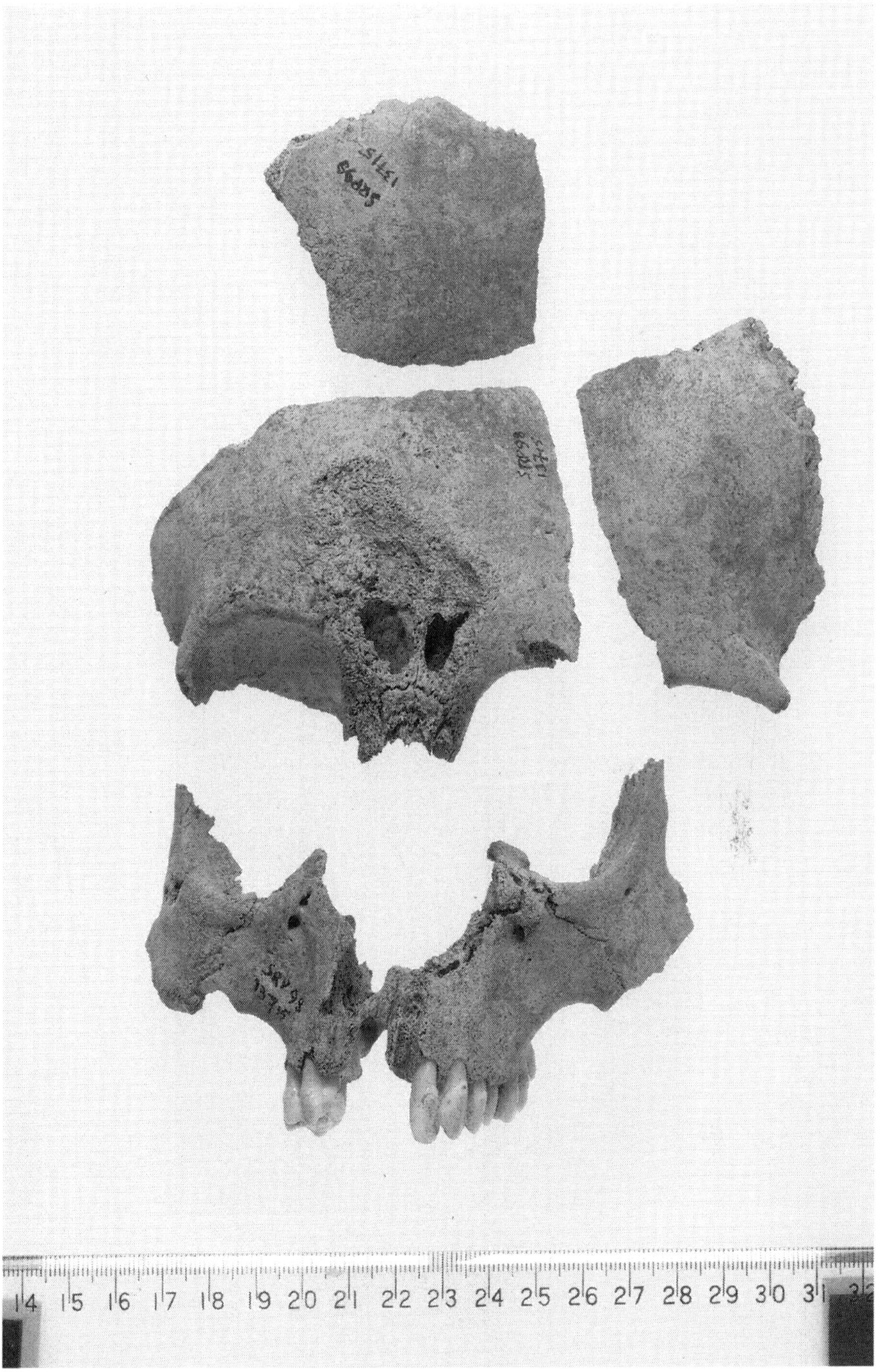

Figure 3.11. Extensive syphilitic changes to the frontal, maxillary, and zygomatic bones of a seventeen-year-old from St. Mary Spital. © Museum of London Archaeology.

medicine, and drugs, in addition to abnormal semen, absence of sperm, testicular disorders, sterilization, ejaculation disorders, and hypogonadism. The relative fertility of both sexes is also influenced by whether they are smokers, their weight, the presence of existing STIs, stress levels, and occupational and environmental factors.[66]

Estimating modern population fertility rates is described by Andrew Chamberlain, but key areas that present problems for bioarchaeologists considering this relationship include estimating accurate ages at death for adult skeletons; assessing whether females with and without VS have borne children; evaluating the cause of the (rare) presence of fetal remains buried in association with female skeletons; reflecting on beliefs about VS in the past (including how VS was transmitted) and how that may have affected reproductive behavior; and trying to produce a sensible answer to the question of frequency rates of VS compared to the number of skeletons excavated and analyzed, when so few skeletons have been diagnosed with the infection, such that frequency rates for VS cannot be realistically estimated.[67]

Nonetheless, this is an interesting question, and there is plenty of clinical evidence to show that VS affects fertility. It can seriously complicate pregnancy ("gestational syphilis") and lead to spontaneous abortion, stillbirth, intrauterine growth retardation, perinatal death, and premature delivery. For example, 5 percent of pregnancies in Ethiopia each year are lost through VS, and stillbirth in seropositive women is five times more common than in seronegative women; this has also been reported for the Americas.[68] Clearly. this is an issue with which populations with VS have to contend. How prevalent this was in the past is at present unknown.

Overview and the Way Forward

This chapter has provided a general introduction to the study of bioarchaeology, including paleopathology, the diagnosis of treponemal disease in archaeological human remains and its challenges, and the current debates about the origin of treponemal diseases. It has also placed the archaeological data into the clinical context of STIs today and considered the current relationship between VS and fertility. What it has not done is provide a commentary on the relationship between VS and fertility in the past. If it is not possible to estimate with any precision the frequency of VS from archaeological human remains, or indeed from early written historical sources, we must ask whether it is actually possible to assess the impact of this condition on fertility in the premodern past. As the paleopathological evidence is beginning to be linked to stable isotope data that might show how VS was transmitted around the world via migration, for various reasons, this might be a small step toward solving the jigsaw puzzle of the history of VS.[69]

The Columbian and pre-Columbian hypotheses for treponemal disease origin and transmission have been keenly debated for many years, but they have to be tested using direct evidence for the treponemal diseases in archaeological human remains. While there can be challenges in diagnosing and differentiating the three syndromes that affect the skeleton, it is perhaps only over the past twenty years that paleopathological analyses have intensified on this infection, especially in Europe. Newly diagnosed skeletons with accurate radiocarbon dates, and the dating and reevaluation of ones excavated and diagnosed years ago across the world, are allowing us to rethink and reflect on these theories. The current data from skeletal remains from archaeological sites do in fact indicate that treponemal disease was present in both Europe and the Americas prior to 1492, but the evidence from the Americas is currently more abundant.

We should now return to the five original hypotheses outlined earlier and consider the skeletal evidence at hand. The following summarizes where the debates are with respect to those hypotheses (apart from the discredited unitarian theory):

- Columbian: there is pre-Columbian dated skeletal evidence in the Americas.
- Pre-Columbian: there is pre-Columbian dated skeletal evidence in Europe, including in Britain and Ireland (e.g., St. Mary Spital). However, most diagnoses and dating have been contested, although these opinions are being debated currently.

In both of these cases some of the evidence is very clear, but other evidence is less convincing, and there are some clear (and less clear) pre-Columbian radiocarbon dates. Indeed, Harper and colleagues claimed that there were only three sites in the United Kingdom where the radiocarbon date was acceptable as pre-Columbian, and only three sites where the skeletal evidence was specific (not consistent or suggestive) for treponemal disease (Blackfriars in Gloucester, Hull Magistrates Court, and St. Margaret's, Norwich). However, there are five other sites that were not considered by Harper and colleagues, some of which had not been published at the time of their paper (see table 3.1). The authors' opinion regarding the British and Irish evidence is that there are a few more sites that have produced undoubted pre-Columbian treponemal disease evidence (individual skeletons from the sites of

London Road, Gloucester; East Smithfield, London; and St. Mary Spittle, London—although archaeologically dated—and All Saints, York, along with the twenty-five skeletons from St. Mary Spital, London); the Apple Down skeleton has also now been dated to 427–634. Virtually all the diagnoses of the skeletons listed in table 3.1 can be upheld. While Harper and colleagues suggested that nine of the UK sites they considered showed suggestive or specific skeletal evidence of treponemal disease, only three sites had clear pre-Columbian dates that also supposedly had marine-reservoir-effect corrected dates (Castle Mound, Huntingdon, St. Margaret's, Norwich, and St. Mary Spital). The numbers still do not reach those in the Americas, but they do add to extant skeletons of pre-Columbian dates in other parts of Europe.

However, to take a fair and transparent approach to this field of study, all the skeletal evidence in both Europe and the Americas needs to be reassessed for diagnosis and dating (beyond Harper and colleagues' 2011 report). Nevertheless, both diagnosis and dating may be impossible if skeletons have been reburied, and the latter may be impossible if destructive analysis is not allowed (e.g., for Native American skeletons). An evaluation of the totality of the (non-British and non-Irish) European and American evidence similar to that provided here for the data from Britain and Ireland was beyond the scope of this chapter. To sum-up the current theoretical viewpoints,

- Evolutionary theory: that pinta may be the earliest manifestation of treponemal disease and VS the latest may hold true, but this cannot be tested because pinta does not affect the skeleton. At the time of this writing, aDNA analysis for treponemal disease appears to be becoming viable, and eventually it is likely to be able to separate out the four different syndromes. We may be in a better position to test this theory as long as, again, acceptable dating can be achieved,
- Evolutionary theory variation: the possibility that non-venereal syphilis was endemic prior to 1492 in the Americas and was then taken to Europe to then mutate into VS in urban environments remains a viable hypothesis.

In summary the extant skeletal data for treponemal disease and dates for sites in Britain and Ireland have been presented and interrogated, revealing that there remains much more work to do to resolve the hypotheses presented in relation to this enigmatic infection. It may be that as biomolecular methods develop for detecting and sequencing ancient DNA of the different pathogens causing treponemal disease, this may help us better understand the impact of this infection. Research has established for the first time three historical *Treponema pallidum* genomes in skeletons from a convent dated to between the seventeenth and nineteenth centuries in Mexico City, two from the subspecies *pallidum* and one from the subspecies *pertenue*.[70] As Ortner stated fifteen years ago, "The history of treponematosis continues to be one of the most contentious issues in science," and this remains the case today.[71] Bioarchaeology is contributing much to learning more about treponemal disease in the past. No data from any discipline are perfect when attempting to reconstruct the origin, evolution, and history of diseases, but bioarchaeology has the ability to contribute to understanding health and well-being in the past if approached in a rigorous manner.

Notes

Rebecca Redfern wishes to thank the Spitalfields Osteology Team and MoLA for their work on the cemetery of St. Mary Spital. We are most grateful to David Bowsher and Andy Chopping (MoLA) for allowing us to use their images and to Lizzy Craig-Atkins, Lauren McIntyre, and Bruce Graham (OSA) for permission to include the Anchoress burial in this work. Jeff Veitch of the Department of Archaeology at Durham University is thanked for converting the JPEG images into TIFFs for the first author.

1. "Sexually Transmitted Infections (STIs): Fact Sheet," World Health Organization, accessed November 14, 2016, www.who.int/mediacentre/factsheets/fs110/en. The greatest incidence of STIs today are linked to the bacteria chlamydia, gonorrhea, syphilis, and trichomoniasis and to the viruses HIV, hepatitis B, herpes simplex virus, and human papillomavirus (HPV).

2. "Sexually Transmitted Diseases (STDs)," Centers for Disease Control and Prevention, accessed November 14, 2016, www.cdc.gov/std/.

3. Public Health England, "Sexually Transmitted Infections and Chlamydia Screening in England 2014," *Infection Report* 9, no. 22 (2015), https://assets.publishing.service.gov.uk/government/uploads/system/uploads/attachment_data/file/437433/hpr2215_STI_NCSP_v6.pdf.

4. For scholars who focus on historical documents, see, for example, Piers Mitchell, "Integrating Historical Sources with Paleopathology," in *A Companion to Paleopathology*, ed. Anne Grauer (Chichester: Wiley-Blackwell, 2012), 310–23; and many other chapters in this volume. For those who research human remains, see Sharon DeWitte and Christopher Stojanowski, "The Osteological Paradox 20 Years Later: Past Perspectives, Future Directions," *Journal of Archeological Research* 23, no. 4 (2015): 397–450; and James Wood et al., "The Osteological Paradox: Problems of Inferring Prehistoric Health from Skeletal Samples," *Current Anthropology* 33, no. 4 (1992): 343–70.

5. Jane Buikstra and Lane Beck, eds., *Bioarcheology: The Contextual Analysis of Human Remains* (Oxford: Elsevier, 2006); Jane Buikstra and Charlotte Roberts, eds., *A Global History of Paleopathology: Pioneers and Prospects* (Oxford: Oxford University Press, 2012); Charlotte Roberts, *Human Remains in Archaeology: A Handbook* (York: Council for British Archaeology, 2009).

6. Wood et al., "Osteological Paradox."

7. See the relevant chapter in Charlotte Roberts and Keith Manchester, *Archaeology of Disease*, 3rd ed. (Stroud: Sutton, 2010).

8. Randolph Nesse and George Williams, *Why We Get Sick: The New Science of Darwinian Medicine* (New York: Vintage Books, 1994); Wenda Trevathan, Euclid. O. Smith, and James McKenna, eds., *Evolutionary Medicine and Health: New Perspectives* (Oxford: Oxford University Press, 2008); Molly Zuckerman, Bethany Turner, and George Armelagos, "Evolutionary Thought in Paleopathology and the Rise of the Biocultural Approach," in Grauer, *Companion to Paleopathology*, 34–57.

9. Roberts, *Human Remains Handbook*, 55–71.

10. Buikstra and Roberts, *Global History of Paleopathology*; Roberts, *Human Remains Handbook*; Roberts and Manchester, *Archaeology of Disease*.

11. Roberts and Manchester, *Archaeology of Disease*; Wood et al., "Osteological Paradox."

12. Lorenzo Giacania and Sheila Lukehart, "The Endemic Treponematoses," *Clinical Microbiology Reviews* 27, no. 1 (2014): 89–115.

13. Ellis Herndon Hudson, "Treponematosis in Perspective," *Bulletin of the World Health Organization* 32, no. 5 (1965): 735–48.

14. Cecil Hackett, "On the Origin of the Human Treponematoses: Pinta, Yaws, Endemic Syphilis and Venereal Syphilis," *Bulletin of the World Health Organization* 29, no. 1 (1963): 7–41; Arturo Centurion-Lara et al., "Molecular Differentiation of *Treponema pallidum* Subspecies," *Journal of Clinical Microbiology* 44, no. 9 (2006): 3377–80.

15. Skin lesions may be identified in preserved bodies in the future. At present aDNA work has been able to identify only congenital syphilis successfully in neonate remains; see Rafael Montiel et al., "Neonate Human Remains: A Window of Opportunity to the Molecular Study of Ancient Syphilis," *PLOS One* 7, no. 5 (2012): e36371.

16. Marjorie Bauer and Charles Carvati, "Osteolytic Lesions in Early Syphilis," *British Journal of Venereal Disease* 43, no. 3 (1967): 175; Donald Resnick and George Niwayama, "Osteomyelitis, Septic Arthritis, and Soft Tissue Infection: Organisms," in *Diagnosis of Bone and Joint Disorders*, ed. Donald Resnick (Edinburgh: Saunders, 1995), 2448–2558.

17. World Health Organization, "Control of Tropical Diseases," *WHO Map Production* (Geneva: World Health Organization, 2012); Giacania and Lukehart, "Endemic Treponematoses."

18. Tibiae is often "sabre shin"–shaped due to additional new bone formation on the anterior of the large lower-leg bones.

19. Resnick and Niwayama, "Osteomyelitis," in Resnick, *Diagnosis*, 2448–2558.

20. Giacania and Lukehart, "Endemic Treponematoses."

21. Resnick and Niwayama, "Osteomyelitis," in Resnick, *Diagnosis* 2448–558.

22. See Mary Lucas Powell and Della Collins Cook, "Treponematosis: Inquiries into the Nature of a Protean Disease," in *The Myth of Syphilis: The Natural History of Treponematosis in North America*, ed. Mary Lucas Powell and Della Collins Cook (Gainesville, FL: University Press of Florida, 2005), 9–62.

23. Resnick and Niwayama, "Osteomyelitis," in Resnick, *Diagnosis*, 2448–558.

24. Roger G. Finch et al., "Infectious Diseases, Tropical Medicine and Sexually Transmitted Diseases," in *Clinical Medicine*, ed. Parveen Kumar and Michael Clark, 5th ed. (Edinburgh: Saunders, 2002), 21–151, 125.

25. Finch et al., "Infectious Diseases," in Kumar and Clark, *Clinical Medicine*, 21–151, 125.

26. Finch et al., "Infectious Diseases," in Kumar and Clark, *Clinical Medicine*, 21–151, 125.

27. Resnick and Niwayama, "Osteomyelitis," in Resnick, *Diagnosis*, 2448–558. Gummas are tumorlike growths in soft tissues that can affect the underlying bones as a result of focal destruction.

28. Symptoms include a runny nose and lesions on the skin in the mucous membranes.

29. Metaphyseal irregularities affect the end of the main shaft of the bone. Resnick and Niwayama, "Osteomyelitis," in Resnick, *Diagnosis*, 2448–558.

30. Simon Hillson, Caroline Grigson, and Sandra Bond, "Dental Defects of Congenital Syphilis," *American Journal of Physical Anthropology* 107, no. 1 (1998): 25–40.

31. Cecil Hackett, *Diagnostic Criteria of Syphilis, Yaws and Treponarid (Treponematoses) and of Some Other Diseases in Dry Bone* (New York: Springer, 1976).

32. Darlene Weston, "Non-specific Infection in Paleopathology: Interpreting Periosteal Reactions," in Grauer, *Companion to Paleopathology*, 492–512; Darlene Weston, "Investigating the Specificity of Periosteal Reactions in Pathology Museum Specimens," *American Journal of Physical Anthropology* 137, no. 1 (2008): 48–59.

33. Donald Ortner, *Identification of Pathological Conditions in Human Skeletal Remains* (London: Academic Press, 2003).

34. The human papillomavirus was also revealed in a lesion in the inguinal region of the mummy using biomolecular study, see Gino Fornaciari, "The Aragonese Mummies of the Basilica of Saint Domenico Maggiore in Naples," *Medicina Nei Secoli* 18, no. 3 (2006): 843–64; and Gino Fornaciari et al., "Syphilis in a Renaissance Italian Mummy," *Lancet* 334, no. 8663 (1989): 614. This is the most common STI in the United States today (see "Genital HPV Infection: Fact Sheet," Centers for Disease Control and Prevention, accessed November 14, 2016, www.cdc.gov/std/hpv/stdfact-hpv.htm), but the mummy is the only evidence in past human remains, to date.

35. Tanya von Hunnius et al., "Histological Identification of Syphilis in Pre-Columbian England," *American Journal of Physical Anthropology* 129, no. 4 (2006): 559–66.

36. Abigail Bouwman and Terence Brown, "The Limits of Biomolecular Palaeopathology: Ancient DNA Cannot Be Used to Study Venereal Syphilis," *Journal of Archeological Science* 32, no. 5 (2005): 703–13.

37. Montiel et al., "Neonate Human Remains"; Verena J. Schuenemann et al., "Historic *Treponema pallidum* from Colonial Mexico," *PLOS: Neglected Tropical Diseases*, June 21, 2018, https://doi.org/10.1371/journal.pntd.0006447.

38. Elizabeth Miller, Bruce Ragsdale, and Donald Ortner, "Accuracy in Dry Bone Diagnosis: A Comment on Palaeopathological Methods," *International Journal of Osteoarchaeology* 6, no. 3 (1996): 221–29.

39. Alfred Crosby, "The Early History of Syphilis: A Reappraisal," *American Anthropologist*, n.s., 71, no. 2 (1969): 218–27.

40. Richmond Holcomb, "Christopher Columbus and the American Origin of Syphilis," *U.S. Naval Bulletin* 32, no. 4 (1934): 401–30; Hackett, "Human Treponematoses," 7–41.

41. Hudson, "Treponematosis in Perspective."

42. Centurion-Lara et al., "Molecular Differentiation."

43. Hackett, "Human Treponematoses"; Mary Lucas Powell and Della Collins Cook, "Treponematosis: Past, Present and Future," in Grauer, *Companion to Paleopathology*, 472–91.

44. Piers Mitchell, "Pre-Columbian Treponemal Disease from 14th Century AD: Safed, Israel, and Implications for the Medieval Eastern Mediterranean," *American Journal of Physical Anthropology* 121, no. 2 (2003): 117–24; see also note 59.

45. For monographs, see Olivier Dutour et al., eds., *L'origine de la syphilis en Europe: Avant ou après 1493?* (Toulon: Centre Archeologique du Var, Errance, 1994); and Mary Powell and Della Cook, eds., *Myth of Syphilis: The Natural History of Treponematosis in North America* (Gainesville, FL: University Press of Florida, 2005). For journal papers, see Brenda Baker and George Armelagos, "Origin and Antiquity of Syphilis: A Paleopathological Diagnosis and Interpretation," *Current Anthropology* 29 no. 5 (1988): 703–37. For the meta-analysis, see Fernando Lucas de Melo et al., "Syphilis at the Crossroad of Phylogenetics and Paleopathology," *PLOS: Neglected Tropical Diseases* 4, no. 1 (2010): e575, https://doi.org/10.1371/journal.pntd.0000575.

46. Buikstra and Roberts, *Global History of Paleopathology.*

47. For the most recent survey and reevaluation, see Powell and Cook, *Myth of Syphilis.*

48. Donald Brothwell, "North American Treponematosis against the Bigger World Picture," in Powell and Cook, *Myth of Syphilis*, 481. This is the most recent synthesis, as of 2019.

49. For England, see Garrard Cole and Tony Waldron, "Apple Down 152: A Putative Case of Syphilis from the Sixth Century AD Anglo-Saxon England,"

American Journal of Physical Anthropology 144, no. 1 (2011): 72–79, table 1. For France, see György Pálfi et al., "Pre-Columbian Congenital Syphilis from the Late Antiquity in France," *International Journal of Osteoarchaeology* 2, no. 3 (1992): 245–61. For Israel, see Mitchell, "Pre-Columbian Treponemal Disease." For Iraq, see F. Kail and A. de Froe, "The Zakho Cranium: An Early Christian Cranium from Northern Iraq with Remarkable Pathological (Syphilitic?) Changes," *Hautarzt* 4, no. 2 (1953): 82. For South Africa, see Maryna Steyn and Maciej Henneberg, "Pre-Columbian Presence of Treponemal Disease: A Possible Case from Iron Age Southern Africa," *Current Anthropology* 36, no. 5 (1995): 869–73. For Turkey, see Yılmaz S. Erdal, "A Pre-Columbian Case of Congenital Syphilis from Anatolia (Nicaea, 13th Century AD)," *International Journal of Osteoarchaeology* 16, no. 1 (2006): 16–33.

50. Dutour et al., "L'origine de la syphilis"; Kristin Harper et al., "The Origin and Antiquity of Syphilis Revisited: An Appraisal of Old World Pre-Columbian Evidence for Treponemal Infection," *Yearbook of Physical Anthropology* 146, no. S53 (2011): 99–133.

51. Data has been reported from Egypt, Kenya, South Africa, and Sudan; China, India, Guam, Iraq, Israel, Kazakhstan, Russia, and Turkey; and Belarus, England, France, Germany, Ireland, Italy, Poland, and Ukraine.

52. Alexandra Bayliss et al., "The Potential Significance of Dietary Offsets for the Interpretation of Radiocarbon Dates: An Archeologically Significant Example from Medieval Norwich," *Journal of Archeological Science* 31, no. 5 (2004): 563–75. Having a diet that includes marine resources, as many people in the late medieval period had, means that radiocarbon dates need to be corrected for the "marine reservoir effect" so that they represent an accurate representation of the actual age of the analyzed sample. This is therefore important with respect to the period of interest here and to dating skeletons with treponemal disease from the pre- or post-Columbian period; see Philippa L. Ascough, Michael J. Church, and Gordon T. Cook, "Marine Radiocarbon Reservoir Effects for the Mesolithic and Medieval Periods in the Western Isles of Scotland," *Radiocarbon* 59, no. 1 (2017): 17–31.

53. Harper et al., "Origin and Antiquity," table 2.

54. Harper et al., "Origin and Antiquity," 124.

55. Standardized accurate descriptions and diagnoses (including differential diagnoses) and AMS radiocarbon dating, as indicated by Harper et al., "Origin and Antiquity."

56. Theya Molleson and Margaret Cox, *The Spitalfields Project*, vol. 2, *The Anthropology: The Middling Sort*, Research Report 86 (York: York Council for British Archaeology, 1993); Megan Brickley, Adrian Miles, and Hilary Stainer, *The Cross Bones Burial Ground, Redcross Way, Southwark, London*, Museum of London Archaeology Monograph Series 3 (London: Museum of London, 1993).

57. Jane Sidell, Christopher Thomas, and Alexandra Bayliss, "Validating and Improving Archeological Phasing at St. Mary Spital, London," *Radiocarbon* 49, no. 2 (2007): 593–610.

58. Brian Connell et al., *A Bioarchaeological Study of Medieval Burials on the Site of St Mary Spital: Excavations at Spitalfields Market, London E1, 1991–2007*, Museum of London Archaeology Monograph Series 60 (London: Museum of London, 2012).

59. Ortner, *Identification of Pathological Conditions*, 280–83; see also Christina M. Marra, "Update on Neurosyphilis," *Current Infectious Disease Reports* 11, no. 2 (2009): 124–34; and Lorna Tilley, *Theory and Practice in the Bioarchaeology of Care* (Cham: Springer International, 2015).

60. A four-year-old child with Hutchinson's incisors and Mulberry molars, indicative of congenital syphilis, has been observed in the Black Death sample from East Smithfield. Ian Grainger et al., *The Black Death Cemetery, East Smithfield, London*, Museum of London Archaeology Monograph Series 43 (London: Museum of London, 2008), 2, table 1.

61. Sandra R. Arnold and E. Lee Ford-Jones, "Congenital Syphilis: A Guide to Diagnosis and Management," *Paediatric Child Health* 5, no. 8 (2000): 463–69.

62. Arnold and Ford-Jones, "Congenital Syphilis."

63. Donald Walker et al., "Evidence of Skeletal Treponematosis from the Medieval Burial Ground of St. Mary Spital, London, and Implications for the Origins of the Disease in Europe," *American Journal of Physical Anthropology* 156, no. 1 (2015): 90–101.

64. Walker et al., "Evidence of Skeletal Treponematosis," 95–97.

65. Gwen Robbins, "Don't Throw Out the Baby with the Bathwater: Estimating Fertility from Subadult Skeletons," *International Journal of Osteoarchaeology* 21, no. 6 (2011): 717–22.

66. "Causes of Infertility," NHS Choices, accessed September 3, 2017, www.nhs.uk/Conditions/Infertility/Pages/Causes.aspx.

67. For estimating accurate ages, see Molleson and Cox, *Spitalfields Project*. In relation to the age at death of individuals with and without venereal syphilis–related bone disease, see Andrew Chamberlain, *Demography in Archaeology* (Cambridge: Cambridge University Press, 2006), 35–36. For assessing whether females have borne children, see Margaret Cox, "Assessment of Parturition," in *Human Osteology in Archaeology and Forensic Science*, ed. Margaret Cox and Simon Mays (Cambridge: Cambridge University Press, 2000), 131–42. Note that the reliability of parturition scars as being indicators of pregnancy and delivery has been heavily critiqued, as there is no accurate or reliable method. Douglas Ubelaker and Jade De La Paz, "Skeletal Indicators of Pregnancy and Parturition: A Historical Review," *Journal of Forensic Sciences* 57, no. 4 (2012): 866–72. For evaluating the cause fetal remains buried with female skeletons, see Charlotte A. Roberts and Margaret Cox, *Health and Disease in Britain: From Prehistory to the Present Day* (Stroud: Sutton Publishing, 2003), 166, fig. 4.1.

68. Mehmet Genç and William Ledger, "Syphilis in Pregnancy," *Sexually Transmitted Infections* 76, no. 2 (2000): 73–79; L. Arnesen, S. Serruya, and P. Duran "Gestational Syphilis and Stillbirth in the America: A Systematic Review and Meta-Analysis," *Revista Panamericana de Salud Pública* 37, no. 6 (2015): 422–29.

69. Charlotte Roberts et al., "Isotopic Tracing of the Impact of Mobility on Infectious Disease: The Origin of People with Treponematosis Buried in Hull, England, in the Late Medieval Period," *American Journal of Physical Anthropology* 150, no. 2 (2013): 273–85.

70. Schuenemann et al., "Historic *Treponema pallidum*."

71. Ortner, *Identification of Pathological Conditions*, 273. For instance, the keen debate over offsetting for the so-called marine reservoir effect of fish-based diets when using radiocarbon dating has been subject to an important development in nuancing the methods used for dating in "treponema diseases contexts." This was presented just as this volume went to press: M. Dee, "Radiocarbon Evidence Pertaining to the Origin and Spread of Treponemal Disease." Abstract of paper presented at the Annual Meeting of the American Association of Physical Anthropologists, Cleveland, Ohio, March 2019, p. 55.

Chapter Four

A Long-Standing Evolutionary History between *Chlamydia trachomatis* and Humans

Visible Ocular and Invisible Genital Variants

Ian N. Clarke and Hugh R. Taylor

Chlamydiae

The most frequently asked questions about *Chlamydia trachomatis*, commonly known as "chlamydia," are (1) what is it? and (2) where did it come from? The capricious and cryptic nature of genital infections caused by *C. trachomatis* and the difficulties in isolating the pathogen have led to many misconceptions about its origins and how infection occurs. The first question is now easy to answer. There is no doubt: chlamydiae are not viruses, nor are they protozoan parasites; they are bacteria.[1] However, they are not free-living bacteria and so cannot be cultivated on conventional media such as agar plates. Chlamydiae are highly specialized bacteria, which can be grown only within living cells; thus they are obligate intracellular pathogens.

Chlamydiae also have a complex developmental cycle.[2] The name is derived from *Chlamydozoa*, which means "cloaked organisms," because they develop within an inclusion membrane within the cytoplasm of the cell and initially in the infection process are not visible.[3] These gram-negative bacteria have a unique development cycle that includes the repeated division of a replicating stage, called an RB, or reticulate body. RBs increase in number to a point where they can be seen under the microscope as moving specks within a defined membrane structure known as an inclusion in the host cell's cytoplasm. With time the inclusion ruptures out of the cell and releases the smaller nonreplicating infectious forms called "elementary bodies."

The genus is also known as *Chlamydia*; it is a proper noun written in italics, with no plural. The genus *Chlamydia* currently contains nine species and no doubt, more will be added. The species *C. trachomatis*, the focus of our discussion, is made up of a number of serovars, differentiated by surface antigens that induce specific antibodies. It has four ocular serovars that cause blinding endemic trachoma, A, B, Ba, and C and at least eight serovars, D to K, which typically cause genital tract infections. There are additionally the three L serovars that cause the condition known as lymphogranuloma venerum. Closely related species are *C. muridarum*, which infects mice and hamsters, and *C. suis*, which is endemic in pigs.

In this chapter we review what is known about the origins and molecular phylogeny of *C. trachomatis* and focus on the history of ocular disease. The social history of the science of urogenital infection caused by *C. trachomatis* is covered by Michael Worboys in chapter 5. In addition, we discuss the interaction between the parasite and the host. We draw attention to the long evolutionary history of chlamydiae and the recognition of the range of clinical manifestations of infection, answering the question, "where did it come from?"

Host Parasite Coevolution

The second question—"where did it come from?"—is the main topic of this chapter. This question has been visited before.[4] While some of these concepts still hold, our ideas on the evolution of bacteria and specifically *C. trachomatis* have grown rapidly in the past few years. Our understanding of the diversity and evolution of *C. trachomatis* has been very limited mainly because of the difficulties in obtaining relevant historical samples.[5] The subsequent application of new advanced sequencing techniques has led to an explosion of new genome sequences and data.[6]

The comparison of genes from all living organisms indicates they share a common ancestor termed LUCA, the "last universal common ancestor."[7] Life on earth can be divided into three distinct domains: bacteria, archaea, and eukarya.[8] The very earliest fossilized microbes found in hydrothermal vents from the earth's primitive crust date up to 4.28 billion years ago, suggesting life on earth first arose (abiogenesis) before this time.[9] Since the domains archaea and eukarya evolved from the bacteria, the development of the relationship between chlamydiae and their host eukaryotic cells must have arisen after or at the earliest time of the emergence of the first eukaryotic cells (eukaryotic cells ultimately evolving to form complex multicelled organisms, i.e., animals and plants). Studies of microfossils in Proterozoic sedimentary rocks suggest single-celled eukaryotes developed at least 1.8 billion years ago.[10]

Much larger than bacteria, eukaryotes are characterized by individual cells with internal "organelles." These structures include cell nuclei, plastids, and mitochondria. The mitochondria are now generally held to be the remnants of endosymbiotic bacteria that were involved in the primary colonization of the eukaryotic cells. Mitochondria are present in nearly all eukaryotic cells. However, the mitochondria, unlike chlamydiae, are not infectious and have been subverted for use as energy-generating powerhouses for their eukaryotic host cell. Plastids are found in plants and also developed from different bacterial endosymbionts and are now typified by chloroplasts, which are needed for photosynthesis. The early, single-celled eukaryotic ancestors from which plants and animals evolved no longer exist, so it was a huge surprise in 1997, when chlamydia-like microorganisms were first found in single-celled, free-living environmental acanthamoebae.[11]

While primitive, single-celled organisms remain abundant within the environment, such as amoebae, some examples are considered "living fossils," which have been on the planet for at least fifty million years.[12] So it is possible that some ancient chlamydia-like microorganisms could have piggybacked through the ages within such dormant forms of single-celled eukaryotes, and those chlamydiae and chlamydia-like microorganisms found today are representative of both modern and ancient forms.

The chlamydia-like microorganisms can infect free-living acanthamoebae (which have been cured of their original infection by treatment with antibiotics), so the chlamydia-like organisms are not symbionts.[13] They possess a similar developmental cycle to human *C. trachomatis*, and they are limited to the acanthamoebal cell cytoplasm, but they do not kill their host amoebae. We now know that these chlamydiae (which have been assigned to a new family known as *Parachlamydiaceae*) are distantly related to *C. trachomatis*.[14] Detailed studies of their genes show that the last common ancestor of both was already well adapted to survive within eukaryotic cells some seven hundred million years ago, which is also coincident with the time when the first multicellular organism might have arisen. Thus, it seems possible that chlamydial evolution was intimately intertwined with their host cells from the most primitive unicellular eukaryotes to the formation of multicellular organisms.[15] The unexpected presence of genes that appear to have a plant origin in *C. trachomatis* may be accounted for by a hypothesis that their distant ancestors were involved in the process of plastid endosymbiosis in the development of early plants over a billion years ago.[16] The most likely explanation for the presence of plant genes in chlamydiae is that these observations are artifacts because lateral gene transfer from prokaryotes to eukaryotes is unidirectional.[17] Thus, the observation of "plant" genes in chlamydial genomes is better explained by gene transfer among bacteria in a process that occurred before the evolution of plant cells, and the presence of these genes is not a result of their direct acquisition by chlamydiae from plants. Health education campaigns have been run to inform the public about chlamydia and sexual health, and the most notable slogan, "Chlamydia is not a flower," is now, with our new evolutionary knowledge, more confounding than the intended verbal irony.

The Classification of Chlamydial Species and Early Phylogenetic Studies

Phylogenetics is the study of the evolutionary history among organisms either as individuals or groups. Since the 1970s the increasing availability of protein and DNA sequences obtained through advances in modern molecular biology has proved particularly useful in understanding and deducing the relationships between organisms over evolutionary time. The ability to relate mutation rates in DNA or protein sequences to events in the past has led to the development of the concept of a molecular clock.[18] In this approach it is possible to deduce when life forms diverged. The time scale is calibrated against independent measures of time, such as the fossil record or, for shorter time spans, archaeological samples.

The advent, availability, and rapid deployment of gene-sequencing technology has allowed systematic analysis of evolutionary relationships among many different species, including bacteria. This began with only gene fragments, then whole genes, and subsequently has progressed to complete genomes. These molecular approaches have confirmed the biological observations that indicated there were many different chlamydiae and chlamydia-like species, of which *C. trachomatis* is only one example. The early studies of chlamydial evolution—phylogeny and taxonomy that relied on using a single gene or even a gene fragment—have been superseded by the use of complete genome sequences.[19]

For many years since their discovery, chlamydiae were thought to be unique microorganisms with no near relatives.[20] Once they were recognized as bacteria, there was only one order, *Chlamydiales*, with one family, *Chlamydiaceae*, and only one genus, *Chlamydia*, which contained two species, *C. trachomatis* and *C. psittaci* (a pathogen of psittacine birds). The number of recognized chlamydial species in this genus has since increased. In addition, there has been a massive expansion in the discovery and knowledge of other chlamydia-like organisms; there are now nine family-level lineages including the *Chlamydiaceae*. These all share the property of having a similar developmental cycle, and the bacteria are totally reliant on the eukaryotic host cell for replication and survival. These discoveries are consistent with the notion that all the chlamydia-like microorganisms share a common ancestor that had established the characteristic developmental cycle some seven hundred million years ago.[21]

Some considerable confusion was introduced by the reclassification of the two genera within the *Chlamydiaceae*. Some of this incorrect nomenclature still persists in the literature. The confusing study was based on limited data related to a small set of critical genes, known as 16S rRNA, that are highly conserved and used as a marker in phylogenetic analysis of bacteria.[22] This study and the subsequent classification based on diversity in the 16S rRNA genes divided the *Chlamydiaceae* family into two genera. Unfortunately, the analysis was premature and did not take into account or give sufficient weight to biological features; it also muddled the use of species names, causing further confusion both in terminology and in the estimation of the evolutionary distance between *C. trachomatis* and *C. psittaci*.[23] The taxonomical record and the way chlamydiae are classified has now been corrected. Currently there is one genus, *Chlamydia*, which contains nine recognized species, with more awaiting official approval by the international committee that oversees the taxonomy of bacterial species.[24] Only two of these species infect humans as their natural host, *C. trachomatis* and *C. pneumoniae*. While *C. pneumoniae* is an important cause of pneumonia in humans, it is also responsible for a wide range of infections in animals and reptiles, including snakes, iguanas, chameleons, frogs, and turtles. Of the remaining seven species *C. muridarum* infects mice and hamsters, and *C. suis* infects pigs, as mentioned earlier. *C. psittaci* is predominantly an avian infection. *C. pecorum* affects mammals, including cattle, sheep, goats, pigs, and koalas. *C. abortus* is common among ruminants but also occurs in horses, rabbits, guinea pigs, mice, pigs, and humans.[25] Infection is frequently associated with abortion. *C. felis* is endemic among cats and causes feline conjunctivitis, rhinitis and respiratory infection. *C. caviae* infects guinea pigs and has been used as a model for human infection.

Essentially every vertebrate species seems to have its own chlamydiae, and infection is highly prevalent in animals. Not only are over 70 percent of domestic cattle and pigs infected, but also nearly 60 percent of feral pigs are polymerase chain reaction positive (on PCR, see below, p. 170). Most calves are infected within two weeks of birth, and the prevalence and intensity of infection increases exponentially with crowding. Among cats 12 percent carry *C. felis*. In many cases animal infection is endemic and asymptomatic, although serious epidemics of manifest infection do occur, particularly in birds, if they are stressed or crowded together. More typically, the asymptomatic infection has a marginal effect, making the animals more susceptible to other infections. Chronic latent or persistent infection may have important implications in animals raised for food production, decreasing growth rates, fertility, and milk production.[26]

Australian marsupials are unique animals and have been geographically isolated from the rest of the world for millennia. These animals also have infections caused by *C. pneumoniae* and *C. pecorum* as well as new strains still to be classified.[27] One study found *C. psittaci* present in 70 percent of koalas, with only 9 percent showing symptoms.[28] Thus, as more genome-sequence data for different chlamydial species has accumulated, it has become clear that they are highly complex intracellular pathogens that have been interacting with the hosts of many species.[29]

Biology, Genomes, and Genomic Interactions

Here our purpose is to consider only *C. trachomatis*. Consistent with other sexually transmitted pathogens, *C. trachomatis* is highly species-specific, and humans are the natural host. It can be forced to infect other host species (e.g., rodents and nonhuman primates) and indeed infect cells from other species in vitro, but these are unnatural situations, and all are poor substitutes for studying disease caused by *C. trachomatis* in its human host.[30] On the basis of biological and clinical observations, *C. trachomatis* infections are divided into three clear types: ocular, genital, and LGV that primarily infect the genital tract but cause a disseminating infection involving the lymph glands.[31] While there are phenotypic differences between the *C. trachomatis* that cause these three types of infection, the accumulating molecular data indicates that variations are minimal and mainly restricted to minor sequence differences on variable surface proteins.[32]

The first genome sequence for *C. trachomatis* was published in 1998.[33] It was a revelation since it provided new insights into the evolutionary history of this microorganism. In one review it was considered as an autobiography, "an ancient text reflecting the entire evolutionary history of chlamydiae."[34] Consistent with other intracellular pathogens, it has a reduced genome size. *C. trachomatis* has a genome of approximately a million base pairs and encodes close to a thousand genes (a quarter the size of the genome of the free-living bacterium *E. coli*). Loss of genome-coding capacity through evolution in intracellular pathogens is generally explained by the exploitation of eukaryotic host biosynthetic pathways and the disappearance of corresponding pathways in the intracellular bacteria. The genome sequence also dispelled some myths, for example, an established belief that *C. trachomatis* was an energy parasite obtaining its energy solely in the form of ATP (adenosine triphosphate) from the eukaryotic host cell. The discovery of all the genes necessary for the biosynthesis pathways that make ATP completely defeated this notion.[35]

As sequencing technologies developed and became faster, more accurate, and cheaper, the ability to sequence the complete genetic blueprint of microorganisms, or indeed all living organisms, has revolutionized biological sciences. The development of next-generation sequencing technologies has fueled an explosion of data, such that the comparison of multiple genomes rather than individual genes has shed light on the details of genome diversity at the highest resolution.[36] In addition—and very surprisingly—individual *C. trachomatis* interact with one another when they infect the same cell and can exchange DNA by a process known as recombination.[37] This is now well established as a way by which this highly specialized and evolutionarily isolated species naturally generates diversity.[38]

Ecological Niches and Origins of *C. trachomatis*

In humans *C. trachomatis* occupies two ecological niches, the eye and the genital tract, although chlamydiae can infect the rectum and pharynx with no apparent symptoms.[39] Ocular infections, leading to trachoma if occurring in children, may ultimately lead to blindness. By contrast sexually transmitted chlamydial infections are diseases of adults or, at least, sexually active individuals. The presence of two clear disease forms leads naturally to the simple question, which came first? Was *C. trachomatis* an eye or mucosal infection that later changed its mode of transmission from nongenital to genital, or was it a genital infection that expanded to other mucosal surfaces?

An early study on genomic phylogeny with only six genomes showed that the species *C. trachomatis* is divided into two distinct clades representing LGV and the ocular and genital tract isolates; the latter two are collectively termed the "trachoma clade."[40] This has been substantiated with a further fifty genomes, and these data indicate that this split occurred early in the evolutionary history of the species.[41] The deep split between these two clades suggests there were severe bottlenecks in evolution and that, if there were other lineages, they have become extinct. Therefore, we can only speculate about how *C. trachomatis* reached its current specialization and the properties of their common ancestor.

Genome sequences within the LGV clade show much less diversity, and the L2b isolates have extremely low-level variation and a worldwide distribution, indicating they are part of a new epidemic that has slowly emerged since the early 2000s.[42] However, it has not been possible to construct an accurate timeline for the emergence of the *C. trachomatis* species in general because of the absence of archaeological isolates, making it difficult to determine the mutation rate of the genome. By contrast, a number of classic LGV isolates with accurate data on their date of isolation from the 1960s and 1970s were sequenced in a study published in 2017.[43] A Bayesian evolutionary analysis of the phylogenetic tree of these isolates suggests a most recent common ancestor between 200 and 1430 CE. Given the very limited time window (fifty years) and the small number of samples used to generate this time line, the confidence limits of the estimate are wide. Nevertheless, these data suggest expansion of the LGV lineage is occurring over a time scale of hundreds to a few thousands of years.

The trachoma clade is made up of two lineages (T1 and T2). Clade T1 is composed of prevalent urogenital isolates, whereas T2 contains rarer urogenital isolates and ocular strains, which form a cluster, indicating that these ocular isolates emerged from a urogenital ancestor. Thus, it seems that chlamydiae have expanded from a genital ecological niche to infect the eye and cause trachoma. The genomic phylogeny indicates that the sexual transmission of *C. trachomatis* is, unusually, the ancestral state rather than this pathogen having arrived from another external source to infect humans. Origination in the genital tract and subsequent tropism for the eye has been explained simply by the dependence of *C. trachomatis* on the amino acid tryptophan.[44] The final step in the biosynthesis of tryptophan is the conversion of indole to tryptophan. Urogenital isolates can utilize indole, which is produced in abundance by the vaginal microbiota.[45] This ability has been lost in ocular strains (consistent with their specialization), which, when tryptophan becomes depleted due to the immune response, are forced into a persistent state (i.e., "dormant" in common parlance, unable to develop further in their cycle but not dying). Thus, urogenital *C. trachomatis* can grow readily both in the genital tract using indole and in the eye, whereas ocular strains cannot compete in the genital tract.[46]

Analysis of 563 complete *C. trachomatis* genomes has given further insight into the history of the species and indicates that there were two phases of *C. trachomatis* evolution: deep variation and contemporary mixing. The time frames for these processes are impossible to pinpoint, with current evaluative methodology, since, unlike LGV, there is a complete absence of isolates from the past. However, it has been speculated that the divergent lineages have "expanded over the last few thousand years."[47]

The History of Trachoma

Given that serovars A–C have the capacity to cause the blinding human disease of trachoma, they have left their mark in recorded history, though the precise bacterial cause was not known until the twentieth century. A key issue to bear in mind, however, is that, even under conditions where effective treatment is lacking, as was the case throughout most of human history, a single episode was not enough to cause sufficient damage to result in functional blindness. Mathematical modeling suggests that about 100 episodes of infection may be needed to cause marked scarring, and around 150 or more to cause trichiasis (in-turned eyelashes that lead to blindness).[48] Animal and human studies also suggest that repeated episodes of infection may be needed to cause fertility-damaging tubal occlusion.[49]

It seems most likely, therefore, that trachoma was first seen in the early settlements in Mesopotamia, the so-called Fertile Crescent, about ten thousand years ago, as people aggregated in settlements and towns.[50] The increased crowding and poor hygiene in these early settlements permitted the sharing of infected ocular secretions and the frequent episodes of reinfections leading to trachoma—the endemic blinding disease that clinically appears to be a chronic "infection." Blinding trachoma differs from the occasional and eventually self-limiting episodes of chlamydial-inclusion conjunctivitis that still continue to occur around the world, even in the most developed countries. Trachoma would also have accompanied the spread of early settlements around the Mediterranean and along the four great river valleys: the Yangtze in China, the Indus and Ganges in South Asia, the Euphrates and Tigris in the Middle East, and the Nile in Egypt. References to trachoma surgery in China date back to 27 BCE.[51] Bronze Age epilation forceps from around 2000 BCE were found in Ur in Sumeria.[52] Trachoma was apparently common in ancient Egypt, and its treatment is described in the Ebers Papyrus (1553 and 1550 BCE). Many of these ancient remedies were still in use in Egypt in the early twentieth century.[53] Written descriptions of trachoma and its treatment also come from India, dating from no later than 500 CE.[54] The term *trachoma* comes from the Greek "rough," to describe the roughness of everted eyelids.[55]

There are scattered reports of trachoma in western Europe from Roman times and throughout the Middle Ages.[56] However, trachoma really came to the attention of Western medicine during the Napoleonic Wars (1798–1815), starting with the Battle of the Nile and the Egyptian Campaign (1798–1802).[57] At times over one-third of French and British troops in Egypt were incapacitated by "Egyptian ophthalmia," with many becoming blind. During the Napoleonic Wars massive armies were hurriedly recruited and quartered in temporary barracks; they marched across Europe and fought with and against soldiers from many countries. The armies had 100,000 or more men who slept rough or crowded in barns without any real access to clean water or good hygiene. This led to huge problems: 25,000 Prussian troops developed trachoma, and 1,100 became bilaterally blind. Similar outbreaks occurred in the Austrian army, and later the Russian army had 80,000 Russian soldiers affected.[58] At the end of the conflict, the regiments were disbanded and the soldiers took the infection home to the civilian populations. This was at the start of the Industrial Revolution, when the overcrowded slums in Europe were at their worst; hygiene was deplorable, and trachoma rapidly became a major public health problem.[59]

Egyptian ophthalmia forced a reconsideration of the role and importance of eye disease as it spread throughout the United Kingdom and other countries.[60] The army formed separate eye hospitals for their soldiers with ophthalmia. Then eye hospitals for civilians started to be founded. The Royal Infirmary for the Diseases of the Eye and the London Dispensary for Curing Diseases of the Eye and Ear were founded in 1805 and later became the world-famous Moorfields Eye Hospital.[61] The new eye hospitals needed specialists to work in them, and this led to ophthalmology being the first recognized specialty area, often coupled with otolaryngology services. A further major epidemic occurred in the Belgian army in 1834, with 4,000 soldiers "totally blind" and another 10,000 partially blinded.[62] To solve this problem, all the affected soldiers were discharged, and so trachoma rapidly spread through the civilian population. This disaster in Belgium led to the First International Congress of Ophthalmology, in Brussels in 1857.

The ophthalmia or trachoma epidemics occurred during the Industrial Revolution. People were flooding into the industrializing cities and living in appalling conditions in crowded tenements and workhouses in the developing urban slums.[63] The number of people who became blind from ophthalmia also led to the founding of specific homes and institutions for the blind and later schools for blind children or those with trachoma.[64] Children were housed in small groups, washed frequently, and treated with copper sulfate or silver nitrate. Not until the 1930s did sulfonamides start to be used to treat the last cases.[65] The last trachoma school in the United Kingdom finally closed in 1944, although the trachoma clinic in the docks area of Glasgow ran until the 1960s.[66]

With the changing socioeconomic conditions and the associated migration to the developing urban slums, it seems likely that the genital transmission of chlamydia, and probably gonococcus as well, increased, as did the ocular transmission. There is no documented evidence for the increase of genital chlamydia infection, although rates of ocular trachoma clearly increased, but a 2017 study has shown rates of treatment for pox (syphilis) eight times higher in Chester City in the 1770s than in the surrounding rural countryside.[67] Gonorrhea is frequently asymptomatic in women, and chlamydia in both sexes. The two diseases were also basically indistinguishable clinically and of course very often would have occurred together as dual infections; either or both would have been called "the clap" in the early modern period. Similarly, with ocular infection of the newborn, ophthalmia neonatorum, there could be no differentiation between that due to chlamydia, the gonococcus, or other organisms until the advent of microbiological diagnoses from the later nineteenth century onward.

The history of trachoma in the United States is also relevant. By the late nineteenth century, trachoma was seen as a major problem for newly arriving immigrant groups, especially those from eastern Europe.[68] Between 1897 and 1924, over twenty-one million immigrants were examined for trachoma, and significant numbers were sent back after having had the letter *T* marked in blue chalk on their clothes.[69] Although trachoma had been widespread in the United States for nearly a century, a survey conducted by the US Public Health and Marine Hospital Service in 1911 defined what became known as the "trachoma belt."[70] The widespread occurrence of trachoma led the US Congress in 1913 to allocate $25,000.[71] Trachoma outreach teams and trachoma hospitals were established in many areas of the Midwest. By the early 1950s trachoma had ceased to be a major problem, and the last program wound up in Missouri.[72] However, trachoma continued to be a problem in the indigenous populations in the Southwest, and the US Indian Health Service ran trachoma-control programs until the 1980s.[73] Trachoma disappeared from the towns and cities of Australia in the early 1900s, but to this day continues to occur and cause blindness in outback Australian Aboriginal communities.[74]

The World Health Organization was founded in 1947, and in 1948 it established a trachoma program and quickly moved to using the newly discovered tetracycline.[75] Tetracycline ointment was messy and labor-intensive, as it had to be applied twice a day for six weeks, but nevertheless it was a significant breakthrough. Working with UNICEF, the WHO initiated trachoma-control programs in eleven countries, including Morocco, Tunisia, Algeria, Taiwan, Burma, India, Oman, Vietnam, Brazil, Libya, and Sudan and by 1962 had treated 7.5 million people. Other programs were run in Argentina, Uruguay, Poland, Hungary, Yugoslavia, the Soviet Union, Turkey, Palestine, Japan, China, Thailand, Egypt, and South Africa.[76] Some of these programs were highly successful, but others were less so.[77] In the 1970s the WHO moved from vertical intervention programs to a more horizontal primary health care approach, and specific disease programs, such as the trachoma programs, gradually disappeared.

Consequently, there has been a dramatic reduction in the estimated number of people with active trachoma.[78] In 1981 500 million people were thought to be affected, but by 2003 the global estimate was 84 million.[79] There had also been a marked drop in the amount of blindness attributable to trachoma, from an estimate of 6–7 million in 1980 to 1.6 million in 2003 in fifty-six countries surveyed.[80]

This progressive decrease in trachoma has been associated with a general improvement in environmental living conditions linked to socioeconomic development.[81] These changes also led to the disappearance of trachoma in the past in western Europe and North America.[82] They included a broad range of improvements in family and community hygiene: piped water, sewage systems, garbage collection, and fly reduction or protection. Close contact with animals was also reduced, with cattle in the country and with horses in the towns, where they were replaced by bicycles, cars, buses, and trucks.[83] Paved roads and dust reduction also contributed, as did electrification, the separation of bedrooms from living and cooking areas, less crowding in bedrooms with fewer children sharing beds (from reduced family size and new forms of heating), adequate hot water, and indoor bathrooms. Education, especially maternal education with an emphasis on hygiene and facial cleanliness, also contributed. One way or another each of these changes facilitated the reduction in the ease and frequency of the transmission of infected ocular secretions from one child to another.[84]

However, trachoma has remained a major problem in many areas of the world, and to address this the WHO resolved in 1998 to reinvigorate efforts to eliminate blinding trachoma as a public health problem.[85] The WHO recommended a four-pronged strategy, the SAFE Strategy: the use of surgery to correct the in-turned eyelashes; antibiotic treatment to reduce or eliminate infection; facial cleanliness to reduce transmission; and environmental improvement to promote better hygiene.[86] The WHO established the Global Alliance for the Elimination of Trachoma by the year 2020 (GET2020) to bring together key NGOs, researchers, representatives of national governments, the corporate sector, and WHO experts. Pfizer initiated a major donation program to provide azithromycin for trachoma-control programs in endemic areas. Since 2013 trachoma has been thought to have been eliminated in eleven countries—Morocco, Oman, Ghana, Iran, China, Nepal, Mexico, Gambia, Myanmar, Laos, and Cambodia—but it remains endemic in forty-five others.[87]

A major effort has been made in the past two years to map nearly 1,500 districts in thirty-four countries to finally define the total population at risk. This doubles the known endemic districts, which contain some 232 million people.[88] At the 2015 GET meeting it was reported that nearly 250,000 trichiasis surgeries had been performed in 2014, 130 million doses of azithromycin committed for distribution in 2016, and nearly half of the previously endemic districts were no longer endemic. With the development of the Neglected Tropical Diseases program, which addresses seventeen tropical diseases, including trachoma, and the global mobilization of resources following the London Declaration, there is optimism that trachoma will be well on the way to being eliminated as a public health problem by 2020.

Diagnosis of Trachoma

Since ancient times diseases of the eye have been diagnosed by simple clinical examinations. It is easy to evert the eyelid, and with hindsight it is possible to see that the features, now codified in the various trachoma classifications, were all described more than two thousand years ago.[89] The system most used now, the WHO simplified grading system, was designed for use by field staff.[90] It was designed so that the signs were well established and clear, so as not to be confused with other conditions. They were meant for public health or population-based work and not necessarily for making individual diagnoses.

They certainly were not designed for use in studies exploring immunopathogenesis or the specificity of lab-based tests. The earlier, more detailed clinical grading systems are much better suited to such studies.[91] In fact, in some settings about half the children with active clinical trachoma may fall below the criterion set for trachomatous inflammation–follicular), the WHO-signified lowest threshold in its grading system.[92] In the early nineteenth century, *ophthalmia* was the term doctors mainly used for the roughening of the inner surface of the eye, some types of which were found to be transferred by the inoculation of ocular discharge from one eye to another, or from an eye to a urethra.[93] As mentioned earlier, at this time there had not been a distinction made between the acute gonococcal and chlamydial infections of either the eye or the genital tract. Clinically, a single ocular infection with chlamydiae causes a self-limited conjunctivitis, now termed *inclusion conjunctivitis*, which is usually less severe than acute gonococcal conjunctivitis. Trachoma was differentiated on clinical grounds with the presence of follicles, scarring, and so forth. Albert Neisser identified the gonococcus *Neisseria gonorrhea* in 1879, but it was many decades before doctors routinely differentiated gonococcal infections and non-gonococcal or nonspecific genital tract infections. In 1884 Albert Neisser and Robert Koch studied trachoma in Egypt and identified the Koch-Weeks bacillus, later renamed *Hemophilus egyptius*. Then Victor Morax identified *Neisserria catarrhalis*, later called *Moraxella catarrhalis*.[94] However, trachoma was thought to be a distinct, viral disease because a specific bacteria could not be identified.[95]

In 1907 Ludwig Halberstaedter and Stanislaus von Prowazek worked with Neisser in Indonesia and identified chlamydiae in trachoma for the first time by identifying the Giemsa-stained intracytoplasmic inclusions.[96] Giemsa cytology has a high specificity but a low sensitivity and so could not demonstrate organisms in every case of clinical trachoma.[97] They followed their discovery with a series of studies in orangutans and reproduced the conjunctival infections and defined the life cycle of chlamydiae. Later that year these findings were confirmed by Charles Nicolle and his colleagues in Tunis as they undertook a range of quite sophisticated studies in monkeys and humans.[98]

The notion that chlamydiae caused these infections was controversial, as the characteristic inclusions were also found in cases clinically diagnosed as ophthalmia neonatorum and gonococcal ophthalmia, and many questioned the specificity of the conclusions. By 1913 the life cycle of chlamydiae was known, although there was still much confusion, as the clinical presentations of the ocular and genital infections caused by chlamydial and gonococcal infection commonly occurred together.[99] The picture began to change in 1909, when doctors were able to differentiate when inclusions were present in patients with ophthalmia neonatorum, inclusion conjunctivitis, or urethritis from those in whom the gonococcus could not be isolated.[100] From then until the 1950s there was much uncertainty about the role of these organisms, which could be seen inside cells but could not be cultured, despite many efforts and blind alleys.[101] Chlamydiae were successfully cultured using chick embryos for the first time from patients with trachoma in 1957 in Beijing.[102]

The ability to culture chlamydiae from the 1950s onward spurred research.[103] Cultured chlamydiae also provided antigens that paved the way for a range of serologic tests, including the detection of specific antibodies against chlamydiae; and enabled the serotyping and the identification of specific serovars.[104] However, the correlation of antibodies in patients' tears and active trachoma was not strong and was less specific than cytology.[105] Nevertheless, serology was widely used for diagnosing genital tract infections, as Giemsa cytology in heavily contaminated specimens was difficult and very time consuming.[106]

Serology testing was largely abandoned with the development of the monoclonal-based, direct immunofluorescent antibody cytology.[107] Immunofluorescent cytology was much more sensitive than Giemsa staining or culture and much easier and quicker than Giemsa cytology. With time this, too, was supplanted in many labs by the direct antigen detection using enzyme immunoassays, which were in turn replaced by nucleic acid amplification tests to identify the unique chlamydial DNA or RNA. PCR (to make multiple copies of a segment of DNA) has now become the standard method for detecting chlamydiae.[108] The PCR tests are highly specific, but they are so sensitive that great care has to be taken to ensure that the specimen is not contaminated. This usually requires double gloving and a meticulous no-touch technique both in specimen collection and in specimen processing. This may not be an insurmountable proposition in an STI clinic, but often it can be a major logistical problem in field studies. The PCR tests are also highly sensitive if infection is present. However, in clinically well-established trachoma, the lab tests are frequently negative, even though the clinical disease is beyond doubt.[109] How can this be the case?

Although there is no doubt that chlamydiae are the cause of trachoma, it is equally clear that the disease itself is an immune response to the chlamydial antigens.[110] In fact, the evidence from extensive animal studies shows that exposure of previously sensitized animals to a purified chlamydial antigen stimulates the clinical disease. The antigen HSP60 stimulates an allergic reaction called delayed-type hypersensitivity reaction (DTH). This reaction causes the appearance of lymphoid follicles and intense inflammation in the surrounding tissues both in the eye and the genital tract, and these cause the observable disease and interference with normal body function.[111] This has been likened to the DTH reaction seen with other antigens, for example, poison ivy, where the mere touching of the skin of a sensitized person with a leaf will stimulate a painful DTH response that will take two to three weeks to resolve, even if the skin is washed right away and the antigen is removed. In a similar way in trachoma the repeated but occasional exposure to chlamydial infection will stimulate and maintain the clinical inflammation and disease even though the actual presence of chlamydiae may be detected only from time to time.[112]

Thus, even in the most severe cases of inflammation in active trachoma, only three-quarters of children will be PCR positive at any given time.[113] With less severe disease or inflammation, this may drop to as low as one-quarter or so and be much less after antibiotic treatment.[114] Given this, the diagnosis of trachoma really depends on the presence of clinical disease and not the result of laboratory testing. With genital tract infection, the diagnosis is made only on the basis of laboratory findings, and so it is highly likely that a large proportion of genuine clinical disease caused by chlamydial infection is actually much higher. The ocular findings, possibly up to four times as many clinical cases, may be present as are detected by the presence of infection (i.e., these are false-negative results from the laboratory, in terms of the disease damage occurring in the patient, but not strictly speaking a false negative in terms of the presence or absence of chlamydiae at the time the assay or swab was taken).

With trachoma the key to the long-term adverse sequelae, the scarring that leads to distortion of the eyelid and the in-turning of the lashes with resultant corneal scarring and blindness are due to the prolonged inflammation sustained by repeated episodes of reinfection. If the transmission of chlamydiae is interrupted and the episodes of reinfection stop, the active inflammation will slowly resolve, leaving whatever structural damage and scarring that may have occurred. All the evidence from animal and clinical studies would suggest that infection and disease in the genital tract follows the same pattern as in the eye.[115] The repeated episodes of reinfection—often asymptomatic and entirely unknown to the victim and possibly even undetected by laboratory testing as well—cause prolonged surface epithelial-cell infection with chlamydiae with replication releasing HSP60, which in turn stimulates and maintains an intense inflammatory response that in turn leads to scarring, tissue distortion, and tubal occlusion.

Given all this, one would expect that chlamydial infection has been with humans since they first evolved. With only occasional or infrequent exposure to infection, little severe tissue damage would be induced. However, with frequent and repeated episodes of infection, the severity of the disease increases. While trachoma has been known and recognized for millennia, chlamydial genital tract infection—and its population prevalence—has come to be gradually recognized as such only in the course of the twentieth century, through a protracted scientific process closely bound up with a series of transformations in clinical practice and laboratory diagnostic technologies, described in full for the first time in chapter 5, in this volume. As the diagnostic tests have become more sensitive and much more widely used, chlamydial genital tract infection has been diagnosed with increasing frequency. In routine screening of sexually active young adults, many of those who are PCR positive are in fact asymptomatic, which further complicates the understanding of the distribution of chlamydial genital tract infection.[116]

Infertility and *C. trachomatis*

C. trachomatis is commonly associated with serious complications such as pelvic inflammatory disease (which leads to infertility), ectopic pregnancy, and tubal infertility.[117] Pelvic inflammatory disease (PID) occurs where *C. trachomatis* ascends from the cervix to the upper genital tract to involve the endometrium, fallopian tubes, and pelvic cavity. Following PID, the risk of tubal infertility has been estimated at around 10 percent in a cohort study of 1,844 women with laparoscopically verified PID.[118]

Sexually transmitted infections tend to cause infertility rather than death.[119] Thus, sexually transmitted pathogens have a better chance of transmission and survival if they coexist with their respective host rather than cause its demise. Keeping the host alive and sexually active increases the chances of transmission, and causing infertility may also be of value to the pathogen, as failure to conceive results in increased mating frequency. Moreover, infections tend to persist, and sexually transmitted pathogens like *C. trachomatis* can enter a persistent state of infection, as clearly demonstrated in vitro; by adopting this approach it is thought that they can evade and subvert the immune response in vivo.[120]

Sexually transmitted infections caused by *C. trachomatis* are characterized by few overt symptoms. While the infection is generally and popularly reported to be in a large percentage of people, the best current estimates are 70–80 percent of infected women and 40–50 percent of men are asymptomatic.[121] Thus genital inspection would not reveal the infection, and the absence of any symptoms will also conceal potential infertility, which otherwise might prevent an individual being selected as a partner. A comprehensive meta-analysis designed to indicate the prevalence and incidence of *C. trachomatis* in the United Kingdom along with its sequelae of PID concluded that the risk of PID in women with an untreated *C. trachomatis* infection is 17.1 percent.[122] PID is a clinical entity, and there is no steadfast or absolute definition; nevertheless, variations in clinical diagnosis were taken into account by the study. It was concluded that for every one thousand contemporary *C. trachomatis* infections in women aged sixteen to forty-four, there were 171 episodes of PID, 2 ectopic pregnancies, and 5.1 women with TFI at age forty four.

Syphilis and gonorrhea have overt symptoms and long-standing diagnostic tests, for example, the Wassermann test for syphilis or culture for gonorrhea, which has allowed evaluation of their role in infertility. By contrast, the absence of reliable tests before the 1990s introduction of commercial nucleic acid amplification tests means there is a paucity of data on the prevalence of *C. trachomatis* in populations before the 1980s. Thus, we can only speculate about the role of infertility due to *C. trachomatis* in these earlier times. Furthermore, there are several significant and complex variables to consider; average age at first birth declined by two and a half years in the United Kingdom from 26.1 years in 1944 to 23.7 years in 1970 and has since increased again to 28.8 years in 2017.[123] The introduction of the oral contraceptive pill in the early 1960s had multiple impacts on social and sexual aspects of women's lives.[124] However, a unique study in Sweden indicated that the frequency of salpingitis (infection and inflammation of the fallopian tubes) closely reflected the prevalence of *N. gonorrhea* and *C. trachomatis* and that ectopic pregnancy could illuminate past patterns of infection, since these sequelae shadow the profile of the primary infections in earlier years. The frequency of salpingitis and ectopic pregnancy may reflect the prevalence of a preceding *C. trachomatis* infection, and, as the high incidence of salpingitis cases decreased in the 1970s, this suggested that the incidence of *C. trachomatis* may have declined since the 1970s.[125]

Emerging Strains of Chlamydiae and New Hypotheses

C. trachomatis is the most commonly reported sexually transmitted infection in the United Kingdom and Europe. The rate of reported cases continues to increase relentlessly despite attempts to impose control programs. Its role in reproductive complications and infertility is well established. *C. trachomatis* is not a single stable entity; the bacterial species is composed of a complex population of different strains, which can evolve through genetic exchange by recombination and mutation. *C. trachomatis* should not be considered a relatively benign infection, even though most cases do not display symptoms and resolve infection naturally. Vigilance is needed, as evidenced by the current ongoing endemic of the so-called LGV "L2b."[126] This causes mainly proctitis among men who have sex with men (MSM), although cases of anorectal infection in women have also been reported. Prior to 2003 LGV was considered a tropical disease, yet the new L2b strain presented predominantly as an anorectal syndrome characterized by severe proctitis in Western MSM.

In 2006 a new strain of *C. trachomatis* also emerged in Sweden, the "Swedish new variant," which is not an LGV strain but a seemingly regular genotype E urogenital isolate. The Swedish new variant carries a mutation within a gene located on its plasmid, which was used for the diagnosis of infection with commercial nucleic acid amplification tests. This mutation or, more accurately, a deletion within the gene targeted for diagnosis—allowed explosive expansion of the strain in the population because the tests in use failed to detect the new variant. It is a classic case of selection by failure to diagnose and treat. Brilliant detective work by Swedish workers Torvald Ripa and Peter Nilsson led to the rapid deployment of new tests, and the Swedish new variant was brought under control.[127] Searching past collections of strains indicated that it was not present before 2003, so it must have arisen in the couple of years before the new variant was identified.[128] It is a good example of how a bottleneck (diagnosis by detection of a plasmid gene) was escaped and how the population of chlamydiae expanded once selection by treatment posttesting was removed. A large-scale longitudinal study has not indicated that the Swedish new variant has an enhanced role in PID.[129] Expansion of the genotype E strains (including the Swedish new variant) has been speculated to occur owing to increased fitness associated with this specific ompA gene (and proximal sequences) preventing recombinations becoming fixed in this part of the genome. Interestingly, while nearly all humans are becoming resistant to antimicrobial treatments, and treatment failure occurs quite frequently, there is no genetic evidence that this is due to antibiotic-resistant strains of *C. trachomatis.*[130]

A study in Australia from 2016 has shed new light on the relationship between trachoma strains and urogenital strains of *C. trachomatis.*[131] The prevailing belief was that chlamydial isolates that cause trachoma are a separate and ancient lineage, but genetic analyses of eye swabs taken from children and their mothers from isolated and remote Aboriginal communities in northern Australia have found that only one or two gene variants are required to change a urogenital-causing strain into a so-called trachoma strain. Since chlamydiae can exchange DNA, this raises the possibility that there is continued potential for new strains of *C. trachomatis* to emerge.

Persistent gastrointestinal infections are prevalent in the animal species; thus, it was speculated that human gastrointestinal infections could act as a reservoir for urogenital infection, especially in women.[132] It has been long established that infants exposed to chlamydiae at birth can asymptomatically shed rectal chlamydiae for years.[133] A hypothesis proposed in 2017 that *C. trachomatis* could be transmitted to the gastrointestinal tract through oral sex.[134] Hence, receptive oral sex in women may contribute to ectopic pregnancy, pelvic inflammatory disease, and tubal factor infertility. This hypothesis is predicated on the assumption that chlamydiae can successfully traverse the hostile acidic environment of the adult stomach while retaining infectivity and then establish a persistent gastrointestinal infection.

The diversity of *C. trachomatis* genomes has allowed new high-resolution methods to be developed that can be used to track and monitor individual strains. These technologies will help in surveillance for new emerging strains and are being used to investigate the distribution of *C. trachomatis* in different populations (heterosexual and MSM) and to examine behavioral factors and social and sexual networks that may give new insights into the role of individual strains of *C. trachomatis* in infertility.

We are now starting to understand the clinical significance of this ancient infection. Exciting and rapid advances in molecular biology are casting light on its origins. We have seen that trachoma is a disease of ocular promiscuity, which starts in young children. They have no capacity to act independently or make their own choices to control infection. Improvements in living standards and hygiene in Western countries, where trachoma was once endemic, have led to its disappearance. By contrast, urogenital infections have soared; here participants, mainly young adults, have agency over exposure and spread of infection. Eliminating trachoma and controlling urogenital chlamydial infections are global public health goals.

Notes

1. William G. Weisburg, Thomas P. Hatch, and Carl R. Woese, "Eubacterial Origin of Chlamydia," *Journal of Bacteriology* 167, no. 2 (1986): 570–74.

2. Michael Ward, "Chlamydial Classification, Development and Structure," *British Medical Bulletin* 39, no. 2 (1983): 109–15.

3. Ludwig Halberstaedter and Stanislaus von Prowazek, "Über zelleinschlüsse parasiätarer natur beim trachom [On cell inclusions of a parasitic nature in trachoma]," *Arbeiten aus dem Kaiserlichen Gesundheitsamke* 26 (1907): 44–47.

4. Richard Stephens, "Chlamydial Evolution: A Billion Years and Counting" (lecture, Tenth International Symposium on Human Chlamydial Infection, Antalya, Turkey, June 16–21, 2002).

5. Ian Clarke, "Evolution of *Chlamydia trachomatis*," *Annals of the New York Academy of Sciences* 1230, no. 1 (2011): E11–E18.

6. Astrid Collingro et al., "Unity in Variety: The Pan-Genome of the Chlamydiae," *Molecular Biology and Evolution* 28, no. 12 (2011): 3253–70; Alexandra Nunes and João Gomes, "Evolution, Phylogeny, and Molecular Epidemiology of Chlamydia," *Infection Genetics and Evolution* 23 (2014): 49–64.

7. Madeline Weiss et al., "The Physiology and Habitat of the Last Universal Common Ancestor," *Nature Microbiology* 1, no. 9 (2016): 16116.

8. Carl Woese, Otto Kandler, and Mark Wheelis, "Towards a Natural System of Organisms: Proposal for the Domains Archaea, Bacteria, and Eucarya," *Proceedings of the National Academy of Sciences of the United States of America* 87, no. 12 (1990): 4576–79.

9. Matthew Dodd et al., "Evidence for Early Life in Earth's Oldest Hydrothermal Vent Precipitates," *Nature* 543, no. 7643 (2017): 60–64.

10. Andrew Knoll et al., "Eukaryotic Organisms in Proterozoic Oceans," *Philosophical Transactions of the Royal Society B: Biological Sciences* 361, no. 1470 (2006): 1023–38.

11. Rudolf Amann et al., "Obligate Intracellular Bacterial Parasites of Acanthamoebae Related to Chlamydia spp.," *Applied and Environmental Microbiology* 63, no. 1 (1997): 115–21.

12. Kenneth Mertens et al., "Living Fossils in the Indo-Pacific Warm Pool: A Refuge for Thermophilic Dinoflagellates during Glaciations," *Geology* 42, no. 6 (2014): 531–34.

13. Amann et al., "Obligate Intracellular Bacterial Parasites."

14. Matthias Horn et al., "Illuminating the Evolutionary History of Chlamydiae," *Science* 304, no. 5671 (2004): 728–30.

15. Richard Stephens et al., "Genome Sequence of an Obligate Intracellular Pathogen of Humans: *Chlamydia trachomatis*," *Science* 282, no. 5389 (1998): 754–59.

16. Jingling Huang and Johann Gogarten, "Did an Ancient Chlamydial Endosymbiosis Facilitate the Establishment of Primary Plastids?," *Genome Biology* 8, no. 6 (2007): R99.

17. Chuan Ku et al., "Endosymbiotic Origin and Differential Loss of Eukaryotic Genes," *Nature* 524, no. 7566 (2015): 427–32.

18. Sudhir Kumar, "Molecular Clocks: Four Decades of Evolution," *Nature Reviews Genetics* 6, no. 8 (2005): 654–62.

19. Alexandra Nunes et al., "*Chlamydia trachomatis* Diversity Viewed as a Tissue-Specific Coevolutionary Arms Race," *Genome Biology* 9, no. 10 (2008): R153; Alexandra Nunes et al., "Adaptive Evolution of the *Chlamydia trachomatis* Dominant Antigen Reveals Distinct Evolutionary Scenarios for B- and T-Cell Epitopes: Worldwide Survey," *PLOS One* 5, no. 10 (2010): e.13171; Naraporn Somboonna et al., "Hypervirulent *Chlamydia trachomatis* Clinical Strain Is a Recombinant between Lymphogranuloma Venereum (L2) and D lineages," *mBio* 2, no. 3 (2011): e00045–11; Simon Harris et al., "Whole-Genome Analysis of Diverse *Chlamydia trachomatis* Strains Identifies Phylogenetic Relationships Masked by Current Clinical Typing," *Nature Genetics* 44, no. 4 (2012): 413–19; Helena Seth-Smith et al., "Co-evolution of Genomes and Plasmids within *Chlamydia trachomatis* and the Emergence in Sweden of a New Variant Strain," *BMC Genomics* 10 (2009): 239; Sandeep Joseph et al., "Population Genomics of *Chlamydia trachomatis*: Insights on Drift, Selection, Recombination, and Population Structure," *Molecular Biology and Evolution* 29, no. 12 (2012): 3933–46.

20. Patrik Bavoil, Bernard Kaltenboeck, and Gilbert Greub, "In Chlamydia Veritas," *Pathogens and Disease* 67, no. 2 (2013): 89–90.

21. Horn et al., "Illuminating the Evolutionary History."

22. Karin Everett, Robin Bush, and Arthur Andersen, "Emended Description of the Order *Chlamydiales*, Proposal of *Parachlamydiaceae* Fam. Nov. and *Simkaniaceae* Fam. Nov., Each Containing One Monotypic Genus, Revised Taxonomy of the Family *Chlamydiaceae*, Including a New Genus and Five New Species, and Standards for the Identification of Organisms," *International Journal of Systematic Bacteriology* 49 (1999): 415–40.

23. J. Schachter et al., "Radical Changes to Chlamydial Taxonomy Are Not Necessary Just Yet," *International Journal of Systematic and Evolutionary Microbiology* 51, no. 1 (2001): 249.

24. Richard Stephens et al., "Divergence without Difference: Phylogenetics and Taxonomy of Chlamydia Resolved," *FEMS Immunology and Medical Microbiology* 55, no. 2 (2009): 115–19.

25. Bernard Kaltenboeck, "Recent Advances in the Knowledge of Animal Chlamydial Infections, in *Chlamydial Infections: Proceedings of the Eleventh International Symposium on Human Chlamydial Infections, Niagara-on-the-Lake, Ontario, Canada, June 18–23, 2006*, ed. Max Chernesky, Harlan Caldwell, and Gunna Christiansen (San Francisco: International Chlamydia Symposium, 2006), 399–408.

26. Kaltenboeck, "Recent Advances," in Chernesky, Caldwell, and Christiansen, *Chlamydial Infections*, 399–408.

27. Tracey Bodetti et al., "Wide Range of Chlamydiales Types Detected in Native Australian Mammals," *Veterinary Microbiology* 96, no. 2 (2003): 177–87.

28. Ben Weigler et al., "Aspects of the Epidemiology of Chlamydia Psittaci Infection in a Population of Koalas (*Phascolarctos Cinereus*) in Southeastern Queensland, Australia," *Journal of Wildlife Diseases* 24, no. 2 (1988): 282–91.

29. Collingro et al., "Unity in Variety."

30. Isao Miyairi, Kyle Ramsey, and Dorothy Patton, "Duration of Untreated Chlamydial Genital Infection and Factors Associated with Clearance: Review of Animal Studies," supplement 2, *Journal of Infectious Diseases* 201 (2010): S96–103.

31. Ward, "Chlamydial Classification."

32. Nicholas Thomson et al., "*Chlamydia trachomatis*: Genome Sequence Analysis of Lymphogranuloma Venereum Isolates," *Genome Research* 18, no. 1 (2008): 161–71.

33. Stephens et al., "Genome Sequence."

34. Richard Stephens, "Genomic Autobiographies of Chlamydiae," chap. 2 in *Chlamydia: Intracellular Biology, Pathogenesis, and Immunity* (Sterling, VA: American Society for Microbiology Press, 1999), 9–27.

35. Emma Iliffe-Lee and Grant McClarty, "Glucose Metabolism in *Chlamydia trachomatis*: The 'Energy Parasite' Hypothesis Revisited," *Molecular Microbiology* 33, no. 1 (1999): 177–87.

36. Nicholas Thomson and Ian Clarke, "*Chlamydia trachomatis*: Small Genome, Big Challenges," *Future Microbiology* 5, no. 4 (2010): 555–61.

37. Robert DeMars et al., "Lateral Gene Transfer in Vitro in the Intracellular Pathogen *Chlamydia trachomatis*," *Journal of Bacteriology* 189, no. 3 (2007): 991–1003.

38. João Gomes et al., "Evolution of *Chlamydia trachomatis* Diversity Occurs by Widespread Interstrain Recombination Involving Hotspots," *Genome Research* 17, no. 1 (2007): 50–60.

39. Roger Rank and Laxmi Yeruva, "'Hidden in Plain Sight': Chlamydial Gastrointestinal Infection and Its Relevance to 'Persistence' in Human Genital Infection," *Infection and Immunity* 82, no. 4 (2014): 1362–71.

40. Seth-Smith et al., "Co-evolution of Genomes."

41. Harris et al., "Whole-Genome Analysis."

42. Harris et al., "Whole-Genome Analysis"; Joke Spaargaren et al., "Slow Epidemic of Lymphogranuloma Venereum L2b Strain," *Emerging Infectious Diseases* 11, no. 11 (2005): 787–88.

43. James Hadfield et al., "Comprehensive Global Genome Dynamics of *Chlamydia trachomatis* Show Ancient Diversification Followed by Contemporary Mixing and Recent Lineage Expansion," *Genome Research* 27, no. 7 (2017): 1220–29.

44. Allan Shaw et al., "Genetic Differences in the *Chlamydia trachomatis* Tryptophan Synthase Alpha-Subunit Can Explain Variations in Serovar Pathogenesis," *Microbes and Infection* 2, no. 6 (2000): 581–92.

45. Christine Fehlner-Gardiner et al., "Molecular Basis Defining Human *Chlamydia trachomatis* Tissue Tropism: A Possible Role for Tryptophan Synthase," *Journal of Biological Chemistry* 277, no. 30 (2002): 26893–903.

46. Harlan Caldwell et al., "Polymorphisms in *Chlamydia trachomatis* Tryptophan Synthase Genes Differentiate between Genital and Ocular Isolates," *Journal of Clinical Investigation* 111, no. 11 (2003): 1757–69.

47. Hadfield et al., "Comprehensive Global Genome Dynamics."

48. Manoj Gambhir et al., "The Development of an Age-Structured Model for Trachoma Transmission Dynamics, Pathogenesis and Control," *PLOS Neglected Tropical Diseases* 3, no. 6 (2009): e462.

49. Dorothy Patton et al., "Distal Tubal Obstruction Induced by Repeated *Chlamydia trachomatis* Salpingitis Infection in Pig-Tailed Macaques," *Journal of Infectious Diseases* 155, no. 6 (1987): 1292–99; A. R. Thurman and D. E. Soper, "Sequelae," in *Pelvic Inflammatory Disease*, ed. Richard Sweet and Harold Weisendfeld (London: Taylor and Francis, 2006), 69–84.

50. Hugh Taylor, *Trachoma: A Blinding Scourge from the Bronze Age to the Twenty-First Century* (Melbourne: Centre for Eye Research Australia, 2008), 1–5.

51. Yaozhen Chen, "Ramble in Chinese Ophthalmology, Past and Present," *Chinese Medical Journal* 94, no. 1 (1981): 1–4.

52. Richard Siebeck, "The Global Distribution of Trachoma 1930–1955," in *World Atlas of Epidemic Diseases*, ed. Ernst Rodenwaldt and Helmut Jusatz (Hamburg: Falk, 1961).

53. Marcia Inhorn Millar and Sandra Lane, "Ethno-Ophthalmology in the Egyptian Delta: An Historical Systems Approach to Ethnomedicine in the Middle East," *Social Science and Medicine* 26, no. 6 (1988): 651–57.

54. Julius Hirschberg, *The History of Ophthalmology*, 11 vols. (Bonn: Wayenborg, 1982–94); Dominic Wajustyk, *The Roots of Ayurveda: Selections from Sanskrit Medical Writings* (London: Penguin Classics 1998).

55. For Pedanius Descorides, 40–90 CE, see Taylor, *Trachoma*, 6; and Lily Beck, *De materia medica*, by Pedanius Dioscorides (Hildesheim, Germany: Olms-Weidmann, 2005), 1.64. I am grateful to Rebecca Flemming for the information that the most extensive surviving discussions of eye diseases in classical medicine come in a range of pseudonymous and encyclopedic texts, which, though it is argued they go back to Demosthenes Philalethes "Ophthalmikos," probably in fact originate from the early or mid-first century CE. Most easily accessible online in English is Paul of Aegina's seventh-century CE summary of all medical knowledge, including at 3.22 on eye diseases (from Galen). Francis Adams, trans., *The Medical Works of Paulus Aeginata*, vol. 1, European Libraries Collection, accessed February 28, 2019. https://archive.org/details/medicalworkspau00paulgoog.

56. Bavoil et al., "In Chlamydia Veritas."

57. Max Meyerhof, "A Short History of Ophthalmia during the Egyptian Campaigns of 1798–1807," *British Journal of Ophthalmology* 16, no. 3 (1932): 129–52.

58. Julius Boldt, *Trachoma* (London: Hodder and Stoughton, 1904).

59. Meyerhof, "Short History of Ophthalmia."

60. Arnold Sorsby and Max Sorsby, *A Short History of Ophthalmology* (London: Staples, 1948).

61. Edward Treacher Collins, *The History and Traditions of the Moorfields Eye Hospital: One Hundred Years of Ophthalmic Discovery and Development* (London: Lewis, 1929).

62. Boldt, *Trachoma.*

63. Taylor, *Trachoma*, 8–15.

64. Treacher Collins, *History and Traditions.*

65. Barrie Jones, "Changing Concepts of Trachoma and Its Control," *Transactions of the Ophthalmological Societies of the United Kingdom* 100, no. 1 (1980): 25–29.

66. Arnold Sorsby, "The Treatment of Trachoma: With Special Reference to Local Sulphonamide Therapy," *British Journal of Ophthalmology* 29, no. 2 (1945): 98–102; Wallace Foulds, pers. comm., Singapore, 2007.

67. Simon Szreter, "Treatment Rates for the Pox in Early Modern England: A Comparative Estimate of the Prevalence of Syphilis in the City of Chester and Its Rural Vicinity in the 1770s," *Continuity and Change* 32, no. 2 (2017): 1–41.

68. Howard Markel, "The Eyes Have It: Trachoma, the Perception of Disease, the United States Public Health Service, and the American Jewish Immigration Experience, 1897–1924," *Bulletin of the History of Medicine* 74, no. 3 (2000): 525–60.

69. John McMullen, "Trachoma: Its Prevalence and Control among Immigrants," *Journal of the American Medical Association* 61 (1913): 1110–13.

70. Harry Gradle, "Trachoma in the United States of America," *Revue internationale du trachome* 16 (1939): 143–48.

71. Shannen Allen and Richard Semba, "The Trachoma 'Menace' in the United States, 1897–1960," *Survey of Ophthalmology* 47, no. 5 (2002): 500–509.

72. Arthur Siniscal, "The Trachoma Story," *Public Health Reports* 70, no. 5 (1955): 497–507.

73. Ronald Friederich, "Eye Disease in the Navajo Indians," *Annals of Ophthalmology* 14, no. 1 (1982): 38–40.

74. Taylor, *Trachoma*, 232–35; National Trachoma Surveillance and Reporting Unit, ed., *Australian Trachoma Surveillance Report 2013*, March 2014, https://kirby.unsw.edu.au/report/australian-trachoma-surveillance-report-2013; Hugh Taylor and Mitchell Anjou, "Trachoma in Australia: An Update," *Clinical and Experimental Ophthalmology* 41, no. 5 (2013): 508–12.

75. World Health Organization, *Summary Report on the 1st Session of the Joint OIHP: WHO Study Group on Trachoma* (Geneva: World Health Organization, 1948).

76. Roger Nataf, *Organization of Control of Trachoma and Associated Infections in Underdeveloped Countries* (Geneva: World Health Organization, 1951), 1–21.

77. André Negrel, "The Winning Hand to Defeat Trachoma," *Revue internationale du trachome* 76e Annee nouvelle serie (1999): 71–125; Kazuichi Konyama,

"History of Trachoma Control in Asia," *Revue internationale du trachome* (2004–5; 1981–82): 107–68; Taylor, *Trachoma*, 17–30.

78. Andrew Solomon et al., "The Global Trachoma Mapping Project: Methodology of a 34-Country Population-Based Study," *Ophthalmic Epidemiology* 22, no. 3 (2015): 214–25.

79. World Health Organization, *Report of the 2nd Global Scientific Meeting on Trachoma* (Geneva: World Health Organization, 2003), 1–27.

80. Serge Resnikoff et al., "Global Data on Visual Impairment in the Year 2002," *Bulletin of the World Health Organization* 82, no. 11 (2004): 844–51; World Health Organization, *2nd Global Scientific Meeting.*

81. Muluken Melese et al., "What More Is There to Learn about Trachoma?," *British Journal of Ophthalmology* 87, no. 5 (2003): 521–22.

82. Allen and Semba, "Trachoma 'Menace'"; Barrie Jones, "The Prevention of Blindness from Trachoma (Bowman Lecture)," *Transactions of the Ophthalmological Societies of the United Kingdom* 95 (1975): 16–33; Taylor, *Trachoma*, 26–31.

83. Nigel Morgan, "Infant Mortality, Flies and Horses in Later-Nineteenth-Century Towns: A Case Study of Preston," *Continuity and Change* 17 (2002): 97–132.

84. Taylor, *Trachoma*, 97–136.

85. "Global Elimination of Blinding Trachoma," World Health Organization, accessed September 11, 2017, www.who.int/blindness/causes/WHA51.11/en/index.html.

86. Victoria Francis and Virginia Turner, *Achieving Community Support for Trachoma Control: A Guide for District Health Work* (Geneva: World Health Organization, 1993), 1–40.

87. World Health Organization, *Report of the 19th Meeting of the WHO Alliance for the Global Elimination of Trachoma by 2020: 28–29 April 2015, Hammamet, Tunisia* (Geneva: World Health Organization, 2016).

88. Solomon et al., "Global Trachoma Mapping Project."

89. Taylor, *Trachoma*, 35–52.

90. Bjorn Thylefors et al., "A Simple System for the Assessment of Trachoma and Its Complications," *Bulletin of the World Health Organization* 64, no. 4 (1987): 477–83. The current WHO grading system for trachoma classifies the disease in 5 grades: trachomatous inflammation–follicular, which requires mostly topical treatment; trachomatous inflammation–intense, during which topical and systemic treatments are considered; trachomatous scarring, when scars are visible, as in tarsal conjunctiva, and which may obscure tarsal blood vessels; trachomatous trichiasis, when an individual is referred for eyelid surgery; and corneal opacity, during which a person is irreversibly blind. See "What Is Trachoma," World Health Organization, accessed August 10, 2017, www.who.int/trachoma/disease/en/.

91. Chandler Dawson, Barrie Jones, and Mario L. Tarizzo, *Guide to Trachoma Control* (Geneva: World Health Organization, 1981).

92. Claude-Edouard Michel et al., "Correlation of Clinical Trachoma and Infection in Aboriginal Communities," *PLOS Neglected Tropical Diseases* 5, no. 3 (2011): e986.

93. Thomas Benedek, "Gonorrhea and the Beginnings of Clinical Research Ethics," *Perspectives in Biology and Medicine* 48, no. 1 (2005): 54–73.

94. John Whitcher and Vicky Cevallos, "Moraxella, Down but Not Out: The Eye Bug That Won't Go Away," *British Journal of Ophthalmology* 90, no. 10 (2006): 1215–16.

95. Boldt, *Trachoma.*

96. Halberstaedter and von Prowazek, "Uber zelleinschusse parasitarer."

97. Julius Schachter and Chandler Dawson, *Human Chlamydial Infections* (Littleton, MA: PSG, 1978).

98. Charles Nicolle, Auguste Cuenod, and Ludovic Blaizot, "Étude experimentale du trachoma," *Archives de L'Institut Pasteur de Tunis* 4 (1913): 157–82.

99. Karl Lindner, "Zur Biologie des Einschlussblennorrhoe (Trachom) Virus," *Archiv für Ophthalmologie* 84 (1913): 1.

100. Karl Lindner, "Zur Trachomforschung," *Zeitschrift fur Augenheilkunde* 22 (1909) 547–50; Phillips Thygeson et al., "Inoculation of Human Volunteer with Egg-Grown Inclusion Conjunctivitis Virus," *American Journal of Ophthalmology* 53, no. 5 (1962): 786–95.

101. Taylor, *Trachoma*, 65–69.

102. Fei-Fan T'ang et al., "Studies on the Etiology of Trachoma with Special Reference to Isolation of the Virus in Chick Embryo," *Chinese Medical Journal* 75, no. 6 (1957): 429–47.

103. These developments are discussed in detail in Michael Worboys, chap. 5, in this volume.

104. World Health Organization, "Fourth WHO Scientific Group on Trachoma Research," in *World Health Organization Technical Report*, series no. 330 (Geneva: World Health Organization, 1966), 24; San-Pin Wang et al., "Serodiagnosis of *Chlamydia trachomatis* Infection with the Micro-Immunofluorescence Test," in *Nongonococcal Urethritis and Related Infections*, ed. Derek Hobson and King K. Holmes (Washington, DC: American Society for Microbiology, 1977), 237–48.

105. Hugh Taylor et al., "The Epidemiology of Infection in Trachoma," *Investigative Ophthalmology and Visual Science* 30, no. 8 (1989): 1823–33.

106. Sohrab Darougar, "The Humoral Immune Response to Chlamydial Infection in Humans," *Reviews of Infectious Diseases* 7, no. 6 (1985): 726–30.

107. Roger Nichols and Dorothy McComb, "Immunofluorescent Studies with Trachoma and Related Antigens," *Journal of Immunology* 89 (1962): 545–54.

108. Julius Schachter, "Diagnosis of *Chlamydia trachomatis* Infection," in *Chlamydial Infections: Proceedings of the Thirteenth International Symposium on Human Chlamydial Infections*, ed. Julius Schachter et al. (San Francisco: International Chlamydia Symposium, 2014), 187–96.

109. Michel et. al., "Correlation of Clinical Trachoma."

110. Taylor, *Trachoma*, 137–65.

111. Hugh Taylor et al., "Pathogenesis of Trachoma: The Stimulus for Inflammation," *Journal of Immunology* 138, no. 9 (1987): 3023–27; Anne Lichtenwalner et al., "Heat Shock Protein 60 Is the Major Antigen Which Stimulates Delayed-Type Hypersensitivity Reaction in the Macaque Model of *Chlamydia trachomatis* Salpingitis," *Infection and Immunity* 72, no. 2 (2004): 1159–61.

112. Taylor, *Trachoma*, 137–65.

113. Michel et. al., "Correlation of Clinical Trachoma"; Jeremy Keenan, Takele Lakew, and Wondu Alemayehu, "Slow Resolution of Clinically Active Trachoma Following Successful Mass Antibiotic Treatments," *Archives of Ophthalmology* 129, no. 4 (2011): 512–26, 512–13; Beatriz Munoz et al., "Can Clinical Signs of Trachoma Be Used after Multiple Rounds of Mass Antibiotic Treatment to Indicate Infection?," *Investigative Ophthalmology and Visual Science* 52, no. 12 (2011): 8806–10.

114. Jeremy Keenan et al., "Diagnostic Characteristics of Tests for Ocular Chlamydia after Mass Azithromycin Distributions," *Investigative Ophthalmology and Visual Science* 53, no. 1 (2012): 235–40.

115. Lichtenwalner et al., "Heat Shock Protein 60"; Roger Rank, M. Melinda Sanders, and Dorothy Patton, "Increased Incidence of Oviduct Pathology in the Guinea Pig after Repeat Vaginal Inoculation with the Chlamydial Agent of Guinea Pig Inclusion Conjunctivitis," *Sexually Transmitted Diseases* 22, no. 1 (1995): 48–54.

116. Anna Yeung et al., "Chlamydia Prevalence in Young Attenders of Rural and Regional Primary Care Services in Australia: A Cross-Sectional Survey," *Medical Journal of Australia* 200, no. 3 (2014): 170–75.

117. Lars Weström and Per-Anders Mårdh, "Chlamydial Salpingitis," *British Medical Bulletin* 39, no. 2 (1983): 145–50.

118. Lars Weström et al., "Pelvic Inflammatory Disease and Fertility. A Cohort Study of 1,844 Women with Laparoscopically Verified Disease and 657 Control Women with Normal Laparoscopic Results," *Sexually Transmitted Diseases* 1992, no. 4 (1992): 185–92.

119. Janis Antonovics et al., "Biology and Evolution of Sexual Transmission," *Annals of the New York Academy of Science* 12301, no. 1 (2011): 12–24; Péter Apari, João Dinis de Sousa, and Viktor Rall Müller, "Why Sexually Transmitted Infections Tend to Cause Infertility: An Evolutionary Hypothesis," *PLOS Pathogens* 10, no. 8 (2014): e1004111.

120. Priscilla Wyrick, "*Chlamydia trachomatis* Persistence in Vitro: An Overview," supplement 2, *Journal of Infectious Diseases* 201, no. 12 (2010): S88–S95.

121. Richard Pattman et al., eds., *Oxford Handbook of Genitourinary Medicine, HIV, and Sexual Health*, 2nd ed. (Oxford: Oxford University Press, 2010), 150.

122. Malcolm Price et al., "The Natural History of *Chlamydia trachomatis* Infection in Women: A Multi-Parameter Evidence Synthesis," *Health Technology Assessment* 20, no. 22 (2016): 1–250.

123. Office for National Statistics, *Births by Parents' Characteristics*, table 4: "Standardised Mean Age of Mother by Birth Order, 1938 to 2017," 2017, accessed February 28, 2019, www.ons.gov.uk/peoplepopulationandcommunity/birthsdeathsandmarriages/livebirths/datasets/birthsbyparentscharacteristics.

124. Louise Tyrer, "Introduction of the Pill and Its Impact," supplement, *Contraception* 59, no. 1 (1999): 11S–16S.

125. Carina Bjartling, Stellan Osser, and Kenneth Persson, "The Frequency of Salpingitis and Ectopic Pregnancy as Epidemiologic Markers of *Chlamydia trachomatis*," *Acta Obstetetricia et Gynecologica Scandinavica* 79 (2009): 123–28.

126. Nynke Hesselina de Vrieze and Henry John de Vries, "Lymphogranuloma Venereum among Men Who Have Sex with Men: An Epidemiological and Clinical Review," *Expert Review of Anti-infective Therapy* 12, no. 6 (2014): 697–704.

127. Torvald Ripa and Peter Nilsson, "A Variant of *Chlamydia trachomatis* with Deletion in Cryptic Plasmid: Implications for Use of PCR Diagnostic Tests," *Eurosurveillance* 11, no. 45 (200): E061109.

128. Margaretha Jurstrand, Hans Fredlund, and Magnus Unemo, "The New Variant of *Chlamydia trachomatis* Was Present as Early as 2003 in Örebro County, Sweden, but Remained Undetected until 2006," *Sexually Transmitted Infections* 89, no. 7 (2013): 607–8.

129. Carina Bjartling et al., "Clinical Manifestations and Epidemiology of the New Genetic Variant of *Chlamydia trachomatis*," *Sexually Transmitted Diseases* 36, no. 9 (2009): 529–35.

130. Hadfield et al., "Comprehensive Global Genome Dynamics."

131. Patiyan Andersson et al., "*Chlamydia trachomatis* from Australian Aboriginal People with Trachoma Are Polyphyletic Composed of Multiple Distinctive Lineages," *Nature Communications* 7 (2016): 10688.

132. Rank and Yeruva, "Hidden in Plain Sight."

133. Julius Schachter et al., "Prospective Study of Perinatal Transmission of *Chlamydia trachomatis*," *JAMA* 255 no. 24 (1986): 3374–77.

134. Patrik M. Bavoil et al., "Does Active Oral Sex Contribute to Female Infertility?," *Journal of Infectious Diseases* 216, no. 8 (2017): 932–35.

Chapter Five

Chlamydia

A Disease without a History

Michael Worboys

Since the late 1990s chlamydia has been the most commonly reported sexually transmitted infection (STI) in Europe and the United States.[1] The infection is caused by the bacterium *Chlamydia trachomatis* (*C. trachomatis*), and its common name follows a pattern established in the late nineteenth century, where an infection is named after its causal pathogen.[2] In England in 2017 there were just over 203,116 new diagnoses, compared to 7,137 of syphilis and 44,676 of gonorrhea.[3] Over 126,000 of the chlamydia diagnoses were made by the National Chlamydia Screening Programme, which targets fifteen to twenty-four-year-olds because the disease, which is asymptomatic in 80 percent of females infected, can lead to infertility due to blocked fallopian tubes. The disease has been equally prevalent in men, and while there has been an expectation of similar effects on seminal vesicles, there is as yet no evidence of a strong correlation between infection and male infertility.[4] The program began in 2004, after a decade in which the reported incidence of chlamydia grew rapidly, and journalists picked up on these reports warnings of a "fertility timebomb."[5] Public health concern about the disease also derived from its seeming novelty and to uncertainties over its pathology. Chlamydia first became recognized as a specific STI in the 1970s, but it took until 1988 for it to become notifiable. Newly diagnosed cases were reported only routinely in STI statistics from 1990, when there were 34,000 new diagnoses. The number began to rise steeply after 1995, reaching 100,000 in 2003. The growing incidence seemed to public health officials to be both "true" and "questionable." The increase seemed to be true because of the increase in the number of couples seeking fertility treatment, plus the pattern of chlamydia's spread seemed to fit with a view that young people were having a greater number of sexual partners.[6] Yet it was also considered questionable because advances in treatments for infertility, notably in vitro fertilization, led to increased demand for services; also more and more cases of chlamydia were identified by improvements in the sensitivity and specificity of testing methods.

Chlamydia as an STI is a disease without a history in two senses: first, it became a clinical entity only in the 1970s, and, second, its medical and social history has still to be written—an absence this chapter begins to correct.[7] Its seeming novelty in the 1970s prompts the question, Was it an infection newly arrived in humans, or had it always been present and was now being recognized for the first time?[8] This is a question that can only be answered, not by a medical historian but by investigations of past populations by epidemiologists, pathologists, and, perhaps most likely, by archaeologists using genomics. However, medical publications and oral testimony reveal that doctors in the 1970s were confident that chlamydia was not a new disease. They believed this new ailment had actually been around for decades and probably centuries, being one, probably the most important, of the infections that had been hidden in that most unsatisfactory disease entity nongonococcal urethritis (NGU), also called nonspecific urethritis (NSU). NGU was defined by what it was not. It required a laboratory diagnosis and had been invented by clinicians when, in patients with gonorrhea-like symptoms, the gonococcus could not be found in genital discharges. NGU was unaffected by antibiotics used to treat gonorrhea, which became further negative diagnostic confirmation. The laboratory was also crucial to the creation of chlamydia as a clinical entity, which came from the development of new techniques in the 1960s and 1970s, which enabled doctors to differentiate NGU into component infections: *C. trachomatis*, lymphogranuloma venereum (LGV, which was later shown to be caused by different strains of *C. trachomatis* from those causing chlamydia), *Mycoplasma genitalium*, and trichomoniasis (caused by the protozoan *Trichomonas vaginalis*).[9]

While there is little or no historical scholarship on chlamydia as an STI, there are some studies of the bacterium's other pathological effects, the eye infection trachoma, caused by the same bacterium; and psittacosis, a type of pneumonia caused by *Chlamydia psittaci*, which bird fanciers catch from infected animals.[10] Trachoma is the leading cause of infectious blindness in the world and now the subject of control efforts by several agencies.[11] There are short histories of NGU, written by STI specialists, which discuss chlamydia along with the other diseases into which the entity has now been broken down; however, these tend to be presentist and teleological, portraying this differentiation as inevitable.[12] The great challenge for historians writing the history of any disease, but especially one that is newly identified, is captured in Charles Rosenberg's provocative claim that "a disease does not exist until we have agreed that it does, by perceiving, naming, and responding to it."[13] Or, as Peter Sedgwick put it, "There are no illnesses or diseases in nature"; rather, illnesses and diseases are the labels and action humans construct about the experiences, meanings, and implications of natural phenomena.[14] Rosenberg qualifies the radical relativist implications of his statement by prefacing it with "in some ways" and applies it only to disease as a "social phenomenon." His realist stance is clear in his view that disease is also a "biological event little modified by the particular context in which it occurs."[15] In this chapter I chart how the social and the biological were brought together by different historical actors to coproduce both NGU and chlamydia. For example, one distinctive feature of the biology of chlamydia—that it is largely symptomless in women—shaped social responses and clinical interventions, and these altered the epidemiology and perhaps the pathology of the infection. Indeed, STIs doctors since the 1990s have debated whether early antibiotic treatment has actually worsened the problem, leading to "arrested" immune responses and persistent vulnerability to infection.[16]

In this chapter I follow the more radical version of Rosenberg's approach, with a narrative that details how chlamydia as a disease entity was *constructed* rather than *discovered*. I show how it was coproduced in the interactions of microbes, patients, doctors, scientists, public health agencies, and other actors, in the context of changing laboratory technologies, attitudes toward STIs and infertility, and health policies. My focus is on Britain, but the story was similar in other industrialized countries and increasingly internationally owing to shared research and comparisons of national policies. I begin with the construction of another clinical entity, nongonococcal urethritis, in the 1930s, which, as the name indicates, was closely linked to medical and social ideas, practices, and policies for gonorrhea. A key difference was that NGU was framed as a condition that affected only men and, unlike gonorrhea, was not associated with ill health and sterility in women.[17] NGU was unusual in being defined by what it was not and, for the time, in having its positive diagnosis dependent on laboratory testing.

I next consider medical and social responses to the growing incidence of NGU in men, from 1951, when new cases were first reported, to the early 1970s. In Britain gonorrhea lost its status as the most prevalent venereal disease to NGU in 1975, prompting new interest in the latter. The incidence of chlamydia in women had been first reported in 1971 and soon became linked to infertility, pelvic inflammatory disease (PID), and chronic ill health. The manner in which chlamydia, as a component of NGU, changed from a one- to two-sex disease echoed how the pathology of gonorrhea was remade in the early twentieth century.[18] My focus in this chapter is on the disease in women, but from the mid-1990s doctors reported that chlamydia could lead to infertility in men, albeit at a lower rate, by damaging sperm and causing epididymitis (and this has not since been confirmed).[19] Finally, I discuss the changing profile of chlamydia from the mid-1970s to the 2010s, the key feature of which was the public health focus on the infection in women, reversing the previous situation. Its incidence in women became a major public health concern, and STI specialists and gynecologists began to talk about its role in creating an infertility crisis. The arrival of HIV/AIDS pushed these concerns aside until the late 1990s, when they were pushed to the fore again and once more linked to fertility and PID. Since then a number of initiatives have been developed to determine the level of incidence in young women, the most vulnerable group, and develop preventive and therapeutic policies and programs.

Gonorrhea and Nongonococcal Urethritis, 1900–1945

Until the late nineteenth and early twentieth century, gonorrhea was a disease understood to affect mainly men. It was a specific type of urethritis, with a characteristic discharge from the penis and inflammation of the genitourinary system caused by the bacterium *Neisseria gonorrhoeae*. The infection typically "cleared up" in three or four weeks, though in many cases there were long-term effects, the most common being inflammation of the joints. Gonorrhea was thought to be less common and less serious in women. However, doctors were clear that women could harbor the gonococcus without symptoms, from the number of babies whose eyes were infected at birth and developed ophthalmia neonatorum, then a major cause of blindness.[20] Some estimates are that a third of all blindness in the nineteenth-century era was due to this infection, a proportion that fell from the 1890s, when it became more common but by no means universal to irrigate the eyes of newborn babies with dilute silver nitrate.[21] The medical and social recognition that gonorrhea could be serious in women came from work of gynecologists and pathologists from the 1890s and the campaigning of public health doctors and women's groups in the first decades of the twentieth century, with no one more active than Christabel Pankhurst. She set out her claims in *The Great Scourge and How to End It*, published in 1913, which is now best known for its seeming invitation for suffragists to start a "Sex War," but it also had a lot to say about women's health.[22] The "Great Scourge" was venereal disease, but, unusually for the time, Pankhurst gave more space to gonorrhea than syphilis and special attention in a chapter on "The Dangers of Marriage." She maintained that male doctors had concentrated on syphilis, the disease that affected mostly their sex, neglecting gonorrhea, the most serious venereal disease in women. Indeed, she stressed that men escaped lightly from gonorrhea with a short-lived, local infection, while women suffered long-term complications, children were threatened by blindness, and the race weakened by a falling birthrate, due to chronic ill health that led to women having fewer or no children.[23] The principal consequence was salpingitis: "an attack of acute suppurating pelvic peritonitis with a background of genital symptoms due to acute suppuration of one or both Fallopian tubes."[24] In newly married women gynecologists termed it "honeymoon appendicitis," but for those with the condition its consequences could be anything but short-term, with lifelong chronic ill health common. As Anne Hanley has shown, many doctors linked venereal diseases with infertility, but there was no consensus on their importance or what to do.[25] The aim of treatments, when tried, was to prevent the spread of the infection to the abdominal cavity (what would now be termed PID) and restore function to the fallopian tubes where possible, which often required surgery.

Contemporary medical opinion was that Pankhurst had exaggerated the incidence of gonorrhea, but that "the serious nature of the *sequelae* . . . is not exaggerated, and it is probably true that they are, on the whole, more serious in women than in men."[26] In the evidence given to the Royal Commission of Venereal Disease, doctors agreed that gonorrhea was responsible for around a third of all sterility, affecting both men and women. Similar estimates of the impact of gonorrhea could be found in the other industrialized countries.[27] In his book on *Gonorrhea in Women*, published in 1913, the US gynecologist Charles Norris reported "that 30 per cent, to 50 per cent, of all childless marriages are directly caused by gonorrhoea."[28] Interestingly, some doctors suggested that the by then relative rarity of ophthalmia neonatorum in obstetric practice was as much due to (increased) female sterility produced by gonorrhea as much as it was to disinfection of babies' eyes.[29] Through the 1920s and 1930s medical views on infection and sterility divided on gender lines: the condition in men was linked primarily to epididymitis caused by gonorrhea, while in women it was associated with infection of the cervix, salpingitis, and pelvic inflammation, as well as puerperal sepsis.[30] In fact, the gonococcus was not the only pathogen associated with sterility: staphylococci, streptococci, the tubercle bacillus, and as yet unspecified microorganisms such as viruses (first identified in this period) were also all implicated. In 1937 Maeve Kenny, who worked at Queen Charlotte's Maternity Hospital, Hammersmith, published an article on the aftereffects of puerperal infection.[31] Her study was of a hundred women treated in the isolation block of Queen Charlotte's, and her principal finding was "that sterility is a prominent sequel to puerperal infection," though she could only speculate on how the disease affected women's reproductive organs and fertility.

Kenny had pioneered, with Leonard Colebrook, the introduction of sulfonamide drugs, which were transforming the prognosis of women with puerperal sepsis and impacting maternal mortality.[32] Sulfonamides also transformed the treatment of gonorrhea.[33] The sex of the patients in the early trials is rarely mentioned, but the implication is that they were principally men, as success was judged by the absence of clinical symptoms.[34] The improvement in the treatment of gonorrhea, along with the prognoses for patients with syphilis, due to Salvarsan and its derivatives, meant that at the end of the 1930s doctors were more and more challenged by patients with chronic, nonspecific venereal disease and its effects. In a letter to the *Lancet* in September 1937, A. Malcolm Simpson argued, "It seems obvious that the syphilis department of a V.D. clinic should be divorced from the gonorrhoeal one; the director of the former having special experience in dermatology, cardiology, and neurology, and that of the latter in genito-urinary surgery and gynaecology."[35]

The particular success of sulfonamides in the treatment of gonorrhea revealed the number of patients at venereal disease clinics who had "genito-urinary (non-gonococcal) infections."[36] Arthur Harkness, a South African who had qualified at Guy's Hospital in 1914 and then served in the Royal Navy Reserve, had labeled this a disease entity in 1933.[37] Harkness's NGU diagnosis depended on negative bacteriological results from patients with the symptoms of gonorrhea, a group that sulfonamide treatment further differentiated.[38] Apparently, Harkness found NGU only in men, with women mentioned only as sources of male infection; indeed, its sex specificity was another marker of NGU's distinctiveness from gonorrhea.[39]

The first published exploration of a link between NGU and trachoma was in 1939, in a review by Lawrence Harrison, Britain's leading venereologist; and Werner Worms, a German émigré doctor.[40] Their focus was on "Waelsch urethritis," a type of urethritis first identified in 1901, and on the presence of so-called inclusion bodies in a number of inflammatory venereal conditions: trachoma, inclusion blennorrhoea, various types of conjunctivitis, LGV, and NGU. Trachoma had attracted the attention of ophthalmologists in the 1920s, with the International Organization against Trachoma founded in 1930.[41] The agency was created around two appeals: first, the prevention of blindness in infants and, second, halting its spread from the tropics; indeed, trachoma had been made a notifiable disease in Glasgow in 1914 because of fears of its importation.[42] At its meeting in 1935, the organization's president maintained that its work "may deservedly be placed among the campaigns against cancer and tuberculosis."[43] There was agreement among ophthalmologists that trachoma was infectious and was associated with intracellular or inclusion bodies that had been first observed in 1907 by Ludwig Halberstaedter and Stanilaus von Prowazek. These became known as TRIC agents (from *tr*achoma *i*nclusion *c*onjunctivitis), and their presence within cells (intracellular) led many bacteriologists to place them in the new category of viruses; but there were other possibilities: phagocytosed gonococci or rickettsia—intracellular bacterial pathogens.[44] Around 1930 similar inclusion bodies were reported in cases of psittacosis, a disease of birds that had spread to humans in sporadic outbreaks in the 1920s and early 1930s.[45]

In the 1940s textbooks on venereal diseases began to include a chapter on "Other Conditions." Angus McLachlan's *Handbook of Diagnosis and Treatment of Venereal Diseases*, published in 1944, discussed eight such diseases: balanoposthitis, LGV, NGU, thrush, trichomoniasis, ulcus actum vulvae, vaginitis, vulvovaginitis, and warts. He wrote that the most puzzling was NGU, which he also termed "simple urethritis" and "post-gonococcal urethritis" (PGU).[46] Clinicians suggested three causes; typically, each was morally loaded: (1) septic and opportunistic bacterial infection, linked to sodomy or intercourse during menstruation; (2) chemical irritation due to the use of contraceptives; and (3) physical trauma caused by sexual excess.[47] The idea that women were carriers and the primary source of the infection was implied in 1942 by Gerald McElligott, a Royal Air Force medical officer, when he wrote, after a survey of men, that "I have not recently had the opportunity of examining many female consorts." Nonetheless, he suggested that infection from women was likely to be facilitated by previous venereal infection; unclean and careless methods of douching; the growing use of internal menstrual tampons; and previous instrumental interference with the cervix, in other words, induced abortion.[48]

NGU Established, 1945–1975

Investigations of NGU had flourished during World War II because of the attention given to venereal diseases in the armed services and the success of sulfonamides and then penicillin in treating gonorrhea.[49] In January 1948 the first report of the newly formed World Health Organization's Expert Committee on Venereal Diseases drew attention to a number of genitourinary infections of "ill-defined origin," including NGU, and called for more studies of them.[50] The findings were based mostly on evidence submitted by Harkness, which showed that NGU was common worldwide. Two years later Harkness published a book titled *Non-gonococcal Urethritis*, which reviewed the literature on all manner of genitourinary conditions and concluded that NGU was a specific condition, though one for which he was unable to specify a microbial cause or diagnostic test.[51] He mentioned *C. trachomatis* as a possible factor, though he was unclear whether it was a primary cause, secondary consequence, or coincidental contaminant. Harkness's work was largely behind the inclusion of NGU in British statistics of new cases of venereal disease from 1951.[52]

In 1954 Harkness and Claude Nicol, the author of a standard textbook on venereal diseases, spoke on NGU at a joint meeting of the Medical Society for the Study of Venereal Diseases and of the Metropolitan Branch, Society of Medical Officers of Health.[53] The discussion after their talk revealed that doctors remained dissatisfied with accounts of NGU's causation but agreed that bacteria were likely the primary or secondary pathogens, given that the new mycin-based antibiotics cured nearly 90 percent of cases. However, a review in the *British Journal of Venereal Diseases* the following year identified four infective candidates as the cause of NGU—bacteria, viruses (which would have included TRIC agents), pleuropneumonia-like organisms (PPLO), and trichomonads—or that it was non-infective and a primary prostate disorder. They concluded that "infection is the probable cause but has not been proved for the majority of cases." The authors also discussed diagnosis and treatment, typically constructing NGU by exclusion: "(1) Whereas gonorrhoea is promptly cured by penicillin, leaving a negligible number of relapses, the position is different with [NGU,] where treatment is less specific, and relapses are common. . . . (2) The diagnosis of gonorrhoea in the male is straightforward, but that of [NGU] depends on negative properties and is thus less easily definable."[54] Despite the uncertainties and the variety of terms and categories, figures for the reported incidence of NGU continued to be published in annual venereal disease statistics.

When the disease was first reported in 1951, there were 10,764 cases in men; unsurprisingly, no numbers for women were given.[55] That year there were 14,975 new cases of gonorrhea in men and 3,089 in women. The gonorrhea figures for women were known to be underestimates for two reasons: clinics tended to test only the contacts of infected men, and the infection was known to be often symptomless in women. Diagnosis of NGU still followed the two negatives: the absence of gonococci and non-responsiveness to penicillin. An investigation into the aetiology, published in 1954, which considered just men, did mention women as "consorts" but admitted defeat in identifying any specific "virus" for NGU. However, immunological tests suggested that links with LGV, psittacosis, and cat-scratch fever merited further attention.[56] In about three-quarters of cases, NGU responded to treatment with antibiotics such as chloramphenicol, aureomycin, terramycin, and erythromycin.[57] The reported incidence of new cases of NGU in men rose steadily through the 1950s, such that in 1961 there were 24,472 new cases, against 29,519 of gonorrhea.[58]

In a lecture on "Venereal Disease and Public Health" in 1960, McElligott, who had risen to be adviser in venereal diseases to the Ministry of Health, reflected on the new epidemiological picture of venereal diseases: "Today gonorrhoea and, indeed, early syphilis, promptly and properly treated . . . still have a cure rate of not much less than 100%. Our therapeutic problems now for the most part comprise relapsing NGU in men with its occasional complications, and trichomoniasis in women patients, the latter condition being increasingly sent on to us by our gynaecological colleagues."[59]

He worried too about social attitudes to NGU because, "not being a statutory venereal disease," it had been "neglected by the public and the medical profession alike, and is often regarded as a respectable complaint rather than a dirty disease with disgraceful implications."[60] The incidence of new cases of NGU exceeded those for gonorrhea for the first time in 1965, and this spurred greater interest into the condition among venereologists. Ideas on causation were fixed firmly on microorganisms.

In the 1964 edition of their textbook on venereal diseases, Ambrose King and Claude Nicol noted several possibilities: TRIC agents; mycoplasma, or bacteria without cell walls, like those that caused pleuropneumonia (termed pleuropneumonia-like organisms or PPLOs); *Trichomonas vaginalis*; fungi; and a Haemophilus influenza organism.[61] The idea that NGU was an allergic reaction of some type was also mentioned. However, the predominant view was that it was an infection, and the possibility of a link between trachoma and NGU was behind work undertaken by Eric Dunlop, with the Oculogenital Virus group at the Institute of Ophthalmology at Moorfields

Eye Hospital.[62] Nonetheless, the nature of the microorganism remained uncertain, as was only too clear in an article on NGU in the *Lancet* in 1965, in which the authors stated they had been studying "a member of the *Bedsonia* or psittacosis/lymphogranuloma/TRIC group."[63] Bedsonia is now often regarded as an obsolete term for the *Chlamydia* group of microorganisms.[64] The review concluded with suggestions of new names for NGUs in men and, seemingly for the first time, in women: "TRIC agent urethritis" and "TRIC agent cervicitis."[65]

It was not until 1971 that the number of new cases of NGU in women was reported in the annual reports of the chief medical officer in Britain. It had been previously discussed in clinical publications but had not been officially recorded because it was "not a clear-cut clinical entity."[66] However, cases had been included in "other conditions" requiring treatment within the [VD] center, in which now remained LGV, trichomoniasis, candidiasis, scabies, pubic lice, genital herpes, genital warts, genital molluscum and other treponomal diseases.[67] The exclusion of chlamydia from the list of "other sexually transmitted diseases" indicated that doctors had decided that it belonged with NGU.

The figures for 1971 were 14,418 new NGU cases in women compared to 62,498 in men, with population rates of 56.54 per 100,000 in women and 263.55 in men. The report observed,

> Research on the causative agent or agents in this group continues to be supported by the DHSS and MRC. It is encouraging that at least four centres are now investigating the role of *Chlamydia* group A organisms in this condition. However, it is still reasonable to suspect that other infective agents are implicated and the possibility that there may be pathogenic strains of mycoplasma cannot be discarded; their isolation in the upper genital tract in women with pelvic complications has been reported from Sweden. The diagnosis of infection in female sex contacts remains a difficult problem, but their diagnosis and treatment seems indicated when there is evidence of inflammatory changes in the genito-urinary tract.[68]

There was discussion of the "epidemiological" or "blind" treatment of "consorts"—that is, giving antibiotics to asymptomatic women contacts of male sufferers with the aim of preventing the reinfection of men and, secondarily, treating women. This indicated that women were still seen as vectors rather than sufferers of NGU. The women's health movement of the 1960s was dependent on established, mostly male, STD specialists and initially focused on the "venereal diseases" of syphilis and gonorrhea.[69] However, this changed in the 1970s; for example, the 1973 edition of *Our*

Bodies, Ourselves included information on "other non-categorized sexually transmitted diseases," but it was not until the 1980s that discussion of the triad of chlamydia, PID, and infertility was added.[70]

Chlamydia: In Fashion Again?

In 1974 a review article in the *Lancet* on chlamydia began with the statement: "The *Chlamydia* genus is in fashion again."[71] The previous occasion alluded to was work on trachoma, but the new attention was because of evidence of its role in genital infection and PID. The article was prompted by the investigations that were finding a "considerable proportion [up to 45 percent] of 'non-specific' genital infection is due to *Chlamydia*."[72] There was similar evidence from the United States, where a study of 113 men with NGU showed 42 tested positive for *C. trachomatis* and commented that "the cause of chlamydia-negative NGU . . . remains obscure."[73] The reference to "'non-specific' genital infection" reflected a shift in terminology as NGU was replaced by NSGI or the more common NSU, which I use from now on. In Britain the key researcher was Eric Dunlop, who is now remembered as "the person who first put chlamydial genital infection in the medical and general public domain"; this was work published in 1972.[74] He was an ophthalmologist, and his suggestion that *C. trachomatis* was a cause of pelvic inflammatory disease came from observations of the number of mothers, whose babies had chlamydial ophthalmia neonatorum, suffered from salpingitis.[75]

In the 1975 edition of their textbook, King and Nicol still listed seven possible causal agents of NSU but were confident that "*Chlamydia*-subgroup A is, at any rate, one cause of non-specific urethritis."[76] In the same year a study based on patients at Guy's Hospital in London concluded that only 20 percent were "truly non-specific"; the remainder broke down as follows: chlamydia, 40 percent; mycoplasma, 20 percent; trichomoniasis, 15 percent; and candidiasis, 5 percent.[77] The diversity of diseases making up NSU remained a challenge and, according to Robbie Morton, a venereologist based in Sheffield, "In spite of much laboratory and other research, nonspecific genital infection continues to be the venereologist's most perplexing problem, clinically, diagnostically and therapeutically."[78] In 1978, Michael Adler, then at the Middlesex Hospital and following a review of the diagnosis and reporting of NSU, wrote, "It is extremely unsatisfactory that when the disease is discussed, described, diagnosed, and notified no accepted criteria are in existence" and "The commonest diagnosis made in STD clinics [is] the one with the least uniformity."[79] The difficulties in diagnosis were acknowledged in the reports of the chief medical officer, where it was noted that "in the absence of specific diagnostic tests outside the research field, therapy remains empirical and the possibilities of control are therefore less than in other sexually transmitted diseases."[80]

The tests in the "research field" first used cultures grown in hen's eggs and then less cumbersome techniques with McCoy cells.[81] Laboratory diagnostic tests began by measuring anti-*Chlamydial* antibodies using serological methods.[82] At this time there were well established and relatively inexpensive tests for the main STDs: serology with the Wassermann reaction for syphilis and culturing and microscopy for gonorrhea. *Chlamydiae*, like viruses, live inside cells not in the intracellular matrix; hence, their manipulation in the laboratory required the same techniques and materials as those for viruses. Relative to the new methods, cell culturing was technically demanding, time consuming, expensive, and difficult to standardize. It was beyond the capacity of most public health and clinical microbiology laboratories. Adler's survey of diagnostic methods being used in the late 1970s revealed that most clinicians were using microscopy to examine urethral exudates, which were stained and then examined for polynucleated leukocytes—a nonspecific test where the presence of this type of white blood cell is taken as an indicator of an infection.[83] Such deficiencies led to calls for the development of better testing and the creation of a cell culture service to enable accurate diagnosis of the most common STD.[84] In Britain the new diagnostic techniques and new interest in chlamydia led to studies of women attending STD clinics and an association with promiscuity.[85] A study in Manchester, published in 1977, used the new methods and found *Chlamydia* organisms in 26 percent of the "promiscuous women" attending the Special Clinic and 1 percent among the control "non-promiscuous group"; the latter was in fact "two hundred female members of hospital staff." The authors were still cautious about the status of chlamydia as a cause of STDs but worried that "in this investigation, *Chlamydia* were isolated from 20% of asymptomatic females, indicating the possibility of a considerable potential reservoir of infection."[86] Why was this concerning? Principally, concerns were growing about the link between STDs and infertility, as seen in an editorial in the *British Medical Journal* in 1975, titled "Promiscuity and Infertility," which focused on tubal inflammation caused by gonorrhea.[87]

Two wider changes in STDs in the late 1970s and early 1980s impacted the emergence of chlamydia as an important public health problem: HIV/AIDS and the medicalization of infertility. I will not go into these in any detail, as there is a large, now historical, literature on each, though, interestingly, chlamydia is rarely mentioned, if at all.[88] First and most important was HIV/AIDS, which radically altered the profile of STDs in medicine and wider society, and the "safe sex" message led to a reported decline in new cases of chlamydia infection in women.[89] One consequence was that STD services expanded and were better funded, with greater investment in diagnostic services and expertise in viral diseases. Closely related, there was the creation of the new specialism of genitourinary medicine.[90] GUM clinics replaced the still stigmatized venereal diseases or STD departments and tried to normalize STDs by dealing with them alongside other diseases of the reproductive and excretory systems. Second, there was the medicalization of infertility and the development of in vitro fertilization.[91] Among many new approaches, doctors sought ways to correct or circumvent blocked fallopian tubes, which in turn drew attention to the possibilities of prevention, through the early recognition of the factors causing salpingitis and other infections of cervix, uterus, and abdomen.

Infection and Infertility

In the late 1970s medical attention on infection and infertility was focused on intrauterine contraceptive devices as major causes of ectopic pregnancies, salpingitis, and PID.[92] Pelvic inflammation in women had been recognized since the late nineteenth century, but PID as a clinical entity was constructed in the 1960s, first in relation to septic infection and then to STDs. These links were central to the controversy over the Dalkon Shield, an intrauterine contraceptive device associated with a high incidence of internal injuries and infections in its users and perhaps infertility.[93] The leading work on the link between infection and infertility focused on salpingitis—inflammation and obstruction of the fallopian tubes. The leading researchers were in departments of obstetrics and gynecology, such as Lars Weström at the University Hospital in Lund, Sweden, and with the WHO Collaborating Centre for Reference and Research on Trachoma and Other Chlamydial Infections. As early as 1975, they reported a study of 415 women followed over nine and half years: "Tubal occlusion was diagnosed after one infection in 12.8 per cent, after two infections in 35.5 per cent, and after three or more infections in 75 per cent of the women. Tubal occlusion was more common after non-gonorrheal than after gonorrhoeal salpingitis."[94] In 1980 Weström reported on the long-term effects of PID and recent changes: "The prevalence of women in the post-PID state has increased by a factor of about 1.5 since 1960. Women in the post-PID state have a tenfold increased risk for ectopic pregnancy and 25% of the increase in ectopic pregnancy can be accounted for by the increase in post-PID women." The overall picture was alarming: "Infertility after PID ranges between 5.8% and 60% depending on severity of infection, number of infections, and age of the woman. The fraction of women rendered infertile because of PID has increased by a factor of about 1.6 since 1960."[95]

An indication of the new medical importance being given to PID was a meeting in April 1980 of an International Symposium at the Centers for Disease Control in Atlanta solely on the condition.[96] James Curran of CDC explained the problem:

> Pelvic inflammatory disease is the most common serious complication of sexually transmitted infections caused by *Neisseria gonorrhoeae* and *Chlamydia trachomatis*. If PID and ectopic pregnancy rates continue unabated, by the year 2000 there will have been more than one episode of PID and three related physician visits for every two women who reached reproductive age in 1970. Fifteen per cent will require hospitalization, more than 3% will experience an ectopic pregnancy, and more than 10% will involuntarily become sterile because of PID.[97]

Michael Adler, E. H. Belsey, and B. H. O'Connor, from a more limited study than Weström, drew less alarmist conclusions. They focused on gonorrhea and the overall morbidity rather than infertility. However, they noted that the incidence of PID in England and Wales had risen "only" 50 percent between 1968 and 1977, and this would have impacted fertility.[98] A direct linkage between chlamydia, PID, and infertility was first aired by Duncan Catterall in an article in the *Lancet* in February 1981 titled "Biological Effects of Sexual Freedom":

> The radical changes in attitudes to sex and in sexual behaviour during the past 25 years have resulted in a sustained increase in the incidence of STD. Research has led to the recognition of a new generation of STDs many of which cause pelvic inflammatory disease and sterility. Inability to become pregnant usually, leads to frustration and unhappiness, and treatment is often unsuccessful. The new generation of STDs has serious and potentially dangerous effects on expectant mothers and their babies. Damage to the developing tissues can occur in the uterus, infection may be transmitted at birth, or the infant may develop disease during the first few months of life. Their effects on prematurity, birth weight, early rupture of the membranes, and failure to thrive are only just being investigated, and there may be some surprises. The adverse biological effects of sexual freedom on women and their babies are a disappointing development in the second half of the 20th century.[99]

Catterall expected that chlamydia, rather than gonorrhea, as previously thought, was the major cause of PID and ectopic pregnancies.[100] He worried further that the true level of the chlamydia infection and that of other "new" pathogens was unknown, because, "unfortunately, laboratory facilities are totally inadequate and thousands of cases are unrecognised."[101] However, he was concerned there was a major problem of fertility decline in the making.

In their large volume on *Disease and Fertility* (1984), Joseph McFalls and Marguerite McFalls, had separate chapters for NGU and "genital chlamydia" and for the latter detailed experimental and clinical evidence of salpingitis due to chlamydia-impairing conception.[102] A research study published in 1984, using the new method of measuring antibodies rather than cell culture, also found strong indications of *C. trachomatis* infection in 75 percent of women with damaged fallopian tubes, compared with 31 percent of seventy-five infertile women with normal fallopian tubes.[103] High-antibody levels were found in 15 percent of fertile women. The authors concluded that tests for the microorganism "should routinely be part of infertility investigations."[104] There was support from the new GUM specialists about the scale of the problem, evidenced by the increasing number of ectopic pregnancies, and for wider testing.[105] In the same year a review in the *Journal of Obstetrics and Gynaecology* on "*Chlamydia trachomatis* infections and their importance to the gynaecologist" ended by warning of the "tragic sequelae," citing projections from the United States:

> By the year 2000, two out of every three women who had reached reproductive age in 1970 will have had one bout of pelvic inflammatory disease and as a result visited their doctors or sexually transmitted disease clinics three times. Fifteen per cent of this group will have been hospitalised for treatment of pelvic inflammatory disease and of these, one-half will require surgery. Curran (1980) estimates that if one episode of pelvic inflammatory disease confers a 20 per cent chance of infertility then 10 per cent of women in this reproductive age group will have been sterilised by pelvic inflammatory disease alone.[106]

Such apocalyptic warnings diminished through the 1980s, and it is not clear why. One likely factor is that the interests and work of GUM specialists and researchers shifted to HIV/AIDS, where an even greater public health crisis was foreseen.[107] Also, the improved success rate and availability of in vitro fertilization meant that tubal damage or obstruction was no longer an untreatable cause of infertility. Nonetheless, investigations of the incidence of chlamydia infection continued to be made. A study published in 1991 tested swabs from a cervical cancer–screening clinic in Glasgow and found 6–12 percent positive, while a study of all women referred in Lothian by general practitioners to GUM clinics found the microorganism in 3.5 percent of samples tested.[108] In both reports the authors claimed that the incidence was high; though they acknowledged that the number of these infections that led to PID and infertility remained unknown, the implication was that clinical experience pointed to a connection.

Chlamydia: The More You Look the More You Find

In principle there are two methods of diagnosing an infection: either to isolate and identify the actual pathogen by microscopy or culture methods, or to find a proxy indicator of its presence. In the latter case this might be either a marker from the microorganism (a toxin, membrane protein, or genetic material) termed an antigen or a marker from the immune response of the person infected, typically an antibody. The constructed character of such methods was explored in Ludwig Fleck's classic study of syphilis.[109] The difficulties in microscopical identification of its bacterial cause—the *Trepanoma pallida*—led doctors to explore methods that tested the blood serum of the patient for antigens and antibodies. Fleck showed how the accepted method, the Wassermann reaction, was changed from "measuring" antigens to antibodies and, though standardized, produced results that varied between laboratories, influenced by materials, skills, and the meanings attached to results. For example, it was a matter of judgment whether the degree to which a run of tests gave few false positives (a result that indicates that a given condition is present when it is not) or false negatives (a result that indicates that a given condition is absent when it is present). Nonetheless, Fleck showed that the Wassermann reaction, a laboratory test, became as, if not more, important than clinical signs and symptoms in making the diagnosis of syphilis a "fact." The importance of the Wassermann reaction to venereologists meant that they were early adopters, compared to other specialisms, in relying on the laboratory. This was nowhere clearer than with the construction of NGU in the 1930s as the absence of the gonococcus, which was possible because of the routinization of bacteriological investigations in venereal disease clinics, and this has also been the case with chlamydia.

Three ways of diagnosing chlamydia infection were developed: utilizing cell culture, identifying antigens in blood and urine samples, and identifying antibodies in blood. The earliest, cell culturing, was the "gold standard" because the actual organism was "seen," though this required making it visible by staining and fixing, procedures that were demanding, lengthy, and expensive. And, as clinicians had effective antibiotics at hand, their practice was to treat first and then, maybe or maybe not, confirm the diagnosis. Cell culturing was highly specific, but there were questions about its sensitivity and accuracy. Specificity, sensitivity, and reliability are key terms in bacteriological testing. Specificity refers to the degree to which a test identifies only a particular microorganism and not other members of the genus or related bacteria. Sensitivity refers to the probability of actually detecting the specific organism, though how this is judged depends on the assumed gold standard for 100 percent detection. Accuracy relates to sensitivity, in relation to the overall percentage of false positives and false negatives but also to the precision and replicability of the test, not least its independence from the equipment and skill levels of technicians in different laboratories and at different times.

Culture methods were improved in the 1970s, first, with the use of irradiated McCoy cells allowing culturing to be standardized. Second, identification was improved when traditional chemical stains were replaced by fluorescently labeled antibodies that adhered to the bacillus, allowing rapid and specific identification through a microscope with ultraviolet light.[110] This method, developed first for trachoma and LGV, was nearly 100 percent specific, though its laboratory sensitivity was estimated at only 70–85 percent and overall sensitivity lower, at 40–85 percent, due to sampling errors and variable laboratory standards.[111] There remained the question of the quality of the samples tested: might microorganisms have been missed in taking swabs, urine, and blood samples or died between clinic and laboratory?

In the 1980s there was a return to vogue of microscopical identification without culturing, using a technique known as direct fluorescence assay. The test involved attaching specially manufactured antibodies to specific sites on the outer membrane of *Chlamydia*. Specimens taken from the urethra and reproductive organs were allowed to react with antibodies, which also carried luminescence-labeled reagents. After washing, the sample was examined for any antibodies remaining adhered to microorganisms, with clinical pathologists looking for bright spots, typically green, under ultraviolet light. When compared with other methods results were more variable, influenced by many factors, including the recognition that were three strains or serotypes of *C. trachomatis*. Nonetheless, it was used because it was quick and relatively inexpensive.

Advances in molecular biology, many developed by the new biotechnology companies and using monoclonal antibodies, revolutionized the laboratory diagnosis of all diseases, and chlamydia was no exception.[112] There were new tests for antibodies (complement fixation and a microimmunofluorescence) and new antigen tests (direct fluorescence assay and enzyme immunoassay).[113] There was intense competition between the companies producing the tests, as the demand for diagnostic testing and, later, screening for chlamydia grew. Manufacturers made competing claims for specificity, sensitivity, and accuracy, as well as price and speed. All were compared to the gold standard of cell culture, though there were increasing doubts that this was any better than any of the new tests.[114] It was a difficult argument to settle, as the different tests were testing for different things; nonetheless, the public health authorities in England and Wales had sufficient confidence to include new cases of chlamydia in the STI statistics from 1990.

In the 1990s new tests became available that used the new DNA technologies, most notably the polymerase chain reaction technologies, to develop nucleic acid amplification tests (NAATs).[115] In these tests fragments of *Chlamydia* DNA extracted from clinical samples were duplicated in repeating cycles, to produce samples large enough for colorimetric evaluations. The first such test was introduced by Roche in 1993—*Amplicor C. trachomatis*. The following year an evaluation made by doctors in Bordeaux found that it had a sensitivity of 95.3 percent and a specificity of 100 percent and concluded that it was superior to culture methods.[116] Other tests from other companies followed: the ligase chain reaction from Abbott Laboratories Illinois and transcription mediated amplification from Gen-Probe, La Jolla, California. A review of the new tests found that while they were based on different molecular strategies, they had equivalent specificity and sensitivity to Roche Amplicor.[117] In a review in 1998 interestingly titled "*Chlamydia trachomatis*: The More You Look the More You Find; How Much Is There?," Julius Schachter suggested it was time to abandon the old assumptions:

> There has been a revolution in diagnostic methodology in recent years with the introduction of nucleic acid amplification tests (NAAT). These tests are far more sensitive than any of the earlier nonculture tests. For the first time, diagnostic laboratories have a technology that is more sensitive than isolation in tissue culture (TC). TC, which has long been considered the gold standard for diagnosis of C. trachomatis, is recognized as having a specificity approaching 100% but is considered to be less sensitive, with estimates typically being on the order of 75% to 85% sensitivity in expert laboratories. The NAAT have shown that these estimates of the sensitivity of cell culture are overestimates. There is even a wider variability in the performance of culture from laboratory to laboratory, than had been previously surmised.

The new methods had, he argued, completely changed the landscape.

> The nonculture methods led to broad-based testing for *C. trachomatis* and changed chlamydia diagnostics from being a cottage industry into being on the regular public health laboratory menu. But these tests were even less sensitive than culture. The NAAT offered tests that were more sensitive than culture. We became aware that the estimates of prevalence of infection determined in the past by either TC [tissue culture] or early nonculture tests (antigen detection methods or the direct nucleic acid probes) were gross underestimates. The number of infections detected by nucleic acid amplification tests could be higher by up to 80% as compared with the use of the older technology.[118]

The improvement offered by the new DNA-based techniques were indicated in a study published in 1997, where the older enzyme immunoassay methods found a prevalence of 1.6 percent (0.8 to 2.7 percent), with a sensitivity of 60 percent and a specificity of 100 percent, while the ligase chain reaction found 2.5 percent (1.5 to 3.9 percent), with 90 percent sensitivity and 99.8 percent specificity. Not only did the new technologies offer greater specificity, sensitivity, and accuracy; they were cheaper and easier. Hence, it became possible to move beyond diagnostic testing to screening for symptomless chlamydia infection in both men and women. Paradoxically, the NAAT technologies may have been responsible for the continuing increase in reported new cases, as they enabled more tests to be made and with greater sensitivity.[119]

The possibility of large-scale screening became policy in Britain in 1998, when the government accepted the recommendation of the chief medical officer's Expert Advisory Group's report on *Chlamydia trachomatis* that a pilot trial be made.[120] Two groups were tested systematically: women and men attending GUM clinics and women seeking termination of pregnancy; there was also to be opportunistic screening of sexually active women aged under twenty-five, especially teenagers. Why make the trial? First, there was the rising annual rate of new cases of chlamydia, which reached fifty thousand in 1998–99, over three times that for gonorrhea; and, second, so much infection is asymptomatic, and, untreated, its consequences for women were severe and lifelong and had implications for society at large. An editorial in the *British Medical Journal* welcomed the report and stressed the importance of its recommendations. "The role of chlamydia in infertility is well documented: the disease may be implicated in as much as 50% of cases. Many cases of infertility occur in the absence of clinical pelvic inflammatory disease, and when this disease process occurs is unknown. A reduction of the incidence of chlamydia infection in the community may therefore produce a corresponding fall in the related incidence of infertility."[121]

Pilot studies showed high rates—10 percent infected—among young women attending general practitioners and other clinics.[122] This prompted the establishment in September 2002 of the National Chlamydia Screening Programme, by which time new chlamydia cases each year was approaching a hundred thousand. The program "offered" screening to all women and men under twenty-five years of age attending various clinical setting using NAATs. The technical term for this type of screening was "opportunistic"—that is, it was offered, but it was up to patients whether to accept and to practitioners how strongly, if at all, they encouraged participation. Nonetheless, in the first year over 16,000 samples were tested (15,241 women and 1,172 men). Excluding those seen at GUM clinics and assumed to represent the general population of young adults, the program found "chlamydia positivity among people under 25 years of age screened in non-GUM settings was 10.1% (1538/15,241) in women and 13.3% (156/1172) in men."[123] Views on the program were mixed. Some doctors complained that it was hardly a public health measure as long as screening remained opportunistic. The participation of general practitioners was optional and not incentivized; few men were screened and contacts untraced.[124] On the other side there were questions about its cost-effectiveness, in part because of new views on the natural history of the infection:

> Increasing evidence shows that the rate of progression of endocervical chlamydia to pelvic inflammatory disease is lower than previously thought. Population based studies consistently estimate lower incidence rates of pelvic inflammatory disease than clinic-based studies. Infections detected by screening asymptomatic people might therefore have a better prognosis than symptomatic infections, because of differences in the burden of the organism. Descriptions of chlamydial infection and its consequences, and models of the impact of screening, however, nearly always cite the higher estimates.[125]

It was, of course, unsurprising that those who were promoting screening used the data that supported their case, but equally interesting was the redefinition of the problem to be tackling pelvic inflammatory disease rather than infertility. This change may have been due to the impact of gender politics, considering women's health as such, rather than in terms of motherhood, and the impact of in vitro fertilization, but it also reflected less confidence in the extent to which chlamydia is a direct and major cause of infertility. This is borne out by later assessments. A *Cochrane Review* published in 2013 found the following: "In women, chlamydia ascends to the upper genital tract in approximately 10% of cases to cause symptomatic pelvic inflammatory disease (PID). The resulting tubal damage can then cause ectopic pregnancy, tubal infertility and chronic pelvic pain. Although about 45% of tubal infertility might be attributable to chlamydia infection, the probability of tubal infertility in women who have had chlamydia is estimated to be only 1% to 4%."[126]

The range of these population estimates is very wide, and such uncertainties mean that how, and to what extent, *C. trachomatis* infection causes infertility has remained a subject of intense research. A 2015 study of the subject concluded, after discussing the complex interactions of host, immunological, epidemiological, and pathogen factors, that "the actual process of host and pathogen factors that result in infertility remain uncertain and require further investigation."[127]

From Male NGU to Female Chlamydia

Chlamydia as an STI was constructed medically and socially from the breakup of NGU as a clinical entity in the 1970s. There was no eureka moment. Rather, there was a slow buildup of evidence, from laboratory investigations using the new tools of molecular biology, that NGU—which had become an embarrassment to STI specialists as a catch-all, negative diagnosis—was a number of distinct infections. Given that my approach followed Rosenberg's maxim that "a disease does not exist until we have agreed that it does, by perceiving, naming, and responding to it," it might be thought inconsistent that I begin with discussion of the construction of NGU in the 1930s. Does this mean my history is presentist and teleological in assuming that chlamydia was always present in NGU? In part, yes: all history is a dialogue between the present and the past, and we cannot escape our knowledge of the deconstruction of NGU in component parts from the 1970s. But also, no: I discuss the emergence of NGU in its historical context as a disease entity in its own right, not as a mistaken, temporary entity whose demise was inevitable. NGU was modeled as having symptoms like gonorrhea, but also unlike it in not being caused by the gonococcus. However, there was another largely unremarked difference. Venereologists found no place for female disease in the new infection, which leads to questioning how well integrated into their practice was concern about the extent and seriousness of gonorrhea in women shown by gynecologists and pathologists, and championed by the suffragettes, in the early twentieth century. The maleness of NGU was further enshrined by the work of venereal disease services in World War II and medical and social attitudes that saw women as only consorts and contacts.

NGU attracted increased attention in the 1970s from STD specialists and researchers because of its increased incidence and continuing dissatisfaction with its uncertain causes. The application of cell culture techniques made possible the isolation of *C. trachomatis* from patients with GNU. This new modeling of the disease made it similar in aetiology and pathology to gonorrhea, which led clinicians to ask about the consequences of the infection in women more generally. The link between chlamydia and PID was well established by the early 1980s, specifically to salpingitis and ectopic pregnancies. This coincided with new medical interventions and social concern about infertility, which led to the reconstruction of chlamydia as a female disease, as seen in the development of screening programs targeted at women. This was not in terms of incidence—it was assumed to be equal in both sexes—but, because it was symptomatic in men, it was treatable, whereas in women symptomless, untreated infection was linked to infertility and PID. The main prompt for this reconstruction was the rising incidence of new cases of chlamydia in young women and projections of the long-term effects of untreated or repeat infection over childbearing years. The association between chlamydia, infertility, and PID proved to be powerful in mobilizing public health initiatives. However, these programs have come under scrutiny for their cost-effectiveness—future benefits in fertility and cost savings remain projections and easy targets for cuts. Furthermore, while no one doubts that chlamydia is a factor in infection-induced infertility, there continue to be ambivalent findings on how, and to what extent, *C. trachomatis* infection is a direct cause of infertility.

Notes

The research for this chapter was funded by a Wellcome Trust Programme Grant (WT 092782). The initial work for this chapter was undertaken collaboratively with John Craske, whose expert advice on microbiology was invaluable. And, finally, thanks goes to the many colleagues and students with whom I have discussed the work, but especially Ian Burney, Ian Clarke, Simon Szreter, Carsten Timmermann, and Elizabeth Toon.

1. Over the period discussed in this chapter, the terms for different diseases and groups of diseases changed. I employ mostly the terms used by historical actors in their context but sometimes have altered them to aid the clarity of the narrative. *Sexually transmitted infection* (STI) has been preferred since the 1990s to *sexually*

transmitted disease (STD), which in turn replaced *venereal disease* or *diseases* (VD) in the 1970s.

2. Michael Worboys, *Spreading Germs: Disease Theories and Medical Practice in Britain, 1865–1900* (Cambridge: Cambridge University Press, 2000).

3. Public Health England, "Sexually Transmitted Infections and Screening for Chlamydia in England, 2017," *Health Protection Report* 12, no. 20 (2018), https://assets.publishing.service.gov.uk/government/uploads/system/uploads/attachment_data/file/713944/hpr2018_AA-STIs_v5.pdf.

4. W. J. Hellstrom et al., "Is There a Role for *Chlamydia Trachomatis* and Genital Mycoplasma in Male Infertility?," *Fertility and Sterility* 48 (1987): 337–39; M. K. Samplaski et al., "Review Article: Chlamydial Infection and Its Role in Male Infertility," *Advances in Andrology* 2014 (2014): 1–11.

5. Beezy Marsh, "The Girls Facing a Fertility Timebomb," *Daily Mail*, December 12, 2002; M. Thrift, "Britain's Fertility Timebomb," *Independent*, June 20, 2005.

6. C. H. Mercer et al., "Changes in Sexual Attitudes and Lifestyles in Britain through the Life Course and over Time: Findings from the National Surveys of Sexual Attitudes and Lifestyles (Natsal)," *Lancet* 382 (2013): 1781–94.

7. L. O. Guerra et al., "Pathogenesis of *Chlamydia trachomatis* in Humans," in *Human Emerging and Re-emerging Infections: Bacterial and Mycotic Infections*, ed. S. K. Singh, 635–48 (Hoboken: Wiley, 2006).

8. See Ian N. Clarke and Hugh R. Taylor, chap. 4, in this volume.

9. N. S. Galbraith et al., "Changing Patterns of Communicable Disease in England and Wales, Part III: Increasing Infectious Diseases," *British Medical Journal* 281 (1980): 5464–69.

10. Hugh R. Taylor, *Trachoma: A Blinding Scourge from the Bronze Age to the Twenty-First Century* (Melbourne: Centre for Eye Research, 2008); see also Clarke and Taylor, chap. 4, in this volume; and J. Schachter, "*Chlamydia psittaci*: 'Re-Emergence' of a Forgotten Pathogen," *New England Journal of Medicine* 315 (1986): 189–91.

11. S. K. West and P. Courtright, "Trachoma Control: 14 Years Later," *Ophthalmic Epidemiology* 22 (2015): 145–47.

12. D. Taylor-Robinson, "The History of Nongonococcal Urethritis: Thomas Parran Award Lecture," *Sexually Transmitted Diseases* 23 (1996): 86–91; J. D. Oriel, "The History of Non-gonococcal Urethritis," *Genitourinary Medicine* 72 (1996): 374–79.

13. Charles E. Rosenberg, "Framing Disease: Illness, Society and History," in *Framing Disease: Studies in Cultural History*, ed. C. E. Rosenberg and J. Golden (New Brunswick: Rutgers University Press, 1992), xv.

14. Peter Sedgwick, *Psychopolitics* (London: Pluto, 1982), 30–31.

15. Rosenberg, "Framing Disease."

16. R. C. Burnham, "Immunity to *Chlamydia trachomatis*," *Journal of Infectious Diseases* 207 (2013): 1796–97.

17. See Roy F. Scragg, chap. 7, in this volume.

18. Michael Worboys, “Unsexing Gonorrhoea: Bacteriologists, Gynaecologists, and Suffragists in Britain, 1860–1920,” *Social History of Medicine* 17 (2004): 41–59; Elliott Bowen, “Limits of the Lab: Diagnosing ‘Latent Gonorrhea,’ 1872–1910,” *Bulletin of the History of Medicine* 87 (2013): 63–85.

19. L. V. Weström, “Chlamydia and Its Effect on Reproduction,” *Journal of the British Fertility Society* 1 (1996): 23–30.

20. Anne Hanley, “‘Scientific Truth into Homely Language’: The Training and Practice of Midwives in Ophthalmia Neonatorum, 1895–1914.” *Social History of Medicine* 27 (2014): 199–220.

21. There were calls for the infection to be made notifiable, which it was in certain towns, to ensure medical practitioners were called on to treat babies if midwives had not done so. S. Stephenson, *Ophthalmia Neonatorum, with Especial Reference to Its Causation and Prevention* (London: Pulman and Sons, 1907); T. G. Benedek, “Gonorrhea and the Beginnings of Clinical Research Ethics,” *Perspectives in Biology and Medicine* 48 (2005): 54–73.

22. Christabel Pankhurst, *The Great Scourge and How to End It* (London: Pankhurst 1913); Emmeline S. Pankhurst, *The Suffragette Movement* (London: Longmans, 1932), 521.

23. C. Pankhurst, *Great Scourge*, 83–84.

24. Aleck B. Bourne, “Discussion of the Treatment of Salpingitis,” *British Medical Journal* 2 (1923): 399–400.

25. Anne Hanley, “‘The Great Foe to the Reproduction of the Race’: Diagnosing and Treating Infertility Caused by Venereal Disease, 1880–1914,” in *Infertility in History: Approaches, Contexts and Perspectives*, ed. Gayle Davis and Tracy Loughran, 335–58 (London: Palgrave Macmillan, 2016).

26. Simon Szreter, “The Prevalence of Syphilis in England and Wales on the Eve of the Great War: Re-visiting the Estimates of the Royal Commission on Venereal Diseases, 1913–1916,” *Social History of Medicine* 27 (2014): 527–29.

27. R. A. Gibbons, “Sterility: Its Etiology and Treatment,” *Lancet* 176 (1910): 708. See also Christina Benninghaus, chap. 10; and Fabrice Cahen and Adrien Minard, chap. 11, both in this volume.

28. C. C. Norris, *Gonorrhea in Women: Its Pathology, Symptomatology, Diagnosis, and Treatment; Together with a Review of the Rare Varieties of the Disease Which Occur in Men, Women and Children* (Philadelphia: Saunders, 1913), 127.

29. “Antenatal Treatment of Gonorrhoea,” *Lancet* 211 (1928): 757–58.

30. “Gonorrhoea, Epididymitis and Sterility,” *Lancet* 201 (1923): 1017; J. W. Burns, “Chronic Endocervicitis and Its Treatment,” *Lancet* 200 (1922): 796–99; Report on the British Congress of Obstetrics and Gynaecology, “Puerperal Sepsis,” *Lancet* 205 (1925): 919–21; M. Huhner, “The Role of the Gonococcus in Sterility,” *American Journal of Surgery* 4 (1928): 299–303.

31. Maeve Kenny, “Remote Effects of Puerperal Sepsis,” *Lancet* 229 (1937): 14–16.

32. Leonard Colebrook, "The Story of Puerperal Fever: 1800–1959," *British Medical Journal* 1 (1956): 247–52; Irvine Loudon, "Puerperal Fever, the Streptococcus, and the Sulphonamides, 1911–1945," *British Medical Journal* 295 (1987): 485–90.

33. "Chemotherapy of Gonorrhoea," editorial, *British Medical Journal* 2 (1938): 665–66; "The Chemotherapy of Gonorrhoea," editorial, *Lancet* 232 (1938): 381.

34. A. J. Cokkinis, "The Treatment of Gonorrhoea with Oral Sulphanilamide," *British Medical Journal* 2 (1937): 905–9.

35. A. Malcolm Simpson, "Over-Treatment of Gonorrhoea," *Lancet* 229 (1937): 899.

36. A. J. Cokkinis, "Sulphonamide in Genito-Urinary (Non-gonococcal) Infections," *British Medical Journal* 2 (1938): 1151–55.

37. "Obituary Notices: A. H. Harkness, F.R.C.S.," *British Medical Journal* 4 (1970): 562; "Obituary: Arthur Herbert Harkness, F.R.C.S.," *Lancet* 296 (1970): 1145.

38. J. D. Oriel, *The Scars of Venus: A History of Venereology* (London: Springer, 1994), 161–65.

39. A. H. Harkness, "Non-gonococcal Urethritis," *British Journal of Venereal Disease* 9 (1933): 173–86, 187–91.

40. Lawrence W. Harrison and Werner Worms, "The Relation between Some Forms of Non-gonococcal Urethritis, Lymphogranuloma Inguinale, Trachoma, and Inclusion Blennorrhœa: Critical Review," *British Journal of Venereal Disease* 15 (1939): 237–59.

41. R. E. Wright, "The Trachoma Problem," *British Journal of Ophthalmology* 19 (1935): 309–18. See also Clarke and Taylor, chap. 4, in this volume; and Taylor, *Trachoma*, 19.

42. S. S. Meighan, "Trachoma in Glasgow," *British Journal of Ophthalmology* 19 (1935): 326.

43. E. de Grósz, "Campaign against Trachoma," *British Journal of Ophthalmology* 19, no. 6 (1935): 320.

44. S. S. Hughes, *The Virus: A History of the Concept* (London: Heinemann, 1977); Victoria A. Harden, *Rocky Mountain Spotted Fever: History of a Twentieth-Century Disease* (Baltimore: Johns Hopkins University Press, 1990).

45. A. W. Downie, "Bedson, Sir Samuel Phillips (1886–1969)," *Oxford Dictionary of National Biography*, rev. ed. (Oxford: Oxford University Press, 2004), www.oxforddnb.com/view/article/30668.

46. A. E. W. McLachlan, *Handbook of Diagnosis and Treatment of Venereal Diseases* (Edinburgh: Livingstone, 1944).

47. D. Lees, *Practical Methods in the Diagnosis and Treatment of Venereal Diseases*, 3rd ed. (Edinburgh: Livingstone, 1937), chap. 13; A. E. W. McLachlan, *Handbook of Diagnosis and Treatment of Venereal Diseases*, 3rd ed. (Edinburgh: Livingstone, 1947), 232; J. Marshall, *The Venereal Diseases* (London: Macmillan, 1948), 299–323.

48. G. L. M. McElligott, "Non-gonococcal Urethritis," *British Journal of Venereal Disease* 18 (1942): 106–12.

49. I. N. Orpwood-Price, "Non-gonococcal Urethritis," *British Journal of Venereal Disease* 18 (1942): 106–12; R. R. Willcox, "The Etiology of Nongonococcal (Nonspecific) Urethritis," *Journal of Chronic Disease* 1 (1956): 381–91.

50. *Report of the WHO Expert Committee on Venereal Diseases* (Geneva: World Health Organization, 1948). See reports in *British Journal of Venereal Disease* 25 (1949): 206–7; and *Bulletin of the World Health Organization* 2 (1949): 139–54.

51. A. H. Harkness, *Non-gonococcal Urethritis: Including the Genital Manifestations of Local and Systemic Diseases and Infestations of the Urinary Tract with Protozoa, Metazoa and Fungi, Etc.* (Edinburgh: Livingstone, 1950).

52. Ministry of Health, *Report of the Ministry of Health Covering the Period from 1st April 1950 to 31st December 1951*, pt. 2, *On the State of the Public Health, Being the Annual Report of the Chief Medical Officer for the Year 1950*, Parliamentary Papers, 1951–52, Cmd. 8582, at 15:315; and pt. 3, *On the State of the Public Health, Being the Annual Report of the Chief Medical Officer for the Year 1951*, Parliamentary Papers, 1952–53, Cmd. 8787, at 8:302.

53. A. H. Harkness and C. S. Nicol, "Non-gonococcal Urethritis" *Public Health* 68 (1954): 10–12.

54. A. Grimble and G. W. Csonka, "Skin Testing in 246 Patients with Non-specific Urethritis with a Review of the Important Literature," *British Journal of Venereal Diseases* 31 (1955): 228–34.

55. Ministry of Health, *Report*, pt. 2, *On the State of the Public Health, Being the Annual Report of the Chief Medical Officer for the Year 1951*, Parliamentary Papers, 1952–53, Cmd. 8787, at 3:302–3.

56. R. R. Willcox, "Researches in Aetiology of Non-specific Urethritis," *British Medical Journal* 1 (1954): 13–15.

57. R. S. Morton and L. Reed, "Non-gonococcal Urethritis: An Investigation to Determine Factors in the Host Influencing Response to Treatment and Recurrence of Symptoms," *British Journal of Venereal Diseases* 33 (1957): 223–27.

58. Ministry of Health, *Report*, pt. 2, *On the State of the Public Health, being the Annual Report of the Chief Medical Officer*, Parliamentary Papers, 1962–63, Cmnd. 1856, at 19:281.

59. G. L. M. McElligott, "Venereal Disease and Public Health," *British Journal of Venereal Diseases* 36 (1960): 207–15.

60. McElligott, "Venereal Disease," 214.

61. A. King and C. Nicol, *Venereal Diseases* (London: Cassell, 1964).

62. B. Goh, "Obituary: Eric Dunlop," *Sexually Transmitted Infections* 76 (2000): 235.

63. E. Dunlop et al., "Infection of Urethra by TRIC Agent in Men Presenting Because of Non-specific Urethritis," *Lancet* 285 (1965): 1125–28.

64. "Chlamydiaceae," National Center for Biotechnology Information, accessed September 30, 2016, http://www.ncbi.nlm.nih.gov/Taxonomy/Browser/wwwtax.cgi?mode=Tree&id=809.

65. E. Dunlop et al., "Infection of Urethra," 1172.

66. "Venereal Diseases in England and Wales: Extract from the Annual Report of the Chief Medical Officer for the Year 1967," *British Journal of Venereal Diseases* 45 (1969): 67.

67. "Sexually Transmitted Diseases: Extract from the Annual Report of the Chief Medical Officer of the Department of Health and Social Security for the Year 1972," *British Journal of Venereal Diseases* 50 (1974): 75–77.

68. "Sexually Transmitted Diseases: Extract from the Annual Report of the Chief Medical Officer of the Department of Health and Social Security for the Year 1971," *British Journal of Venereal Diseases* 49 (1973): 89–95, 93.

69. Boston Women's Health Collective, *Women and Their Bodies: A Course* (Boston: New England Free Press, 1970), 49–58.

70. K. Davis, *The Making of Our Bodies, Ourselves* (London: Duke University Press, 2007), 28.

71. "Chlamydia and Genital Infection," editorial, *Lancet* 304 (1974): 264–65.

72. Eric M. C. Dunlop, "Some Aspects of Sexually Transmitted Diseases Today," *Proceedings of the Royal Society of Medicine* 68 (1975): 13; Dunlop et al., "Chlamydia and Non-specific Urethritis," *British Medical Journal* 2 (1972): 575–77.

73. K. King et al., "Etiology of Nongonococcal Urethritis," *New England Journal of Medicine* 292 (1975): 1199–205.

74. Goh, "Obituary"; Eric M. C. Dunlop et al., "Chlamydial Infection: Incidence in 'Non-specific' Urethritis," *British Journal of Venereal Diseases* 48, no. 6 (1972): 425–28.

75. Goh, "Obituary."

76. Ambrose King and Claude Nicol, *Venereal Disease* (London: Baillière Tindall, 1975), 259.

77. A. S. Grimble and K. L. Amarasuriya, "Non-specific Urethritis and the Tetracyclines," *British Journal of Venereal Disease* 51 (1975): 204.

78. R. S. Morton and J. R. W. Harris, eds., *Recent Advances in Sexually Transmitted Diseases* (Edinburgh: Churchill Livingstone, 1975), 251.

79. Michael W. Adler, "Diagnostic, Treatment, and Reporting Criteria for Non-specific Genital Infection in Sexually Transmitted Disease Clinics in England and Wales," *British Journal of Venereal Disease* 54 (1978): 422–27.

80. "Sexually Transmitted Diseases" (1972), 73.

81. L. N. Pedersen, B. Herrmann, and J. Kjølseth Møller, "Typing *Chlamydia trachomatis*: From Egg Yolk to Nanotechnology," *FEMS Immunology and Medical Microbiology* 55 (2009) 120–30.

82. Dunlop et al., "Chlamydia and Non-specific Urethritis"; P. Reeve et al., "Serological Studies on the Role of Chlamydia in the Aetiology of Non-specific Urethritis," *British Journal of Venereal Disease* 50 (1974): 136–39.

83. Adler, "Reporting Criteria"; World Health Organization, *The Epidemiology of Infertility*, WHO Technical Report Series Number 582 (Geneva: World Health Organization, 1975); L. Weström and P. A. Mårdh, "Pelvic Inflammatory Disease: Epidemiology, Diagnosis, Clinical Manifestations and Sequelae," *Report of WHO Scientific Group on Non-gonococcal Urethritis and Other Selected Sexually Transmitted Diseases of Public Health Importance* (Geneva: World Health Organization, 1978), 347.

84. J. R. Willcox et al., "The Need for a Chlamydial Culture Service," *British Journal of Venereal Disease* 55 (1979): 281–83; D. Taylor-Robinson and P. E. Munday, "Chlamydia Culture Service," *British Journal of Venereal Disease* 56 (1980): 183.

85. A. S. Hilton, "*Chlamydia* A in the Female Genital Tract," *British Journal of Venereal Diseases* 50 (1974): 1–10.

86. J. M. Woolfitt and L. Watt, "Chlamydial Infection of the Urogenital Tract in Promiscuous and Non-promiscuous Women," *British Journal of Venereal Diseases* 53 (1977): 93–95.

87. "Promiscuity and Infertility," editorial, *British Medical Journal* 3 (1975): 501–2.

88. The literature on HIV/AIDS also makes little mention of other STIs, such as gonorrhea and syphilis. See Virginia Berridge, *AIDS in the UK: The Making of Policy, 1981–1994* (Oxford: Oxford University Press, 1996); and Elizabeth Fee and Daniel M. Fox, *AIDS: The Making of a Chronic Disease* (Berkeley: University of California Press, 1992). There is discussion of infertility due to STIs in Naomi Pfeffer, *The Stork and the Syringe: Political History of Reproductive Medicine* (Oxford: Polity, 1993), 8–12, 49–50.

89. K. Shanmugaratum and R. S. Pattman, "Declining Incidence of *Chlamydia Trachomatis* in Women Attending a Provincial Genitourinary Medicine Clinic," *Genitourinary Medicine* 65 (1989): 400; K. Sivakumar and R. Basu Roy, "Declining Prevalence of *Chlamydia Trachomatis* in Women Attending a Provincial Genitourinary Medicine Clinic," *Genitourinary Medicine* 65 (1989): 400.

90. "Obituary: Duncan Catterall," *Independent*, July 5, 1993.

91. Gayle Davis and Tracey Loughran, "Introduction: Situating Infertility in Medicine," and Anne Hanley, "'The Great Foe to the Reproduction of the Race': Changing Medical Knowledge and Practice; Diagnosing and Treating Infertility Caused by Venereal Diseases, 1880–1914," both in *The Palgrave Handbook of Infertility in History: Approaches, Contexts, Perspectives*, ed. Gayle Davis and Tracey Loughran (London: Palgrave Macmillan 2017), 265–72, 344–49.

92. "Ectopic Pregnancy and the I.U.D.," editorial, *Lancet* 306 (1975): 963.

93. L. Weström, L. P. Bengtsson, and P. A. Mårdh, "The Risk of Pelvic Inflammatory Disease in Women Using Intrauterine Contraceptive Devices as Compared to Non-users," *Lancet* 308 (1976): 221–24; J. R. Daling, "Primary Tubal Infertility in Relation to the Use of an Intrauterine Device," *New England Journal of Medicine* 312 (1985): 937–41; N. J. Grant, *The Selling of Contraception: The Dalkon*

Shield Case, Sexuality, and Women's Autonomy (Columbus: Ohio State University Press, 1992); P. D. Darney, "Time to Pardon the IUD?," *New England Journal of Medicine* 345 (2001): 608–10.

94. L. Weström, "Effect of Acute Pelvic Inflammatory Disease on Fertility," *American Journal of Obstetrics and Gynecology* 121 (1975): 707–13.

95. L. Weström, "Incidence, Prevalence, and Trends of Acute Pelvic Inflammatory Disease and Its Consequences in Industrialized Countries," *American Journal of Obstetrics and Gynecology* 138 (1980): 880–92.

96. "Pelvic Inflammatory Disease, 1980," *American Journal of Obstetrics and Gynecology* 138 (1980): 845–1112.

97. J. W. Curran, "Economic Consequences of Pelvic Inflammatory Disease in the United States," *American Journal of Obstetrics and Gynecology* 138 (1980): 848–51.

98. Michael W. Adler, E. H. Belsey, and B. H. O'Connor, "Morbidity Associated with Pelvic Inflammatory Disease," *Sexually Transmitted Infections* 58 (1982): 151–57. See also Michael W. Adler, "Trends for Gonorrhoea and Pelvic Inflammatory Disease in England and Wales and for Gonorrhoea in a Defined Population," *American Journal of Obstetrics and Gynecology* 138 (1980): 901.

99. R. D. Catterall, "Biological Effects of Sexual Freedom," *Lancet* 317 (1981): 318–19.

100. M. J. Hare, "Pelvic Inflammatory Disease," *British Medical Journal* 4 (1986): 1225–28. See also L. Weström, "Chlamydial Salpingitis," *British Medical Bulletin* 39 (1983): 145–50.

101. Hare, "Pelvic Inflammatory Disease," 1225–28.

102. J. A. McFalls and M. H. McFalls, *Disease and Fertility* (Orlando: Academic Press 1984), 258–307, 377–85.

103. D. Conway et al., "Chlamydial Serology in Fertile and Infertile Women," *Lancet* 323 (1984): 191–93. The authors cited similar findings from investigations in the United States and Finland.

104. Conway et al., "Chlamydial Serology," 192.

105. See correspondence on the question: "Is the Incidence of Ectopic Pregnancy Rising?," *British Medical Journal (Clinical Educational Research)* 291 (1985): 967, 1199–200, 1426.

106. J. L. Lane, "*Chlamydia trachomatis* Infections and Their Importance to the Gynaecologist," *Journal of Obstetrics and Gynaecology* 4 (1984): 253. Lane's comment is based on data from Curran, "Economic Consequences."

107. D. Taylor-Robinson, "*Chlamydia trachomatis* and Sexually Transmitted Disease," *British Medical Journal* 308 (1994): 150.

108. J. R. Smith, "Prevalence of *Chlamydia trachomatis* Infection in Women Having Cervical Smear Tests," *British Medical Journal* 302 (1991): 82–84; J. D. C. Ross et al., "Genital *Chlamydia trachomatis* Infections in Primary Care," *British Medical Journal* 313 (1996): 1192.

109. L. Fleck, *Genesis and Development of a Scientific Fact* (1935; repr., Chicago: University of Chicago Press, 1979); Ilana Löwy, "Ludwig Fleck and the Social Construction of Medical Knowledge," *Sociology of Health and Illness* 10 (1988): 133–55.

110. J. D. Oriel, "Chlamydial Infection: Isolation of *Chlamydia* from Patients with Non-specific Genital Infection," *British Journal of Venereal Diseases* 48 (1972): 429–36.

111. J. T. Grayston and S. Wang, "New Knowledge of *Chlamydiae* and the Diseases They Cause," *Journal of Infectious Diseases* 132 (1975): 87–105.

112. Lara V. Marks, *The Lock and Key of Medicine: Monoclonal Antibodies and the Transformation of Health Care* (New Haven: Yale University Press, 2015).

113. For a review of methods from the 1960s to the 1990s, see C. M. Black, "Current Methods of Laboratory Diagnosis of *Chlamydia trachomatis* Infections," *Clinical Microbiology Review* 10 (1997): 160–84.

114. T. Crowley et al., "The Laboratory Diagnosis of Male *Chlamydia Trachomatis* Infections: A Time for Change?," *Journal of Infection* 25 (1992): 69–75. See also J. W. Newhall et al., "Head-to-Head Evaluation of Five Different Non-culture Chlamydia Tests Relative to a Quality-Assured Culture Standard," *Sexually Transmitted Diseases* 21 (1994): S165–66; and P. E. Hay et al., "*Chlamydia trachomatis* in Women: The More You Look, the More You Find," *Genitourinary Medicine* 70 (1994): 97.

115. Black, "Current Methods," 164–75.

116. B. de Barbeyrac et al., "Evaluation of the Amplicor *Chlamydia trachomatis* Test Versus Culture in Genital Samples in Various Prevalence Populations," *Genitourinary Medicine* 70 (1994): 162–66.

117. J. Schachter, "*Chlamydia trachomatis*: The More You Look the More You Find; How Much Is There?," *Sexually Transmitted Diseases* 25 (1998): 229–31. See also J. Schachter, "DFA, EIA, PCR, LCR and Other Technologies: What Tests Should Be Used for Diagnosis of Chlamydia Infections?," *Immunological Investigations* 26 (1997): 157–61.

118. Schachter, "*Chlamydia trachomatis*, 230.

119. M. J. Rekart and R. C. Burnham, "Epidemiology of Chlamydia: Are We Losing Ground?," *Sexually Transmitted Infections* 84 (2008): 87–91.

120. Chief Medical Officer's Expert Advisory Group, *Main Report of the CMO's Expert Advisory Group on Chlamydia trachomatis* (London: Department of Health, 1998), accessed September 29, 2016, http://webarchive.nationalarchives.gov.uk/20130107105354/http://www.dh.gov.uk/prod_consum_dh/groups/dh_digitalassets/@dh/@en/documents/digitalasset/dh_4062264.pdf.

121. F. Boag and F. Kelly, "Screening for *Chlamydia trachomatis*," editorial, *British Medical Journal* 316 (1998): 1474.

122. J. M. Pimenta et al., "Opportunistic Screening for Genital Chlamydial Infection II: Prevalence among Healthcare Attenders, Outcome, and Evaluation of Positive Cases," *Sexually Transmitted Infections* 79 (2003): 22–27. See also

M. Catchpole et al., "Chlamydia Screening in the United Kingdom," *Sexually Transmitted Infections* 79 (2003): 3–4.

123. D. S. LaMontagne et al., "Establishing the National Chlamydia Screening Programme in England: Results from the First Full Year of Screening," *Sexually Transmitted Infections* 80 (2004): 335–41.

124. R. Jones and F. Boag, "Screening for *Chlamydia trachomatis*," editorial, *British Medical Journal* 334 (2007): 703.

125. N. Low, "Screening Programmes for Chlamydial Infection: When Will We Ever Learn?," *British Medical Journal* 334 (2007): 72. Low's evidence for a new view of the natural history of chlamydia infection drew on A. J. Boeke et al., "The Risk of Pelvic Inflammatory Disease Associated with Urogenital Infection with *Chlamydia trachomatis*: Literature Review," *Nederlands Tijdschrift voor Geneeskunde* 149 (2005): 878–84. See also N. Low et al., "Epidemiological, Social, Diagnostic, and Economic Evaluation of Population Screening for Genital Chlamydial Infection," *Health Technology Assessment* 11 (2007), http://dx.doi.org/10.3310/hta11080; L. A. Wallace et al., "What Is the Excess Risk of Infertility in Women after Genital Chlamydia Infection? A Systematic Review of the Evidence," *Sexually Transmitted Infections* 84 (2008): 171–75; and J. A. Land et al., "Epidemiology of *Chlamydia trachomatis* Infection in Women and the Cost-Effectiveness of Screening," *Human Reproduction Update* 16 (2010): 189–204.

126. N. Low et al., "Screening for Genital Chlamydia Infection," *Cochrane Database Systemic Review* 12 (2013): 1–15. See also M. H. Ahmadi et al., "Association of *Chlamydia trachomatis* with Infertility and Clinical Manifestations: A Systematic Review and Meta-analysis of Case-Control Studies," *Infectious Diseases* 48, no. 9 (2016): 517–23.

127. S. Menon et al., "Human and Pathogen Factors Associated with *Chlamydia Trachomatis*-Related Infertility in Women," *Clinical Microbiological Reviews* 28 (2015): 978–79.

Part Three

Population Decline in the Global South

Chapter Six

Population Decline in Island Melanesia

Aphrodisian Cultural Practices, Sexually Transmitted Infections, and Low Fertility

Tim Bayliss-Smith

Island Melanesia

The Melanesian islands of the Southwest Pacific (Island Melanesia) experienced the effects of European contact somewhat later than islands in Micronesia and Polynesia. There were sporadic contacts in the early nineteenth century, but most places had little sustained impact until whaling ships, traders, missionaries, and labor recruiters arrived in larger numbers after 1850. In consequence the islands of the Bismarck Archipelago (Papua New Guinea), Solomons, and New Hebrides (Vanuatu) experienced growing instability in local politics, increasingly violent interisland relations, epidemics, and a decline in population that became increasingly apparent to outside observers in the last three decades of the nineteenth century. A few islands were altogether depopulated, and most others (not all) saw a fall in numbers, but neither the magnitude of decline nor the reasons for decline were documented, and medical information is almost nonexistent. Apart from the colony of Fiji, even a basic head count of the populations did not take place in these islands until well into the twentieth century.

An exception is Simbo and Vella Lavella, two islands in the western Solomons that were visited by William H. R. Rivers and Arthur Hocart in 1908. The extensive genealogies collected by these pioneer anthropologists enabled Rivers to demonstrate the high proportion of married women living on these islands who had borne no children. Rivers himself came to favor a "psychological" explanation for childlessness, seeing colonialism as a form of trauma or shell shock that affected people's willingness to conceive, carry out abortions, or permit children to survive.[1] The evidence he provided for these assertions was weak, and growing evidence now suggests an alternative explanation.[2] I argue that the introduction and spread of STIs, especially gonorrhea, resulted in miscarriages, stillbirths, and sterility, and it was these effects that caused the severe decline in fertility rates.[3] The resulting fall in population probably started before 1850 and accelerated in the 1880s and 1890s.

I also consider how far we can generalize this model across Island Melanesia, which is a region with very great cultural diversity between and even within islands. Were Simbo and Vella Lavella especially vulnerable to high levels of infection by STIs because they were "Aphrodisian cultures," *sensu* Marshall Sahlins?[4] Did neighboring islands such as Guadalcanal and Malaita experience little or no population decline because their strict sexual codes prevented the influx of STIs like gonorrhea? Perhaps on these neighboring islands, despite heightened mortality following epidemics of diseases such as measles, dysentery, and influenza, the populations maintained high fertility so that communities could recover. This chapter reviews the evidence and concludes that diminished fertility because of high rates of STIs is indeed a factor hitherto underrated and one that can help to explain the geographic variation in the pattern of severe depopulation in the Pacific Islands.

Colonization and Germs

Melanesia was one of the last regions of the world to be affected by the global integration that accelerated in 1492 with the European colonization of the Americas, a process accomplished with the help of "guns, germs and steel."[5] This process spread to Australia and Polynesia in the late eighteenth century, reached Fiji about 1810, and started to affect the islands of western Melanesia in the 1840s. The "scramble for the Pacific" by European colonial powers reached its climax in the 1890s, and, apart from some small isolated pockets, full integration into processes of global epidemiology was completed in the 1930s with the Australian and Dutch expansion into the New Guinea highlands.

In all regions previously isolated from Eurasia and Africa, namely the Americas, Australasia and Oceania, the outcome of contact and colonization was decided not only by "guns and steel" but also by "germs"—by disease pathogens and their demographic impacts.[6] Before 1492 the indigenous peoples of this global periphery had an advantage over Eurasians and Africans in suffering from a smaller number of infectious diseases, but sustained contact transformed their situation. For example, Alfred Crosby listed the following new diseases introduced after 1492 in the Americas: smallpox, measles, chicken pox, whooping cough, typhus, typhoid fever, bubonic plague, cholera, scarlet fever, malaria, yellow fever, diphtheria, and influenza. Whether or not a name should be added or subtracted from this list is relatively unimportant, Crosby suggests, in view of the "avalanche of disease that decimated all native American peoples, and even obliterated many [societies] . . . struck by the micro-invaders and the macro-invaders simultaneously."[7]

The scale of depopulation in the Americas and the process itself have been much studied by historians. The highland populations in the former Aztec and Inca Empires are now estimated to have declined by at least 90 percent in the first post-contact century. Mexico's population, for example, fell from about thirty million in 1492 to less than three million in 1600.[8] The decline in the Amerindian populations of the tropical lowlands and Caribbean Islands is not so fully recorded, but often it was more extreme.

In Polynesia an equivalent catastrophic decline has been proposed by David Stannard for the population of Hawai'i in the century after 1778.[9] Norma McArthur studied the demographic histories of Tonga, Samoa, Cook Islands, and French Polynesia, and she came to more cautious conclusions. Her research suggested that of the Polynesian Island groups that she studied (which excluded Hawai'i), only Tahiti, Marquesas, and Rarotonga suffered really severe post-contact effects. Rarotonga's population was halved, mainly by dysentery, while Tahiti declined from about thirty-five thousand in 1769 to under eight thousand one hundred years later. The Marquesas Islands were probably even more affected, but the pre-contact population estimates may not be reliable.[10] Peter Pirie blamed the gonorrhea spread by the crews of visiting whaling ships for low fertility in eastern Polynesia in the nineteenth century. Sexually transmitted infections (STIs) are particularly implicated in the catastrophic population decline of Hawai'i.[11]

The Depopulation of Island Melanesia

Documenting Population Change

"Island Melanesia" includes the Bismarck Archipelago, Solomon Islands, Vanuatu, New Caledonia, and Fiji (see figure 6.1). This region's engagement with "guns, germs and steel" did not really begin until after 1800, and the process is therefore well documented by comparison with the history of early contact in the Americas. Even so, the information available needs careful interpretation. In the absence of proper medical diagnoses or full and accurate population statistics, very often we are forced to rely on the more casual observations of contemporary observers.

It is only Fiji's population decline from about 1850 up until the 1920s that is relatively well documented.[12] At the time the causes of this decline were poorly understood, so it was almost impossible for officials to devise appropriate countermeasures. Many policies that were justified in the name of "sanitation" seem in fact to have been designed to make Fijians more visible and easier to administer. For example, both colonial government and missionaries urged the creation of larger, nucleated settlements centered on the new (and usually crowded) churches and schools. This new settlement pattern and lifestyle appeared orderly and more civilized to British eyes, but it also facilitated a more rapid transmission of many diseases, as the fortuitous quarantine effects of population dispersal were removed. Infant mortality rates were high, and the evidence is overwhelming that exotic infections were the primary cause rather than neglect by bad mothers, as was claimed by some contemporaries.[13]

In the Melanesian islands west of Fiji, the administrative effort was more feeble, and it is mainly traders, missionaries, and other visitors who provide the primary evidence. In all cases their testimony strongly reflects their positionality. For example, a mission teacher, Florence Coombe, visited the Banks Islands (Vanuatu) on the Melanesian Mission ship *Southern Cross*. At Gaua the people said that formerly there were many large settlements, whereas she found "villages with only 30 to 50 inhabitants apiece, and amongst them not half a dozen babies." She speculated that "magic and poisoned arrows have been doing destruction for generations, and sheer ignorance and laziness account for the scarcity of children."[14] In fact, the regular visits of the *Southern Cross* were themselves a major cause of the rapid transmission of infections, which could now spread direct from New Zealand to what had once been remote islands in Melanesia.[15]

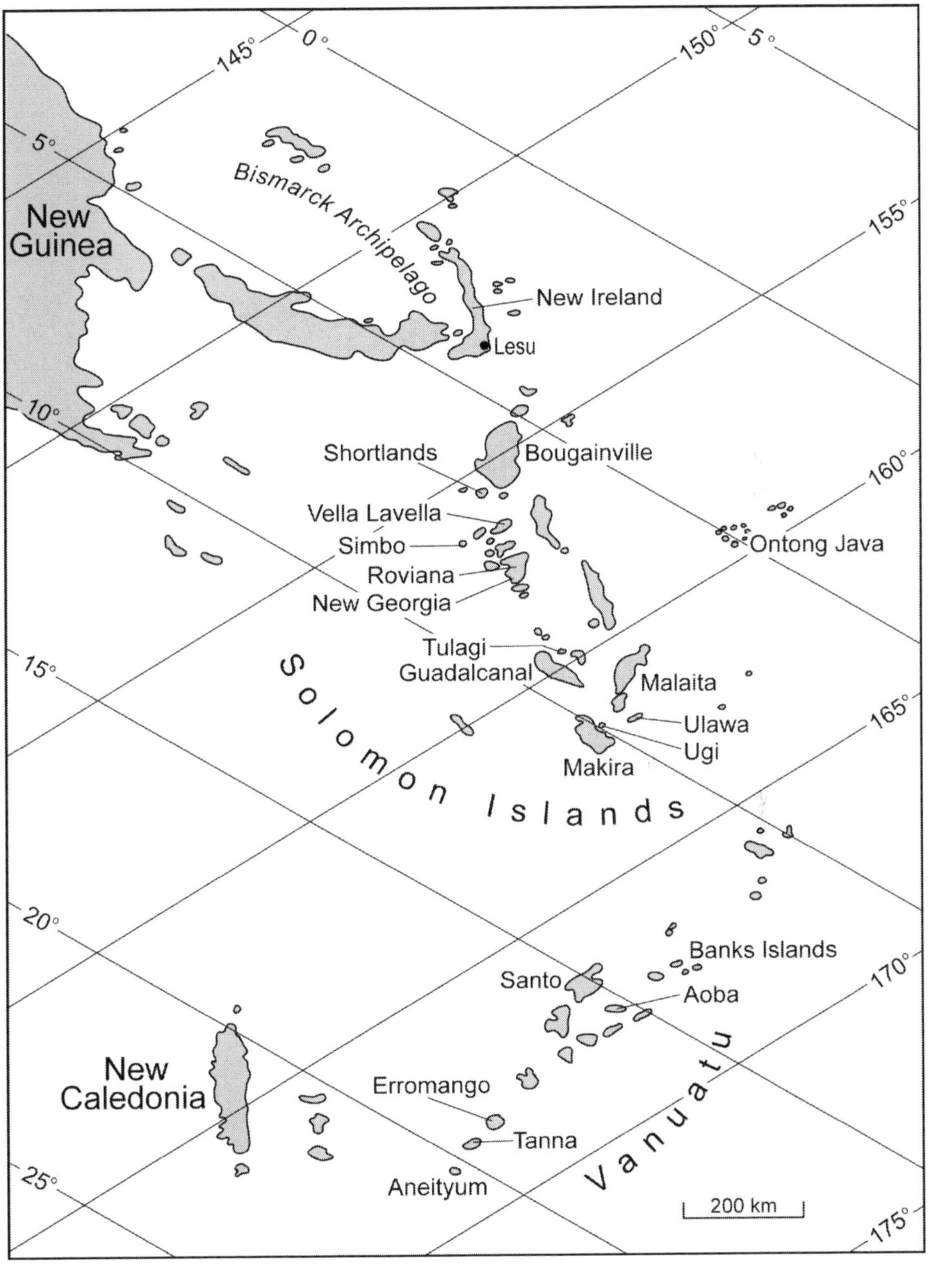

Figure 6.1. Island Melanesia, showing the locations of islands mentioned in the text. Modified after Bayliss-Smith, "Fertility and the Depopulation," 16.

The resident missionaries are generally more reliable than visitors; for example, Walter Ivens, who worked in Solomon Islands from 1895 to 1909 on the islands of Ulawa and South Malaita. Ivens was a skilled linguist and ethnographer, and the supposed effects of "magic" form no part of his analysis. Instead, he blamed the direct and indirect effects of the labor trade known as "blackbirding," which started in the 1860s and continued until 1906. On Ulawa Ivens found that only nine small villages remained with a population of about nine hundred, but oral histories indicate there had been many more people in the recent past. He estimated that dysentery in 1869 killed a quarter of the population: "The epidemic was introduced by some ship, possibly by a vessel seeking labor." On the most populous island, Malaita, where over forty-one thousand people were counted in the first government census in 1931, dysentery and influenza had spread from visiting ships and caused considerable mortality. The numerous deaths among children were "probably owing to hookworm and yaws."[16] Both were diseases already present in the islands, but almost certainly their effects were exacerbated by the population moving from dispersed hamlets into large coastal settlements.

Shorter-term visitors to the islands frequently blamed indigenous practices for population decline, for example Lt. Boyd Somerville, who spent eight months in the Solomons in 1893–94 surveying Marovo Lagoon, New Georgia, for the Royal Navy. Somerville interacted with traders as well as local people, but nowhere does he mention the impact of either the labor trade or disease:

> In the eastern parts [of Marovo] the number of the population has gone down with great rapidity. An old trader of twenty years experience [Frank Wickham] told me that in his recollection the numbers had terribly decreased. This to a large extent is probably due to head-hunting which has . . . almost annihilated some villages. . . . No doubt head-hunting has always been their custom; but . . . rifles and especially tomahawks, during the last forty or fifty years, have largely increased its fatal effects; so that where one man's head was taken in olden times, three or more are taken today.[17]

How damaging were these various effects? In the Solomon Islands, as elsewhere in the Pacific, the earliest visitors usually reported the presence of many more people than were actually counted some years later, but there is sometimes doubt about the accuracy of these early reports. McArthur was particularly skeptical about the reliability of pre-census estimates, for example, those used by Tom Harrisson for the New Hebrides (today's Vanuatu).[18] Harrisson proposed that a total population for the islands of one million had collapsed to six hundred thousand by 1882 and forty-five thousand in 1935 because of new epidemic diseases. The statistical basis for the "one million" appears not to have been published, but its origin was probably an extrapolation from the cases of Erromango and Aneityum in southern Vanuatu. It is still unclear how typical were such islands where early missionary censuses do enable a truly massive decline in population to be reconstructed.[19]

The Chronology of Depopulation

For the Solomon Islands Ivens was the first observer to provide a well-informed chronology of depopulation, based on his long-term residence in the islands. He divided the depopulation process into three overlapping stages, beginning with the onset of labor recruitment (blackbirding) in the 1860s through to the 1890s. He estimated that only about half of the men recruited ever returned home from Australia, Samoa, New Caledonia, or Fiji, and of those who did return, many delayed their marriages or never married at all.[20] He argued, therefore, that not only did the absentees deplete the population, but also fewer children were being born than previously.

The second stage was one of escalating warfare between the 1870s and 1890s. The introduction of rifles by traders and blackbirders led to increasing bloodshed and political unrest. This overlapped with the third stage of increasing epidemic infections between the 1880s and 1920s. The establishment of copra plantations, regular trade, and the migration of large numbers into new coastal villages saw the onset of a new era of high epidemic mortality, in particular from dysentery and influenza. Ivens observed that in the new villages that sprang up on the coast after the return of recruited laborers in 1906–8 "everyone suffered either from malaria or from ulcers [yaws?], and their cemeteries are literally full of children."[21]

After the British Solomon Islands Protectorate was established in 1893, the number of introduced diseases increased. Following fieldwork on Malaita, Guadalcanal, and Ontong Java as well as in New Guinea, the social anthropologist Ian Hogbin noted that the twentieth century saw "periodic outbreaks of chicken-pox, whooping cough, measles and influenza," along with dysentery, while "several new diseases, such as gonorrhoea, tuberculosis, dysentery, and leprosy have also become endemic."[22] He did not observe any precautions being taken against the spread of infection, and he noted the lack of proper nursing or suitable foods. On Malaita birth and death rates did not seem to vary between Christian and pagan areas, contrary to the predictions of anthropologist William H. R. Rivers.[23]

According to the Rivers model, the Christianized areas, being more acculturated, should have had an increased susceptibility to psychological malaise, but Hogbin rejected this idea because he had "never seen a native die of despair." Apart from accidents, all those people whose deaths he witnessed were suffering from disease. He believed that sexual intercourse was, if anything, on the increase, and everywhere he went the people still wanted to have children.[24] These authors all suggest that in both Melanesia and Polynesia it was heightened mortality rates that resulted in population decline in the nineteenth century, with lowered fertility playing a minor role.

The Conventional Model of Depopulation

Thus, for most islands in both Melanesia and Polynesia, the conventional model echoes the modern consensus about the causes of post-Columbian depopulation in the Americas, seeing depopulation as the result of new diseases that increased death rates, while birthrates were rather little affected. In Island Melanesia the chronology of the process (summarized in table 6.1) was somewhat later than in Polynesia. Within this region there were many local variations, and the model probably does not apply to inland New Guinea, where it seems that highlanders were protected from the main onslaught of epidemic disease by the late arrival of Europeans after the 1920s. Except in the New Guinea interior, the initial population decline began in the nineteenth century and was driven primarily by epidemic mortality plus the effects of new endemic infections, particularly tuberculosis. This model suggests that fertility may have fallen in consequence, or it may have been unaffected. In either case the rising birthrates of the twentieth century were too little and came too late to protect these populations from several decades of severe and sometimes catastrophic decline, although extreme cases, like Aneityum's population decline, may not be typical.

Changes in Fertility

In almost all this literature, fertility changes are not regarded as a major factor. There were reports, often anecdotal, that certain customs detrimental to fertility were continuing, such as late marriage and self-induced abortion. Upon closer inspection the evidence for such practices often appears unreliable.[25] There were also reports, seldom supported by clinical diagnosis, that new STIs were reducing fertility.[26] Usually, however, the main focus was on

Table 6.1. The depopulation of Island Melanesia: the conventional model

Period	Demographic processes	Outcome
Pre ca. 1840	High fertility balanced by high mortality	Stability
Ca. 1840–1920	Epidemic mortality much increased; rapid decline, with fertility somewhat reduced by death of spouses and failure to remarry	Rapid decline; depopulation of small islands and outlying areas
Ca. 1920–60s	Control of infectious disease; acquired immunity and rising birthrates as traditional fertility checks are abandoned	Recovery and slow increase
Post-1960s	Further reduction in incidence and effects of infectious disease; control of malaria (not applicable to Fiji)	Rapid increase

Source: Modified after Bayliss-Smith, "Fertility and the Depopulation," in Ulijaszek, *Population, Reproduction and Fertility*, 25.

high epidemic mortality and high endemic levels of infant mortality. It was claimed that the child death rate was being exacerbated by lack of breast-milk supplements, poor hygiene, dirty clothing, and bad mothering. Unless reforms could be instituted, it was suggested, Melanesians would fail to adjust to the new challenges of modernity. Their populations would not replace the numbers lost to the increased mortality rates, and extinction would become inevitable. Where low birthrates were noted, they were often attributed to polygamous marriages, to the men leaving villages to work on plantations, or to the failure of widows or widowers to remarry.[27]

Low Birthrates in Makira

The interaction between epidemic mortality and the subsequent fertility of the surviving population is usually difficult to establish from historical sources. Census data are absent, incomplete, or unreliable, and we are left with anecdotal evidence. An example is a logbook entry by the captain of a Solomon Islands copra boat, John Philp, who appears to have been a perceptive and disinterested observer:

> Wanomi Bay [Wainomi, Makira]. Thursday June 5th 1913. . . . At noon I went across to the Marist Mission. . . . Later I joined the fathers at their evening meal. . . . We were discussing population question. Father B. [Babonneau]

> gave as his experience that the rate of decrease in San Cristoval [Makira] was 60 per cent! Mothers are (before marriage) made sterile in many cases, or again, children are unwelcome to men who wish to have the services of their women wholly at their disposal for work in gardens. . . . In all the villages infanticide or abortion are commonly practiced. So evidently the population must decrease.

As evidence for these assertions Philp records some statistics provided by Father Emile Babonneau. Ten mission girls from Wainomi Bay had all been married for some years. Of these ten, seven were childless, and the other two had borne one child each, of whom only one now survived. Obviously, the sample is small and probably unrepresentative, but it seems very possible that STIs were responsible for this low birthrate. Philp later observed that in most villages on Makira there were "few young children and many couples [are] without issue."[28]

Identifying the STI that might have caused this low fertility is not straightforward. Nonvenereal yaws (*Treponema pallidum* ssp. *pertenue*) was an endemic disease in Solomon Islands and is very closely related to syphilis (*Treponema pallidum* ssp. *pallidum*). As a result the rate of syphilis infection was probably much reduced by acquired cross-immunity.[29] In general, clinicians who have experience of both diseases found that infection with one protected against the other, while the epidemiologists found that in areas where yaws was widespread there was little syphilis. Only after successful campaigns to eradicate yaws using penicillin and other antibiotics did populations see a reduction in their acquired active immunity to *T. pallidum pallidum*.[30]

In the Solomon Islands it is therefore likely that gonorrhea was not only the more prevalent but also the more dangerous STI, but unfortunately the medical evidence to support this claim is sparse. Charles Woodford, a naturalist collector and later the resident commissioner of the protectorate, commented that he never observed STIs on Guadalcanal, where he lived among the people for a total of nine months in 1886–87. He suggested that "such cases, of course, are more common upon those islands where the unbridled and promiscuous licentiousness of the natives render it as a matter of surprise that they are not more universal than they actually are."[31]

The people of Makira (San Cristobal) Island were undoubtedly among those notable for "licentiousness," and there are indeed several contemporary records that suggest that this particular island became heavily infected with STIs, especially gonorrhea but probably including syphilis.[32] The Royal Navy surgeon Henry Guppy blamed the introduction of STIs to Makira on white traders.[33] Usually in Island Melanesia these diseases were hardly noticed, and they were documented sparsely even by medically qualified doctors such as Rivers, but Guppy is an exception. He was described by Woodford as the first medical man to have paid an extended visit to the Solomon Islands.[34] For four months in 1882 Guppy visited many coastal villages on Makira and the nearby island of Ugi, and he wrote at some length about the various diseases that he encountered: "Venereal diseases, both constitutional and local, are said by traders to be very frequent in certain islands, as in Ugi, which have had most intercourse with the outside world. I rarely, however, came upon unequivocal evidence of the constitutional form of these diseases, those observations being of the non-constitutional types which, as in other tropical regions, are often of a rapidly destructive character."[35] Given Guppy's experience of STIs through his work as a naval surgeon, it is likely that the "constitutional form" refers to the symptoms of secondary or tertiary syphilis or possibly yaws, whereas "non-constitutional" or "local" probably refers to the symptoms of gonorrhea or another STI.

Unfortunately, there are only a few anecdotes we can add to Guppy's evidence. For example, a New Zealand copra trader stationed at Hada Bay on Makira recorded in his diary for September 22, 1885, "One native in the house today was very bad with the Veneral [*sic*] disorder and ultimately it will finish him."[36] Was this "disorder" gonorrhea or syphilis, or could it instead have been tertiary yaws? Very little was understood about the etiology of yaws until the early twentieth century, and in the Pacific Islands it was not even recognized as a disease in its own right.[37]

The great missionary ethnographer Robert H. Codrington agreed that it was whalers and traders who had first introduced STIs to Makira, but he suggested that after 1870 there were new agents of spread. He believed that male and female laborers returning from plantation work in Fiji or Queensland had brought back "syphilis, or the venereal disease which was taken for it," whereas previously this disease was unknown at least in those islands visited by the Anglican Mission.[38] What was this newly introduced venereal disease, which was taken by the missionaries to be syphilis? It cannot have been yaws, a disease well known in the islands but almost absent in Queensland. Today the consensus view is that neither gonorrhea nor syphilis were present in Melanesia before the nineteenth century.[39] Therefore, if we can trust Codrington's diagnosis, the newcomer on Makira must have been syphilis.[40]

Codrington's opinion is supported by Henry Welchman, who was based on Santa Isabel Island from 1890 until he died there eighteen years later. Welchman had practiced medicine in the English midlands for thirty years before becoming an Anglican missionary. In 1903 he wrote to Woodford, now the resident commissioner, pointing out that many men were being returned by labor vessels in a diseased condition, sometimes with infectious diseases. Some had been returned to their homes with "syphilis and gonorrhoea which was promptly communicated to their wives and other natives." He himself was giving medical treatment to several such cases.[41] It is possible that Welchman could not distinguish yaws from syphilis, as some symptoms in adults are similar, but if we can trust his account it would appear that the two new STIs had arrived with the labor trade.

Was Each Island Unique?

All this anecdotal evidence suggests that the impact of "guns, germs and steel" was no less severe in the Solomon Islands than elsewhere in the Pacific, but the process was geographically diverse and poorly documented. The weak state of colonial governance can be gauged from the fact that no population census took place until 1931. Estimates around 1900 for the Solomons group as a whole ranged from 100,000 to 150,000 people, all observers agreeing that total numbers were in decline and that some small islands had become depopulated.[42]

Charles Woodford spoke in his public writings only of his fear of labor shortages in the future.[43] However, in 1910 Woodford wrote in a confidential report that "nothing in the way of the most paternal legislation or fostering care, carried out at any expense whatever, can prevent the eventual extinction of the Melanesian race from the Pacific."[44] His "paternal legislation" involved quarantine regulations, while "fostering care" in the protectorate was minimal and barely extended beyond one small hospital in the capital Tulagi, itself a small island with few links to the main centers of population. In this corner of the British Empire, it appears a belief in inevitable "eventual extinction" influenced almost all aspects of colonial administration.

The contemporary literature can be read as suggesting that each place in Island Melanesia has its own unique history of European contact, and to a large extent this may be true. Undoubtedly some islands had early and intense involvement with trading ships, blackbirders, missionaries, and government agents, while other islands were more fortunate in avoiding devastating epidemics, wars, or cultural malaise. After touring the Solomons in 1921, the medical doctor Sylvester Lambert reported as follows to the International Health Board of the Rockefeller Foundation: "The natives from the big islands . . . near the infesting trade routes were much more heavily diseased. Disease diminishes steadily as we moved down toward the less frequented parts. My superficial look . . . verified my theory: epidemics are the fruits of island hospitality." Lambert admitted that the evidence available to test his theory was patchy and often ill-informed or biased. There were no reliable statistics, and in the Solomon Islands, for example, a scattered population that he estimated at a hundred thousand was served by only one government medical officer and "some missionary doctors who strove with bravery against conditions that should have broken their valiant spirits."[45]

In constructing any general model of underlying causes, these problems of data and its interpretation loom large. We need to focus on rigorous microstudies of particular societies, where demography and epidemiology were analyzed in some depth, to get beyond some of the sweeping generalizations of earlier scholarship. The island of Simbo provides such an opportunity.

Simbo and Vella Lavella

Vital Statistics for Simbo and Vella Lavella

While most contemporary observers blamed depopulation on the combined effects of disease, labor recruiting, and warfare, the social anthropologist William H. R. Rivers was one of the few to emphasize instead the low birthrate.[46] Rivers based his opinion on the field data that he collected in 1908 with Arthur Maurice Hocart on the islands of Tanna and Santo in the New Hebrides (Vanuatu) and on Vella Lavella and Simbo in the western Solomons.

Rivers became convinced of the importance of low fertility from his analysis of genealogies. On Simbo these covered the entire population and were collected during four months of careful questioning and cross-checking. For the larger island of Vella Lavella, also in the western Solomons, the genealogies represent "random samples taken from various villages of the coast" and were regarded by Rivers as "less trustworthy." His genealogies from Santo and Tanna (Vanuatu) are based on brief visits and the analysis of single families, but, interestingly, these also show the same patterns.[47] Rivers had proposed at the outset of his career in social anthropology that genealogies not only revealed aspects of social organization but also had the potential to generate "vital statistics."[48] In his Solomon Islands expedition of 1908, his intention was therefore to collect genealogies that were both accurate and complete.

After World War I Rivers returned to these genealogies to calculate "vital statistics." At that point Rivers needed evidence to support his emerging ideas about the links between psychoneurosis, reproductive instincts, and population change. He used the information gained from the genealogies from Simbo and Vella Lavella for what became his last publication on the depopulation of Melanesia.[49] Elsewhere I have discussed his methodology and the validity of his interpretations.[50]

Fertility Rates and Childlessness

The genealogies for the two sample populations in the western Solomons provided Rivers with aggregate data for the number of "marriages," how many children were born per marriage, and the mortality rates for children. He calculated these statistics for three reconstructed generations, called I, II, and III.[51] Rivers did not date these generations, but from the stated ages of sample individuals we can estimate that marriages in Generation I involved women born between about 1830 and 1850, in Generation II about 1850 to 1870, and in Generation III about 1870 to 1890. Unlike the women in Generations I and II, some women in Generation III were still in their reproductive years at the time of the 1908 fieldwork. I have checked the allocation of individuals to generations and the numbers of children born by analyzing the original genealogies, which are all preserved in the Haddon Papers in the Cambridge University Library. I found that Rivers's figures are accurate, apart from a few trivial errors and minor repetitions.

Rivers claimed for Simbo that his genealogies included almost the entire living population of around 400 as well as their ancestors, in a population that numbered about 2,000 individuals during the past three generations. Summary data that he produced appeared to show that the women in Generation I gave birth to 267 sons but only 180 daughters, an imbalance that could be the result of selective infanticide, the neglect of female infants, or simply inaccurate recall—this last being the explanation that Rivers himself favored. He thought the imbalance had arisen because many girls who died young and without issue were forgotten—at least by male informants—and so are left out from the genealogies, whereas the dead boys tended to be remembered.

The daughters of Generation I parents make up the female part of Generation II and consist of 180 women born circa 1850–70. According to Rivers's data, some of them died young (8 persons) or before the age of marriage (16 persons), and 8 were recorded as "unmarried." The remaining 148 females in Generation II became married, the great majority (134 women, 91 percent) having only one marriage, 13 women (9 percent) marrying twice, and 1 with three marriages. The sex ratio of the children born to these 180 women in Generation II is almost balanced (195 sons, 184 daughters, total 379), which suggests that the genealogical data for this period are much more complete than those for Generation I. By 1908 the Generation II women had finished childbearing but were mostly still alive so that they, or more likely their husbands, were in a good position to provide Rivers and Hocart with complete and accurate information.

Rivers calculated an average of only 1.3 children "per marriage" in Generation II (see table 6.2), but an equally revealing statistic is the average fertility per woman. The 180 women in Generation II gave birth to 2.2 children per woman, which is below the replacement rate in a society where at least 13 percent "died young" or before the age of marriage. We have similar data for the women of Lesu in New Ireland, studied in 1929–30 by Hortense Powdermaker, using the same genealogical method. Lesu, also a declining population, had an average fertility of 2.1 children for the generation of women born between about 1855 and 1880, and 2.6 for the generation born in the period circa 1880 to 1905.[52]

As well as demonstrating low fertility, Rivers also showed that childlessness was remarkably common on Simbo, although his data refer to the proportion of childless marriages, not childless women. From his data it appears that in Generation II almost half of all marriages had no children, and the proportion on Vella Lavella was almost as high.[53] Childlessness could therefore explain some of the population decline on Simbo—the fertility rate was simply too low for population replacement.

What about mortality rates? The data for Generation I are clearly incomplete, but in Generation II, although the data may also underestimate the death rate somewhat, we do not find that infant and child mortality rates are dramatically high. Women in Generation II were giving birth mainly in the 1870s and 1880s, and Rivers reported that 69 out of 379 children born had died before the age of marriage, a death rate of 18 percent. The equivalent rate for Generation III, its reproduction still incomplete but with the best record of births and deaths, was higher at 26 percent, probably reflecting the impact of recent epidemics (see table 6.2). We can conclude that in all three generations deaths could have been compensated by more prolific births, but these births were lacking. With this lethal combination of moderate or high mortality and low fertility, the Simbo population was clearly heading for extinction. Changing sexual practices, new medical treatments, and declining infection rates can all help to account for the island's subsequent demographic recovery later in the twentieth century.[54]

What is striking about the 1908 data is the high proportion of childless marriages in Generation II (approximately 1870s and 1880s), within cohorts

Table 6.2. A summary of the vital statistics of Simbo in 1908 and 1953

	Generation I	Generation II	Generation III	Mid-Twentieth Century Repeat Survey
Period of years during which women were fertile (approx.)	1850–70	1870–90	1890–1908	Census in 1953
Total number of marriages	207	295	110	118
Childless marriages (% of total)	40 (19%)	136 (46%)	58 (53%)	9 (8%)
Total number of children born	> 447	379	72	532
Children who died before the age of marriage (% of total)	> 94 (21%)	69 (18%)	19 (26%)	> 22 (4%)

Sources: The data for Generations I, II, and III are reconstructed from genealogies collected jointly by Rivers and Hocart (Rivers, "Psychological Factor," in *Essays on the Depopulation of Melanesia*, 98); the 1908 data are compared to a 1953 survey by the British Solomon Islands Protectorate Medical Department. Statistics shown with ">" are likely to be significant underestimates. The 1908 data are from Bayliss-Smith, "Colonialism as Shell Shock," in Hviding and Berg, *Ethnographic Experiment*, 190, correcting Rivers, "Psychological Factor," in *Depopulation of Melanesia*, 998; the 1953 data are from Allen, *Report*, 18–19.

where Rivers regarded the data as reasonably complete and accurate. An extraordinary 46 percent of Simbo marriages in this period were childless, rising to 53 percent in Generation III (see table 6.2). On the neighboring island of Vella Lavella, the proportion of childless marriages was low in Generation I (12 percent) but rose to 35 percent in Generation II, and the childless proportion rose to an extraordinary 72 percent in Generation III. Of the rather few children born on Simbo between about 1890 and 1908, one in four had died before the age of marriage, and about the same proportion died on Vella Lavella.

Explaining Depopulation

Despite these data, by 1922 Rivers had convinced himself that there was no clear evidence of any severe impact from introduced diseases in the western Solomons: "There is no record of any very severe epidemics. Tubercle and dysentery, the two most deadly diseases in Melanesia, do not appear to be, or to have been, especially active; and though both the chief forms of venereal disease exist on the island, they do not seem to have done any great amount of mischief."[55] Furthermore, he believed that several of the other factors commonly cited in Melanesia, including changes in clothing, house type, alcohol use, and firearms, were also absent on Simbo or were negligible in their effects. Because he downplayed the role of epidemics and was perhaps ignorant of the effects on fertility of STIs, he tried to explain the low birthrates shown by his genealogies by invoking "the psychological factor." The suggested effects of this factor were a reluctance of women to conceive, their eagerness to secure abortions, and their neglect of babies. By the 1870s (Generation II) these practices were seen as having a severe effect on population replacement, as shown by reduced family size and high infant mortality rates.

I have argued elsewhere that Rivers's explanations for the causes of low fertility are simply not credible.[56] By the 1920s Rivers was deeply involved in exploring the impact of the unconscious mind on the psyche and especially on "protopathic" instincts, following his years of clinical practice with shell-shocked soldiers in World War I.[57] Seeing colonialism in the Solomons as a kind of shell shock, he invoked "psycho-neurosis" as a process with severe impacts on the parental instincts. He followed more popular writers such as Robert Louis Stevenson in regarding the cultural impacts of colonialism in the Pacific as leading to fatalism, despair, and the loss of the will to live. Invoking "suggestion" as the way in which such feelings could affect whole societies, he saw population decline as the inevitable consequence.

In addition, Rivers ignored the historical evidence of over a hundred years of European contact with the islands of the western Solomons. Especially after 1870 foreign ships began to visit Simbo more frequently, and blackbird labor was recruited for Queensland.[58] The growing stream of foreigners and returning plantation laborers interacted with a population no longer living inland in scattered hamlets but now clustered in a few coastal villages and thus vulnerable to more effective disease transmission. White men were visiting more regularly, and traders became resident on Simbo after 1896.[59] More trade meant more contact, which in turn increased risks of infection, but medical treatment was almost nonexistent. In 1890 the captain of HMS *Cordelia* left Simbo for Australia and reported, "Am sending two boys [men] suffering from syphilis secondary to same place [Cooktown in Queensland]."[60] This was token treatment indeed.

As well as European visitors, laborers returning from plantation work in Fiji or Queensland could also introduce disease. In nearby Roviana the Methodist leader George Brown noticed in 1899, "a great apparent decrease in the population from that which I had seen twenty years before," an impression that traders like Wickham confirmed.[61] In 1906 the district commissioner reported that "there has been a tremendous amount of sickness among the natives, both in Simbo and Rubiana [Roviana]. They have been dying every day and are still doing so. It is carrying off all the old men and women."[62] There are also missionary reports that confirm the severity of epidemics at this time.[63]

Once introduced, diseases were likely to spread. Edvard Hviding has emphasized the strong links between all islands in this region, seeing the New Georgia group (including Simbo) as a region having "a long history of inter-island exchanges including people, objects, practices and beliefs."[64] We can surely add "diseases" to this list of interisland exchanges, including the STIs so often implicated in fertility declines.

Reasons for Simbo's Fertility Decline

How far can we trust the explanation given by Rivers regarding the "psychological" causes of low fertility? His ethnography seems to have been dominated by particular questions that he could ask of those men who could speak pidgin English. During their fieldwork in Melanesia, neither Rivers nor Hocart had any significant interaction with female informants. Rivers himself focused on Simbo kinship, which was the main reason for his genealogical work, as well as religious belief and sexual behavior.[65] Hocart collected data on ritual, magic, ethnomedicine, and warfare.[66] Although he was a qualified doctor, Rivers seems not to have undertaken medical diagnoses on Simbo in any systematic way, beyond treating a principal informant for pneumonia and himself and Hocart for malaria.

Instead of applying their Western medical knowledge, Rivers and Hocart concentrated their efforts on documenting indigenous beliefs and practices, recording "about a hundred examples of . . . conjoined processes of taboo and medicine." They recorded in detail sixty cases, which included magical spells and ritual practices connected to conditions like insanity and epilepsy as well as remedies for introduced infections like pneumonia and dysentery. Epidemics were attributed to a spiritual power called Ave, whose coming was signaled by broken rainbows, shooting stars, red clouds, raindrops falling during sunshine, and also by the presence of fever, headache, and cough.[67] The impression conveyed by these accounts is of a community in which much effort was invested in protection from many sources of morbidity and mortality.

The impact of STIs was not emphasized by Rivers, but he reported their presence on Simbo ("both the chief forms"), and their symptoms were recorded in clinical detail by Hocart.[68] These graphic descriptions are enough to demonstrate a close knowledge by Simbo men of the effects of both gonorrhea and syphilis.[69] Gonorrhea was probably the more prevalent disease, as in New Ireland.[70] Rivers's own account from Simbo of sexual beliefs and practices before and after marriage indicate that any sexually transmitted infection would have quickly spread through the unmarried population.[71] He considered it "exceptional and almost certainly unknown in the past" that a woman remained a virgin before marriage, and having multiple sexual partners was an accepted and integral part of a young woman's puberty rituals. According to Hocart, if a slave captured in warfare was a woman, then "the owner may hire her out as a prostitute, which is no more than he does with his own daughters."[72]

It seems unlikely that white men in the nineteenth century were excluded in any way from sexual relations with Simbo women. After his 1908 fieldwork Hocart recalled that "one man sent word to a trader that his [female] slave was at his disposal," and many other unmarried women would also have been available for sexual intercourse.[73] As a result, widespread gonorrhea and, perhaps, syphilis infection were the likely outcomes. Whereas Rivers blamed women for securing their childlessness through induced abortion or contraception, it is more likely that STIs were achieving the same result.

We can conclude that in the western Solomons the effects of STIs on sterility and spontaneous abortions (miscarriages) were combined with the effects of epidemic disease on adult mortality. Such deaths resulted in many marriages being terminated by the loss of one spouse. As a result, fewer children were born, and inevitably there was some neglect of orphans. Finally, the high infant mortality rate among the small numbers of children born further reduced the population's capacity for replacement. The result was a decline that probably started before 1850 and accelerated in the last two decades of the nineteenth century.

Aphrodisian Cultures

Peter Pirie was the first scholar to postulate that the "degree of licentiousness . . . is a major geographical variable in the distribution of gonorrhea-related sub-fertility in the Pacific." He tested this idea with evidence from all corners of Polynesia, Micronesia, and Melanesia, concluding that lowered fertility should be added as a cause of population decline with STIs contributing to this process in many places.[74] Pirie's "licentiousness" was later termed "large-scale ritual promiscuity" when described for two societies in lowland New Guinea.[75] In Island Melanesia, ever since Bronislaw Malinowski's classic ethnography, the Trobriand Islands have provided the best-known example of the sexual freedom of unmarried women, especially in ritual contexts.[76] In Polynesia it is only Hawai'i that matches Tahiti in its reputation for ritualized promiscuity, following the rapturous reception extended to James Cook and his crews when they landed there in 1779.

To explain ritualized promiscuity in Hawai'i, Sahlins and Crosby pointed to the "Aphrodisian culture" of those islands.[77] Hawai'ian cosmology, ritual practices, and everyday behavior emphasized the celebration of women's sexuality and fertility, with dramatic effects on the transmission of STIs.[78] Crosby suggested that the white men in Hawai'i invariably misinterpreted sexual generosity as prostitution, which they "soon, by their expectations, made into just that."[79] Syphilis, gonorrhea, infertility, and severe depopulation soon followed.

In Island Melanesia John Cromar was one white man who took full advantage of the sexual freedom that he encountered in some Aphrodisian island societies. Cromar was a young Scottish sailor working on ships returning and recruiting labor for Queensland in the period 1882–86. He noted in relation to Aoba, New Hebrides, that "as in most native islands where customs of free-love exist the scourge of disease had made itself known." He reported that an infected man, or man and woman, would often volunteer as plantation laborers in Queensland (married couples could legally be recruited), in the hope and expectation that they might be cured by the white man's medicines. In Santa Ana, Solomon Islands, he also found "girls . . . whose freedom in matters of love was soon made very evident. . . . I am afraid that few of us were capable of resisting [their] seductive enchantment."[80]

Makira

In addition to Simbo and Santa Ana, there were some other places in the Solomons where the women acquired a reputation among white men for sexual generosity. These included Makira, the Roviana Lagoon in New Georgia, and the Shortland Islands group. On Makira Henry Guppy found in 1882 that "conjugal fidelity is usually preserved," but before marriage chastity was unknown: "For two or three years after a girl has become eligible for marriage, she distributes her favors amongst all of the young men of the village. Should she be unwilling to accept the addresses of anyone, it is but necessary for her admirer to make her parents some present. Fathers offer their daughters to the white man in the hope of a remunerative return."[81] The evidence suggests that whalers, traders, and labor recruiters took advantage of these opportunities on Makira and thereby introduced infections.[82] Woodford agreed with Guppy's STI diagnosis, observing that most STI cases that he saw in 1886–88 were "of a non-constitutional type, aggravated by filthy neglect"—that is, gonorrhea.[83] The Makira case shows that intensive contact with whalers and traders, when combined with puberty rituals in which sexual freedom was sanctioned, provided an effective way for STIs to spread quickly through an island community. As the Simbo case has shown, there were serious consequences for women's sterility, fetal miscarriages, and the birthrate.

Roviana Lagoon

Woodford did not visit Simbo or Makira in 1886–88, but he traveled elsewhere—for example, within the Roviana Lagoon, New Georgia—where he had many discussions with the resident traders. He noted in his diary for October 6, 1886, "The population here is said by the traders to be rapidly decreasing, nor is the reason far to seek. The women for some years before marriage are common property which naturally militates against their having children after marriage."[84] The statement is euphemistic, but the stated cause and supposed effect makes sense if STIs had become endemic in Roviana.

Woodford also noted rites of passage for young women similar to those described for Simbo (Rivers) and Makira (Guppy). His information came from conversations with Frank Wickham, a well-respected Englishman who had lived in Roviana Lagoon since about 1875 and was married to a local woman.[85] Woodford wrote in his diary, "Frank Wickham the trader . . . told me with reference to the treatment of women that when a girl arrives at the age of puberty she is known as Bimbolo having previously been a Vinéke. When she is Bimbolo she is temporarily a prostitute during a periodical feast or festival and is free to [word erased] all the men of the town she may choose. After this, should she be married she becomes a Bakalinge. There is another class of women chiefly slaves from Sambana [Santa Isabel] who are called Mangota and are prostitutes all their lives."[86] Hviding confirms the existence of these categories in both Roviana and Marovo but suggests the term *prostitute* is inappropriate for *bimbolo*.[87]

There was another New Georgia custom that Woodford regarded as problematic for birthrates, in a situation of increased adult mortality: "Neither widow nor widower can marry again without incurring the grave censure of the tribe." In addition, head-hunting was depopulating some islands by the scale of killings alone.[88] Scholars have pointed out that head-hunting escalated in the western Solomons when steel axes and firearms were acquired through trading.[89]

More than twenty years after his first visit, when the protectorate government had pacified the western Solomons by force and the Methodist Church was beginning to have influence, Woodford was pleased to note in the *Annual Report* that populations in the Roviana Lagoon were starting to increase.[90] To what extent did this change reflect a lower rate of transmission of STIs in Roviana following the abandonment of the sexual practices involving bimbolo? It seems more likely that the spread of Methodism was a slow process, and for a long time sexual behavior was unaffected. In 1908, after living there for six years, Rev. John Goldie wrote that "female chastity is not a very common virtue among the unmarried women and girls," although after marriage adultery if discovered was severely punished.[91] It is probable that populations started to increase in the early twentieth century because of fewer epidemics and lower infant mortality rather than an increased birthrate, but without census data we cannot test this idea.

Shortland Islands

Elsewhere, however, there were populations still in steady decline, including the Shortland Islands group. In 1901 Graham Officer, a museum collector from Melbourne, visited Fauro, the largest island in the group, and noted in his diary, "There are very few natives in Fauro although a large island. Disease (venereal) killed them off years ago."[92] Officer had been staying with the Atkinson family at Awa, a small island off Fauro, where Atkinson had been a trader and planter since 1895.[93] The Atkinsons would have been concerned about the local labor supply and probably were also well informed about such matters as STI prevalence. Woodford later alleged that "foeticide, infanticide and indiscriminate intercourse now prevail among the natives [of Shortland Islands] . . . to a terrible extent" and that as a result the population there was still in decline.[94]

The reputation of the Shortland Islands for STIs was long-established. Carl Ribbe reported that in the 1890s copper vitriol crystals (i.e., copper sulfate) were being sold by traders to the islanders to treat their venereal diseases, which, he said, were causing sterility and blindness.[95] In the wider world copper sulfate or bluestone was sometimes used in the treatment of venereal sores, both gonorrheal and syphilitic.[96] Treatment was painful, potentially toxic, and probably ineffective. Sarsaparilla was also widely used as a syphilis treatment before Salvarsan, but only a token amount ("2 cases") was listed among imports to Tulagi from Sydney in 1902–3.[97] We do not know who in Solomon Islands used sarsaparilla, nor for what purpose.

Although no longer a German colony, the Shortland Islands are also mentioned in the Deutsch-Neuguinea *Annual Report* for 1908–9: "The Shortland islands, which have been British since 1900, are infected with syphilis. Scarcely any children are born there any more. In former years there was a lively traffic between these islands and the south coast of Bougainville, mainly for the purpose of buying children for childless Shortland Islanders. Venereal diseases were also introduced [to Bougainville] by this traffic and syphilis is said to occur there fairly frequently."[98] Is it quite possible that some observers mistook yaws symptoms for syphilis, that copper sulfate or sarsaparilla was being used to treat yaws as well as venereal infections, and that a more hidden gonorrhea infection was the main cause of population decline in Shortland Islands. Without a convincing, retrospective medical diagnosis, these questions cannot be properly answered.

Non-Aphrodisian Cultures

Malaita

If Simbo, Makira, Roviana, and the Shortland Islands once had cultures that were, to some degree, Aphrodisian, can we assess the demographic effects of such cultural practices by looking at the experience of non-Aphrodisian cultures in Island Melanesia? The large island of Malaita in the central Solomons provides an obvious test case. In about 1884 John Cromar, who seems to have tried his luck with the girls almost everywhere he went, visited

Langalanga Lagoon, Malaita, where he met a returned Queensland laborer. The man spoke pidgin English and gave him a strong warning that the women of Malaita were "taboo":

> He went on to tell me that the sexual code of the Malaita people was an extremely rigid one, and that any infringement of it meant death to both parties. The single girls must remain virgins until marriage, and adultery was almost unknown on the island. He knew of the looseness of the inhabitants of other islands, and that women could be obtained in some places for a few sticks of tobacco, but the Malaita people held such things in abhorrence. The women occupied different living quarters from the men, even married folk living apart at night, and the women's house could not be entered by members of the male sex.[99]

Beliefs and practices of this kind did not help Malaitans to participate in the new opportunities for trade. With their women unavailable, and lacking local resources of turtle shells or coconut oil, Malaita had nothing to offer the whalers and traders.[100] The island soon gained a reputation for treachery and violence, as their leaders sought to obtain by force the trade goods that other islanders could gain in more legitimate ways.[101]

Later administrators and anthropologists have confirmed the non-Aphrodisian character of Malaitan cultures. In 1933 Ian Hogbin lived for six months among the To'ambaita people in north Malaita. He reported that premarital chastity was the norm for both sexes, partly because of a belief that the sexual act was injurious to men's potency but also because, if an illicit sexual liaison could be proved, the death penalty was imposed on the man who had seduced the girl or woman.[102] From his long experience among the Kwaio, last of the pagan bushmen of central Malaita, Roger Keesing claimed that while violence could erupt for many reasons, "most often killings on Malaita began with a violation of the strict sex code—with seduction or adultery."[103] According to another anthropologist Harold Ross, the Baegu men that he knew in 1966–68 "believe that the rest of the world is peopled by scarlet women and libertine men." Baegu women sometimes accused their husbands of going away not for migrant labor but to philander. The populations that Ross studied were vulnerable to epidemics, especially influenza, pneumonia, and dysentery, as well as endemic malaria, but their fertility rates were sufficient to allow mortality losses to be replaced.[104]

It seems likely that this relative isolation spared Malaita from many introduced diseases, at least until the onset of the labor trade in the late nineteenth century. In particular Malaitans were protected from the STIs that were helping to destroy some populations elsewhere. In the first colonial census of 1931, Malaita, with only 15 percent of the total land area of the protectorate (and much of it barren or mountainous), had over forty-one thousand people, or 44 percent, of its total population.[105] Its strict sexual codes (which still prevail today) seem the best explanation for its more successful engagement with "guns, germs and steel," preventing the influx of the germs of STIs in particular.

Guadalcanal

A second case is Guadalcanal, characterized by Charles Woodford as an island where "the greatest propriety prevails in the intercourse between the sexes."[106] During 1886–88 Woodford visited Guadalcanal three times, residing at Aola, north Guadalcanal, and collecting animal and plant specimens for a total of seven months, but neither in his diary nor in a later book did he report seeing any STI cases during that time.[107] Guadalcanal, like Malaita, retained a vigorous population, including inland groups seldom contacted by Europeans until the mid-twentieth century. Hogbin visited the interior of Guadalcanal several times in the period 1929–45, living with the Kaoka people in 1933. Among the Kaoka he found that premarital chastity was the norm and that married women were not promiscuous.[108] Both the geography of Guadalcanal and its non-Aphrodisian cultures seem to have provided an effective quarantine, at least until the destabilizing effects of the labor trade.

Depopulation and Cultural Practices

Island Melanesia is a region with very great cultural diversity between and even within islands. In this chapter I have argued that islands like Simbo, Makira, and the Shortlands were especially vulnerable to high levels of infection by STIs because they were "Aphrodisian cultures" (*sensu* Sahlins). The evidence compiled by Rivers demonstrated high levels of childlessness and low birthrates on these islands in the period circa 1870–1908, as well as heightened mortality from introduced infections. The "psychological" explanation that he offered for this situation can be rejected as implausible, in the light of historical evidence for the presence of STIs and the likelihood of their rapid spread and damaging effects on fertility. Other islands like Guadalcanal and Malaita experienced much less population decline. Although liable to heightened mortality following occasional epidemics of diseases like measles, influenza, and dysentery, the Malaita population in particular was able to recover because strict sexual codes prevented the influx of STIs, especially gonorrhea. I conclude that diminished fertility because of high rates of STI prevalence is indeed a factor hitherto underrated by historians. It is a process that helps to explain the widespread depopulation following European contact with Island Melanesia, and also why some islands experienced much more severe declines in population than others.

Notes

1. William H. R. Rivers, "The Dying Out of Native Races," *Lancet* 98 (1920): 42–44, 109–11; Rivers, "The Psychological Factor," in *Essays on the Depopulation of Melanesia*, ed. William H. R. Rivers (Cambridge: Cambridge University Press, 1922), 84–113.

2. Roy F. R. Scragg, *Depopulation in New Ireland: A Study of Demography and Fertility* (Port Moresby: Administration of Papua and New Guinea, 1954); Scragg, "Historical Epidemiology of Papua New Guinea," *Papua New Guinea Medical Journal* 20, no. 3 (1977): 108; Tim Bayliss-Smith, "Fertility and the Depopulation of Melanesia: Childlessness, Abortion and Introduced Disease in Simbo and Ontong Java, Solomon Islands," in *Population, Reproduction and Fertility in Melanesia*, ed. Stanley J. Ulijaszek (New York: Berghahn, 2005), 28–30. See also Roy F. R. Scragg, chap. 7, in this volume.

3. Bayliss-Smith, "Fertility and the Depopulation," in Ulijaszek, *Population, Reproduction and Fertility*, 35–37; Tim Bayliss-Smith, "Colonialism as Shell Shock: W. H. R. Rivers's Explanations for Depopulation in Melanesia," in *The Ethnographic Experiment: A. M. Hocart and W. H. R. Rivers in Island Melanesia, 1908*, ed. Edvard Hviding and Cato Berg (New York: Berghahn, 2014), 189–94.

4. Marshall D. Sahlins, *Islands of History* (Chicago: University of Chicago Press, 1985), 9.

5. Jared Diamond, *Guns, Germs and Steel: the Fates of Human Societies* (London: Cape, 1997).

6. Diamond, *Guns, Germs and Steel*, 191–214.

7. Alfred W. Crosby, *Germs, Seeds and Animals: Studies in Ecological History*, 2nd ed. (London: Routledge, 2015), 86.

8. James M. Blaut, *The Colonizer's Model of the World: Geographical Diffusionism and Eurocentric History* (New York: Guilford, 1993), 194.

9. David E. Stannard, *Before the Horror: The Population of Hawai'i on the Eve of Western Contact* (Honolulu: University of Hawai'i Press, 1989), 27–31.

10. Norma McArthur, *Island Populations of the Pacific* (Canberra: Australian National University Press, 1968), 281.

11. Peter Pirie, "The Effects of Treponematosis and Gonorrhoea on the Populations of the Pacific Islands," *Human Biology in Oceania* 1, no. 3 (1972): 202, 192–96. See also Stannard, *Before the Horror*, 69–77; Alfred W. Crosby, "Hawaiian Depopulation as a Model," in *Epidemics and Ideas: Essays on the Historical Perception of Pestilence*, ed. Terence Ranger and Peter Slack (Cambridge: Cambridge University Press, 1995), 175–202; and Patrick V. Kirch, "'Like Shoals of Fish': Archaeology and Population in Pre-Contact Hawai'i," in *The Growth and Collapse of Pacific Island Societies*, ed. Patrick V. Kirch and Jean-Louis Rallu (Honolulu: University of Hawai'i Press, 2012), 53.

12. Nicholas Thomas, *Colonialism's Culture: Anthropology, Travel and Government* (Cambridge: Polity, 1994), 112–23; Margaret Jolly, "Other Mothers: Maternal 'Insouciance' and the Depopulation Debate in Fiji and Vanuatu, 1890–1930," in *Maternities and Modernities: Colonial and Postcolonial Experiences in Asia and the Pacific*, ed. Kalpana Ram and Margaret Jolly (Cambridge: Cambridge University Press, 1998), 193.

13. Jolly, "Other Mothers," in Ram and Jolly, *Maternities and Modernities*, 192–97.

14. Florence Coombe, *Islands of Enchantment: Many-Sided Melanesia* (London: Macmillan, 1911), 67.

15. David Hilliard, *God's Gentlemen: A History of the Melanesian Mission, 1849–1942* (Saint Lucia: University of Queensland Press, 1978), 156–57.

16. Walter G. Ivens, *Melanesians of the South-East Solomon Islands* (London: Paul, Trench, Trubner, 1927), 44–45, 25.

17. Boyd T. Somerville, "Ethnographical Notes in New Georgia, Solomon Islands," *Journal of the Anthropological Institute of Great Britain and Ireland* 26 (1896): 410.

18. Norma McArthur, "The Demography of Primitive Populations," *Science* 167 (1970): 1099; McArthur, "And Behold the Plague Was Begun among the People," in *The Changing Pacific: Essays in Honour of H. E. Maude*, ed. Neil Gunson (Melbourne: Oxford University Press, 1978), 273–84; Tom Harrisson, *Savage Civilization* (New York: Knopf, 1937), 261.

19. Matthew J. T. Spriggs, *The Island Melanesians* (Oxford: Blackwell, 1997), 257–59; Spriggs, "Population in a Vegetable Kingdom: Aneityum Island (Vanuatu) at European Contact in 1830," in Kirch and Rallu, *Growth and Collapse*, 284.

20. Walter G. Ivens, *The Island Builders of the Pacific* (London: Seeley Service, 1930), 42.

21. Ivens, *Island Builders*, 47.

22. Ian Hogbin, *Experiments in Civilisation: The Effects of European Culture on a Native Community of the Solomon Islands* (London: Routledge, 1939), 127.

23. Rivers, "Dying Out"; Rivers, "Psychological Factor," in *Depopulation of Melanesia*, 84–113.

24. Hogbin, *Experiments in Civilisation*, 136; see also Scragg, chap. 7, in this volume.

25. Judith H. Underwood, "The Demography of a Myth: Abortion in Yap," *Human Biology in Oceania* 2, no. 2 (1973): 115–27; Judith A. Bennett, "A Vanishing People or a Vanishing Discourse? William H. R. Rivers's 'Psychological Factor' and Depopulation in the Solomon Islands and the New Hebrides," in Hviding and Berg, *Ethnographic Experiment*, 214–51.

26. Pirie, "Effects of Treponematosis," 188; David Wetherell, *Reluctant Mission: The Anglican Church in Papua New Guinea, 1891–1942* (Saint Lucia: University of Queensland Press, 1977), 224–29.

27. Bennett, "Vanishing People," 227–33.

28. Richard A. Herr, *A Solomons Sojourn: J. E. Philp's Log of the Makira, 1912–1913*, with E. Anne Rood (Hobart: Tasmanian Historical Research Association, 1978), 141, 142.

29. Pirie, "The Effects of Treponematosis," 188–89; Richard W. Hornabrook, in *Encyclopaedia of Papua New Guinea*, vol. 2, *L–Z*, ed. Peter Ryan (Melbourne: Melbourne University Press, 1972), 1108–9.

30. George R. Cannefax, "Immunity in Syphilis," *British Journal of Venereal Disease* 41 (1965): 265; James F. Jekel, "Role of Acquired Immunity to *T. pallidum* in the Control of Syphilis," *Public Health Reports* 83, no. 8 (1968): 632.

31. Charles M. Woodford, *A Naturalist among the Head-Hunters, Being an Account of Three Visits to the Solomon Islands in the Years 1886, 1887 and 1888* (London: Philip and Sons, 1890), 35.

32. Judith A. Bennett, *Wealth of the Solomons: A History of a Pacific Archipelago, 1800–1978* (Honolulu: University of Hawai'i Press, 1987), 29.

33. Henry B. Guppy, *The Solomon Islands and Their Natives* (London: Swan Sonneschein, 1887), 43.

34. Woodford, *Naturalist*, 36.

35. Guppy, *Solomon Islands*, 177.

36. Tim Bayliss-Smith and Judith Bennett, eds., *An Otago Storeman in Solomon Islands: The Diary of William Crossan Copra Trader, 1885–86* (Canberra: Australian National University Press, 2012), 48.

37. Raeburn Lange, "European Medicine in the Cook Islands," in *Disease, Medicine and Empire: Perspectives on Western Medicine and the Experience of European Expansion*, ed. Roy McLeod and Milton Lewis (London: Routledge, 1988), 72–73.

38. Robert H. Codrington, *The Melanesians* (Oxford: Clarendon, 1891), 12.

39. Jenny Hughes, "A History of Sexually Transmitted Diseases in Papua New Guinea," in *Sex, Disease and Society: A Comparative History of Sexually Transmitted Diseases and HIV/AIDS in Asia and the Pacific*, ed. Milton Lewis, Scott Bamber, and Michael Waugh (Westport: Greenwood, 1997), 231; Vicki Luker, "Papua New Guinea: Epidemiological Transitions, Public Health and the Pacific," in *Public Health in Asia and the Pacific: Historical and Comparative Perspectives*, ed. Milton J. Lewis and Kerrie L. MacPherson (Abingdon, UK: Routledge, 2008), 254.

40. Roy Scragg (email message to the author, September 24, 2018) suggests that in the Southwest Pacific endemic yaws provided acquired immunity to syphilis, so

the "syphilis" described in early sources must have been another of the STIs, either lymphogranuloma venerum or granuloma inguinale. Scragg's interpretation assumes that yaws infection in Melanesia was both widespread and pandemic.

41. Cited by Peter Corris, *Passage, Port and Plantation: A History of Solomon Islands Labour Migration, 1870–1914* (Carlton, Victoria: Melbourne University Press, 1973), 116.

42. Bennett, *Wealth of the Solomons*, 151.

43. See, for example, British Solomon Islands Protectorate, *Handbook of the British Solomon Islands Protectorate* (Tulagi: Government of the BSIP, 1911), 47.

44. Cited by Hilliard, *God's Gentlemen*, 157.

45. Sylvester M. Lambert, *A Doctor in Paradise* (London: Dent and Sons, 1941), 110.

46. Rivers, "Psychological Factor," in *Depopulation of Melanesia*, 99–101.

47. Rivers, "Psychological Factor," in *Depopulation of Melanesia*, 100–103.

48. William H. R. Rivers, "A Genealogical Method of Collecting Social and Vital Statistics," *Journal of the Royal Anthropological Institute* 2 (1900): 80–81.

49. Rivers, "Psychological Factor," in *Depopulation of Melanesia*, 97.

50. Bayliss-Smith, "Fertility and the Depopulation," in Ulijaszek, *Population, Reproduction and Fertility*, 27–32; Bayliss-Smith, "Colonialism as Shell Shock," in Hviding and Berg, *Ethnographic Experiment*, 184–95.

51. Rivers, "Psychological Factor," in *Depopulation of Melanesia*, 98.

52. Hortense Powdermaker, "Vital Statistics of New Ireland (Bismarck Archipelago) as Revealed in Genealogies," *Human Biology* 3, no. 3 (1931): 357.

53. Rivers, "Psychological Factor," in *Depopulation of Melanesia*, 98.

54. Colin H. Allen, *Report of the Special Lands Commission: Customary Land Tenure in the British Solomon Islands Protectorate* (Honiara: Western Pacific High Commission, 1957), 18–19; see also Scragg, chap. 7, in this volume.

55. Rivers, "Psychological Factor," in *Depopulation of Melanesia*, 101.

56. Bayliss-Smith, "Fertility and the Depopulation," in Ulijaszek, *Population, Reproduction and Fertility*, 35–38; Bayliss-Smith, "Colonialism as Shell Shock," in Hviding and Berg, *Ethnographic Experiment*, 192–210.

57. Ben Shephard, *A War of Nerves: Soldiers and Psychiatrists, 1914–1974* (London: Cape, 2000), 89–90.

58. Bayliss-Smith, "Colonialism as Shell Shock," in Hviding and Berg, *Ethnographic Experiment*, 191.

59. Bennett, *Wealth of the Solomons*, 386.

60. Harry T. Grenfell, "Australia Station: New Guinea and Solomon Islands, 1890; Correspondence Regarding Outrages by Natives on British Subjects," in *Annual Reports, Western Pacific High Commission* (Suva: Western Pacific High Commission, 1890), 7.

61. George Brown, *George Brown, D. D., Pioneer-Missionary and Explorer: An Autobiography* (London: Hodder and Stoughton, 1908), 516.

62. Thomas W. Edge-Partington, "Ingava, Chief of Rubiana, Solomon Islands: Died 1906; Extract from a Letter," *Man* 7 (1907): 22.

63. John F. Goldie, "News from the Solomon Islands," *Australasian Methodist Missionary Review* 13, no. 12 (1904): 11; John A. Crump, "Brief Mention," *Australasian Methodist Missionary Review* 14, no. 4 (1904): 1.

64. Edvard Hviding, "Across the New Georgia Group: A. M. Hocart's Fieldwork as Inter-Island Practice," in Hviding and Berg, *Ethnographic Experiment*, 85.

65. William H. R. Rivers, *Medicine, Magic, and Religion* (1924; repr., London: Routledge, 2001), 44; Rivers, "Sexual Relations and Marriage in Eddystone Island of the Solomons," in *Psychology and Ethnology*, ed. Grafton Elliot Smith (London: Paul, Trench, Trubner, 1926), 71–94.

66. Arthur M. Hocart, "The Cult of the Dead in Eddystone of the Solomons," pts. 1–2, *Journal of the Royal Anthropological Institute of Great Britain and Ireland* 52 (1922): 71–112, 259–305; Hocart, "Medicine and Witchcraft in Eddystone of the Solomons," *Journal of the Royal Anthropological Institute of Great Britain and Ireland* 55 (1925): 229–70; Hocart, "Warfare in Eddystone of the Solomon Islands," *Journal of the Royal Anthropological Institute of Great Britain and Ireland* 61 (1931): 301–24.

67. Rivers, *Medicine, Magic, and Religion*, 30–45.

68. Rivers, "Psychological Factor," in *Depopulation of Melanesia*, 101; Hocart, "Medicine and Witchcraft," 237.

69. Stanley J. Ulijaszek, letter to the author, 2004.

70. Scragg, *Depopulation in New Ireland*; Scragg, "Historical Epidemiology," 108; see also Scragg, chap. 7, in this volume.

71. Rivers, "Sexual Relations," in Smith, *Psychology and Ethnology*, 71–96.

72. Hocart, "Warfare in Eddystone," 306.

73. Hocart, "Warfare in Eddystone," 306.

74. Pirie, "Effects of Treponematosis," 188, 197.

75. Hughes, "Sexually Transmitted Diseases," in Lewis, Bamber, and Waugh, *Sex, Disease and Society*, 236.

76. Bronislaw Malinowski, *The Sexual Life of Savages in North-Western Melanesia* (London: Routledge and Paul, 1929); Adam Reed, "Contested Images and Common Strategies: Early Colonial Sexual Politics in the Massim," in *Sites of Desire, Economies of Pleasure: Sexualities in Asia and the Pacific*, ed. Lenore Manderson and Margaret Jolly (Chicago: University of Chicago Press, 1997), 49–51; Katherine Lepani, "Fitting Condoms on Culture: Rethinking Approaches to HIV Prevention in the Trobriand Islands, Papua New Guinea," in *Making Sense of AIDS: Culture, Sexuality and Power in Melanesia*, ed. Leslie Butt and Richard Eves (Honolulu: University of Hawai'i Press, 2008), 249–51.

77. Sahlins, *Islands of History*, 9; Crosby, *Germs, Seeds and Animals*, 135.

78. Stannard, *Before the Horror*; Crosby, "Hawaiian Depopulation," in Ranger and Slack, *Epidemics and Ideas*, 175–202.

79. Crosby, *Germs, Seeds and Animals*, 194.

80. John Cromar, *Jock of the Islands: Early Days in the South Seas* (London: Faber and Faber, 1935), 77, 132.

81. Guppy, *Solomon Islands*, 101.

82. Codrington, *Melanesians*, 12; Bennett, *Wealth of the Solomons*, 29.

83. Woodford, *Naturalist*, 35.

84. Charles Morris Woodford, "Diary from 4th August 1886 to November 10th 1886: Chas. M. Woodford F.R.G.S., Gravesend, England," October 6, 1886, Pacific Research Archives, Australian National University, Canberra, ANU 481.

85. Graeme A. Golden, *The Early European Settlers of the Solomon Islands* (Melbourne: privately printed, 1993), 206–7.

86. Charles Morris Woodford, "Diary Beginning 24 January 1887," March 15, 1887, Pacific Manuscripts Bureau, Australian National University, PMB 1290_Reel2_part2_G_Diary.

87. Edvard Hviding, email message to the author, October 2016. According to Hviding, a young girl in Roviana (*vineki*) had the potential to become bimbolo at puberty, but not all did so. Some bimbolo were the daughters of high-ranking men and were sought after as wives subsequent to having been bimbolo. While bimbolo they were treated with herbal medicines to avoid pregnancy but later could have many children once they became married women (Roviana *bari kalengge*). The institution of bimbolo disappeared with the end of head-hunting, as the favors of a bimbolo had been managed by the chief as one of the privileges of returned warriors.

88. Woodford, "Diary," March 15, 1887, Pacific Manuscripts Bureau.

89. John M. McKinnon, "Tomahawks, Turtles and Traders: A Reconstruction of the Circular Causation of Warfare in the New Georgia Group," *Oceania* 45 (1975): 290–307; Edvard Hviding and Tim Bayliss-Smith, *Islands of Rainforest: Agroforestry, Logging and Ecotourism in Solomon Islands* (Aldershot: Ashgate, 2000), 148–49.

90. Charles M. Woodford, *Colonial Reports: Annual; British Solomon Islands: Report to 30th June 1913* (London: His Majesty's Stationery Office, 1913), 5.

91. John F. Goldie, "The People of New Georgia: Their Manners and Customs, and Religious Beliefs," *Proceedings of the Royal Society of Queensland* 22 (1908): 28; David L. Hilliard, "Protestant Missions in the Solomon Islands, 1849–1942" (PhD diss., Australian National University, 1966), 266.

92. David R. Lawrence, *The Naturalist and His Beautiful Islands: Charles Morris Woodford in the Western Pacific* (Canberra: Australian National University Press, 2014), 214.

93. Golden, *Early European Settlers*, 360.

94. Woodford, *Colonial Reports* (1913), 5.

95. Carl Ribbe, *Zwei jahre unter den kannibalen der Salamo-inseln* (Dresden: Bayer, 1903), 67–68, 70, 274; Bennett, *Wealth of the Solomons*, 98–99; Judith A. Bennett, "Gorai and Population Decline in the Shortlands: A Reply to Peter Sack," *Journal of Pacific History* 41, no. 1 (2006): 100; Peter Sack, "Who Wants to Know What 'Really' Happened? 'King' Gorai and the Population Decline in the Shortland Islands," *Journal of Pacific History* 40, no. 3 (2005): 347.

96. Maganlal P. Vora, "Treatment of Venereal Sores," *Medical Bulletin* (Bombay), 8, no. 14 (1940): 466; Corris, *Passage, Port and Plantation*, 58; Peter H. H. A. Dollwet and John R. J. Sorenson, "Historic Uses of Copper Compounds in Medicine," *Trace Elements in Medicine* 2, no. 2 (1985): 80–87; Thomas Power Lowry, *Venereal Diseases and the Lewis and Clark Expedition* (Lincoln: University of Nebraska Press, 2004), 44.

97. Charles M. Woodford, *Colonial Reports: Annual. No. 774; British Solomon Islands: Report for 1902–1903* (London: His Majesty's Stationery Office, 1903), 12.

98. Peter Sack and Dymphna Clark, *German New Guinea: the Annual Reports* (Canberra: Australian National University Press, 1979), 298.

99. Cromar, *Jock of the Islands*, 137.

100. Bennett, *Wealth of the Solomons*, 30–31, 120–21.

101. Clive Moore, "The Misappropriation of Malaitan Labour: Historical Origins of the Recent Solomon Islands Crisis," *Journal of Pacific History* 42 (2007): 214.

102. Hogbin, *Experiments in Civilisation*, 47, 98.

103. Roger M. Keesing and Peter Corris, *Lightning Meets the West Wind: The Malaita Massacre* (Melbourne: Oxford University Press, 1980), 18.

104. Harold M. Ross, *Baegu: Social and Ecological Organization in Malaita, Solomon Islands* (Urbana: University of Illinois Press, 1973), 67, 42, 100–101.

105. Moore, "Misappropriation of Malaitan Labour," 214.

106. Woodford, *Naturalist*, 35.

107. Woodford, "Diary," 1886, Pacific Research Archives; Woodford, "Diary," 1887, Pacific Manuscripts Bureau.

108. Ian Hogbin, *A Guadalcanal Society: The Kaoka Speakers* (New York: Holt, Rinehart and Winston, 1964), 21–22.

Chapter Seven

Community Infertility in Papua New Guinea

Uncovering the Role of Gonorrhea

Roy F. R. Scragg

Population Decline in New Ireland, Papua New Guinea

In this chapter I discuss my own research and clinical experiences in Papua New Guinea, where I worked between 1947 and 1974 and had subsequent visits up until 1987, studying the relationship between community infertility and the prevalence of gonorrhea. Its particular significance for this volume is that this was the first time that a rigorous and systematic clinical and medical examination had been performed on a population suffering from widespread infertility to determine whether psychosocial factors or STIs—and specifically gonorrhea—were the source of the community's infertility. Gonorrhea was, indeed, found to be the cause in the Tabar Islands, and the hypothesis was confirmed by a concurrent program of universal penicillin distribution throughout the Tabar population resulting in a remarkable rebound in fertility and a reversal of the population decline.

I was born in New Zealand, and through to my graduation in medicine had regular contact with Pacific Islanders and missionaries. However, my engagement with New Guinea research began by chance. Medical interns without a family medical background were and are influenced by the role models presented by their teachers. My future career was subtly influenced by Sir John Cleland, professor of pathology, who had studied and written extensively on anthropology and Australian Aboriginal health. He offered me a medical research position in Arnhem Land, but I saw medical positions available in the Territory of Papua and New Guinea. In August 1947 I became the thirteenth medical officer to be appointed after World War II, to a country where the fortunate were receiving medical care from barefoot orderlies, but many others had no medical contact.

There were no numerators or denominators to measure the impact of endemic and introduced diseases on the inhabitants of this tropical environment. In 1948, as medical officer at Sohano on Buka Island, a large island just north of Bougainville Island, I set about establishing medical records and genealogies of two Buka communities: Lemankoa, a large village of the Haku tribe on the northwest coast; and villages of the inland Solas people along the Gagan River. I had access to the birth, death, and marriage records collected by Catholic missionaries since 1915, which were preserved in bound volumes that had been wrapped in banana leaves and hidden in caves during the war.

In 1950 I was in Sydney completing studies at the School of Public Health for my diploma of tropical medicine and hygiene, when Dr. John Gunther, director of public health in Papua New Guinea, wrote, advising me, "You should become District Medical Officer, New Ireland . . . where there has been frank depopulation of 27% in twenty years and such a state of affairs needs early and rapid correction. Much research has been done there recently in a repeat demographic survey by Mr Chinnery."[1]

Ernest W. P. Chinnery and Edwin Holland had done a demographic study of the declining population of the east coast of New Ireland in 1929. Holland reported that "sterility in one or both partners is common. Thus of 3,073 unions investigated in 1929, 835 were fruitless."[2] He knew that an earlier campaign to treat gonorrhea had revealed high levels of infection and suggested that childlessness was one likely outcome, but he also emphasized social factors. He was concerned that "sexual abstinence in early pregnancy and during the long period of lactation . . . is considered to be necessary for the good of the child, [but] as a cause of infidelity in the male is a fertile cause of divorce, and consequently of a low birth rate."[3]

Historical Evidence for Gonorrhea

After Jacques Schouten and Willem Le Maire arrived, followed by Abel Tasman in the early seventeenth century, the coconut-treed islands to the northwest and the northeast of New Guinea were regularly visited by explorers. From the mid-nineteenth century men from the Bismarck Archipelago and particularly New Ireland were blackbirded or recruited to sustain the economic development of New Guinea, Samoa, and North Queensland.

The German government formally annexed northeast New Guinea and the Bismarck Archipelago in 1884. The German and other settlers were mainly unattached men, as the then governing private company considered the conditions too harsh for European married couples and single women. Between 1887 and 1897 deaths of Europeans were 106 males but only 9 females and 4 children, indicating the demographic scene.[4] The Germans also brought in male Chinese and Malay workers to speed their development of mainland New Guinea.

New Ireland was the only district where single women were permitted by law to be indentured to work with single male employers. New Ireland women had a reputation for promiscuous behavior, dating back to the first physical contact with explorers, matching that of the women of Tahiti and Hawai'i. Stewart Firth has shown that from 1905 to 1907 recruiters shipped 475 women from New Ireland for employment in the Gazelle Peninsula of New Britain and in Madang, and another 150 New Ireland women were employed elsewhere in the colony and in Samoa. They worked as plantation laborers, household servants, and concubines.[5] In the official publications of German New Guinea, there is no mention of the recently discovered link between gonorrhea and fertility, but population decline was noted in New Ireland and localities in other colonies with high rates of infection.

It is clear that gonorrhea had significant prevalence in German New Guinea from at least the 1880s. Admissions to the government native hospitals in the Gazelle Peninsula show venereal disease prevalence averaging 5 percent from 1903 to 1909 and 11 percent from 1909 to 1912.[6] The administration's *Annual Report* for 1898–99 records, "As regards venereal disease, it is reported that gonorrhea is the most prevalent and is widespread over the whole [Bismarck] Archipelago. The [German north] Solomon Islands are still comparatively free of this disease. It is extraordinarily difficult to take measures against it."[7]

Statistics on the STIs treated in New Guinea hospitals were collected and published annually from 1903 to 1912.[8] The record is patchy, with no cases reported in some districts in some years. Over the whole nine-year period,

27 Europeans and 118 indigenes were treated for syphilis, and 96 Europeans and 603 indigenes were treated for gonorrhea.[9] The majority of the gonorrhea patients were in Rabaul. The diagnosis of syphilis must be questioned, as yaws was a universal disease, and over my six years there before community-wide penicillin was used, I saw only one European, but no indigenes, with syphilis. Their actual diagnosis must have been either granuloma venereum or yaws.[10]

In 1911–12 the medical statistics collected by Dr. Willi Hoffman showed that syphilis and gonorrhea were much more prevalent in male plantation laborers near Kavieng Station compared to places in New Ireland farther away.[11] Diseases in the village people were rarely reported, and as the 1912 German New Guinea *Annual Report* states, "The white doctor is a figure inspiring not trust but terror. At his approach the patients will flee into the bush."[12] The women hid themselves when they thought they would be examined by the patrolling doctor.

Professor Robert Koch assessed European mortality in German New Guinea in 1899–1900. His protégé, Paul Ehrlich, ensured that German New Guinea received an adequate quantity of salvarsan when he sent the medication worldwide in 1910. British Papua did not receive this medication until 1920. German archives mention an immediate change of attitude of the native people when it was used for the treatment of yaws. The results were dramatic, "contributing greatly to creating trust in European doctors and healing methods so much so that natives suffering from yaws began to seek medical aid without pressure, even people from remote areas with very little contact with whites."[13]

Low birthrates and small family size were common in all villages except those on Buka Island and Gazelle Peninsula. These were ascribed to inbreeding, birth control, infanticide, abortion, and high infant mortality—all the responsibility of New Guineans. On the other hand, venereal disease was reported as being present mainly in laborers living in villages adjoining the settlements. Reports written by the physicians serving the Kokopo and Rabaul communities from 1896 indicate a controversy over the importance of the preexisting conditions and environment as opposed to the diseases, particularly venereal, accompanying colonization.

In 1914 Dr. Ludwig Kulz, as preparation for his appointment as director of health, patrolled extensively in the Gazelle Peninsula and northern New Ireland. Margrit Davies extracted unpublished statistics collated by Kulz as a member of a medico-demographic research team in 1913:

> A sample of 154 women (past childbearing age) had born 394 children. With an infant mortality rate of 35%, a woman raised on average 1.7 children. This low figure clearly indicated that the population was declining. Kulz ascribed this in no uncertain terms to the consequences of excessive recruitment especially that of women, and argued that up to 1909, when mainly single women were recruited from New Ireland, their recruitment had been a form of prostitution. . . . Of 220 married couples, those in which neither partner had been recruited had nearly twice as many children as those where one or both partners have been away on plantations work.[14]

The *Annual Report* of the colony reported in 1909–10 that in Kavieng, the district's capital, "a general program of treatment of the free natives [Melanesians who were not plantation laborers] for venereal disease has been initiated."[15] This program used salvarsan and neosalvarsan that Ehrlich had distributed worldwide. It must be one of the first community-wide campaigns against yaws and syphilis ever attempted, predating anything equivalent in British or French colonies.

It was reported the following year that "Unfortunately there are still signs of a rapid decline in population in the whole of Neu Mecklenberg [New Ireland]."[16]

Dr. Willy Wick, in his 1914 memorandum on the care of workers in German New Guinea, reported that "almost all [unmarried female indigenes] become infected with venereal disease during their contract period—they are actually nothing other than prostitutes (*puellae publicae*)."[17] Recruitment of women from New Ireland did not cease with the end of the German colony; it continued under the Australian administration. An ordinance in March 1917 permitted lonely white men to get special exemptions to employ women; renewal of three-year contracts allowed this behavior to continue until the mid-1920s.[18] These men came from Europe, Southeast Asia, and Australia and would have brought to New Guinea all the then existing STIs from their homelands. At the end of their indenture, the return of these women to their home villages in New Ireland set the scene for the rapid population decline that was found in 1950.

Research in the Interwar Period

In 1914 the German administration was dissolved, and in 1920 the League of Nations Trust Territory became the responsibility of Australia. There was an effective exchange of information on health between the two administrations, and there was also new research.[19] As well as Chinnery and Holland, in 1929 Hortense Powdermaker, a Harvard anthropologist, began work in eastern New Ireland and made her own assessment of the region's historical epidemiology. Based on the reconstructed vital statistics for the village of Lesu, her data showed low birthrates, increasing infant mortality rates, and high levels of childlessness, especially among women in her "Generation II," the cohort born around the 1860s and 1870s. While not discounting the role of other diseases, she pointed out that gonorrhea could have resulted in these women's sterility. She noted that in 1928–29 more than half of the 442 gonorrhea cases reported in the Territory of New Guinea were in New Ireland District. However, these treated cases were mostly male plantation workers seen in "native hospitals," for example, at Kavieng in New Ireland.[20] The first clinical investigations of infertile women in New Guinea ever undertaken were by Dr. Phyllis Cilento in the Western Islands in 1927. Cilento examined 40 women of Auna and reported, "of 40 women inspected 21 showed retroversion, retroflection or other malposition of the uterus, while 13 showed severe transverse tears of the cervix."[21]

In 1949 Chinnery revisited the New Ireland eastern coast and reported no change in the rate of population decline.[22] The general decline of many populations in the Pacific was a phenomenon already known to professors at the Sydney School of Public Health, but they considered it to be a psychosocial problem, not a medical one. The diploma course in tropical medicine and hygiene did not include any lectures from anthropologists or sociologists, but all Australian administration appointees attended lectures given by members of the Sydney University Department of Anthropology.

There had in fact been a long history of official concern about the decline of population in many Pacific Islands. Since the late nineteenth century it had been most obvious in the smaller islands; in the larger ones any local decline was imperceptible, because of replacement migration from nearby villages. Depopulation was most severe in western Melanesia, where there was high mortality from malaria, but it had occurred also in Fiji, the easternmost of the Melanesian Islands.[23] In 1893 the Fijian colonial government set up a commission to inquire into remedies for population decline. Their report included thirty-six recommendations, many of which were directed at socioeconomic problems: those related to health included infant and maternal care, sanitation, and diet. The problem of low fertility is only hinted at in the recommendation to facilitate miscegenation through marriage and the relaxation of laws against fornication and adultery.[24]

Many of the thirty-six socioeconomic measures listed in the Fiji recommendations of 1893 became part of government policy in both Papua and New Guinea. As the Pacific War of 1941–45 came and went, the population decline in New Ireland District continued and social interventions were expanded by the Australian administration in an endeavor to reverse all possible social and environmental causes.[25] The public health service had no special program for the management of STI's before, during, or after the war.

The Influence of William H. R. Rivers

In 1898 Arthur C. Haddon organized the famous Cambridge University Anthropological Expedition to the Torres Strait, which became the first large-scale field study of "primitive" societies.[26] The participants included William H. R. Rivers and Charles Seligman: both left England as physicians and experimental psychologists, and both metamorphosed into anthropologists. Rivers went on to develop strong links between anthropology and psychiatry in his studies of societies in both India and the Solomon Islands. In 1914 he was completing a genealogical and anthropological assessment of the people in depopulating communities in the New Hebrides (today's Vanuatu) when the outbreak of World War I interrupted his studies. He returned to Europe, where he became involved in the pioneer diagnosis and treatment of the psychological damage of "shell shock."[27]

After the war Rivers returned to Melanesian studies, but not to Melanesia, interpreting the infertility he had observed there against Freudian concepts of psychiatry.[28] He decided that under colonialism the contact between cultures had resulted in depression among the indigenous peoples, which caused cohabiting couples to avoid conception and, if conception did occur, to abort the fetus. He did not consider that the depression that he had observed might have resulted from the distress felt by couples when they had no offspring. Rivers's psychosomatic view of the low fertility that he documented did, however, include elements that were close to ideas offered by the peoples themselves, as rationalizations of their infertility.[29]

This bias may reflect the fact that Rivers's medical education had taken place in Britain in the 1880s, when the role of gonorrhea as a cause of infertility was controversial. In 1838 Philippe Ricord had described the clinical difference between gonorrhea and syphilis.[30] In 1857 Gustave Bernutz and Ernest Goupil found gonorrheal infections of the fallopian tubes, ovaries, and the pelvic peritoneum.[31] In 1876 Emil Noeggerath described "latent gonorrhea" damaging women's fertility, and in 1879 Albert Neisser identified the organism causing gonorrhea infection.[32] In spite of these discoveries, there was still in the 1880s a serious controversy, which continued in Britain through to 1910, among gynecologists over the existence of "latent gonorrhea."[33]

It was only these cultural and behavioral aspects of observed infertility, not its physical causes, that came to dominate Rivers's views, reflecting the focus of his overlapping careers in experimental psychology and shell-shock psychiatry.[34] Before he died in 1922, Rivers edited the *Essays on the Depopulation of Melanesia* that included his chapter on *The Psychological Factor*. This study revealed that the scale of the childlessness he had found in certain islands of the New Hebrides and western Solomons was at the same level as that later found by Chinnery and Powdermaker in New Ireland.[35] In Rivers's view involuntary infertility from any cause such as gonorrhea was "trivial or of slight importance":

> It is well known that certain forms of venereal disease will produce sterility. . . . There is little doubt however that if we take Melanesia as a whole, causes of this kind are trivial or of slight importance as compared with voluntary restriction. Throughout Melanesia the people are acquainted with various means of producing abortion and also practice measures which they believe to prevent conception, and processes of this kind almost certainly form the main agencies in lowering the birth rate. We have here only another effect of the loss of interest in life which I've held to be so potent in enhancing mortality. The people say to themselves "Why should we bring children into the world only to work for the white man?" Measures which before the coming of the European were used chiefly to prevent illegitimacy have become the instrument of racial suicide.[36]

In his review of population problems of the Pacific, the historian Stephen H. Roberts mentioned many reasons for decline but concluded, along with Rivers, that "the physical causes were contributory to the wider psychological ones, or agencies through which these latter worked, but the root of the matter lay with that curious despair which dominated the native mind and colored his every thought and action."[37] Another influential armchair theorist was George Pitt-Rivers, who in 1927 pointed to the destruction of rituals and cultural institutions such as magic and gift exchange in Melanesia, resulting in boredom and loss of joie de vivre following European contact. He suggested that, even if indigenous sexual practices were unaffected, women's emotional lives had been disturbed, causing problems of ovulation and conception.[38]

Rivers's theory connected what he thought he had found in Melanesia in his field trips of 1908 and 1914 to what he observed in hospitals that treated patients for shell shock, such as Maghull and Craiglockart. In both cases he believed that the symptoms of disturbance could be reversed only by social rather than physical interventions.[39] Rivers's authority in the academic world persuaded social scientists of all disciplines and many governments. His psychological theory envisaged that women were using their own contraceptives and abortifacients in a manner handed down by the older women. However, in areas with declining population, other anthropologists, physicians, and colonial administrators thought that venereal disease was the main problem, with infertility seen increasingly as being mainly involuntary.[40] There was a suggested link to the prevalence of gonorrhea, but there was no supporting medical evidence.

New Ireland

In 1950 in Port Moresby, en route to Kavieng, I read Dr. Willi Hoffman's report on his medical surveys of 1911–12 among the New Ireland people. He reported that among the 6,781 inhabitants there had been 184 deaths but only 60 births and that it was shocking at the "line-up" of village populations to discover how many marriages of long standing were childless. Even in fruitful marriages the number of children did not usually exceed three, and only one old man had the maximum number of children: seven. The extent of the infertility that Hoffman described indicated to me that the population decline on New Ireland had started at least forty years earlier. Dr. Hoffman in 1912 managed to examine men only, and he found 5 percent infected with gonorrhea and 2.5 percent with syphilis. He reported that salvarsan and neosalvarsan, Ehrlich's "magic bullets," were in use and were an effective treatment for yaws.[41]

I arrived in Kavieng, the district capital at the northeastern tip of New Ireland, in September 1950; at that time Chinese, European, and New Guinean people lived in separate settlements. Kavieng had its own airport, and the 140-mile East Coast Road, the longest road in the territory, linked Kavieng to Namatanai, where there was another doctor (see figure 7.1). I found the New Ireland people to be more westernized than those on the New Guinea mainland or in Bougainville. Most of those attending the Kavieng hospital came from the Tigak villages surrounding the town. I immediately set about collecting comparable demographic data for the Tigak people with that which I already held from the Buka villages. I quickly confirmed the high level of infertility reported by Chinnery.[42]

I had not been there long when a young village woman presented with an ectopic pregnancy. I had not seen this condition in my two years at Lae, Rabaul, and Sohano. Shortly afterward another case presented, and I wrote up these two unusual cases for publication: my first medical communication.[43]

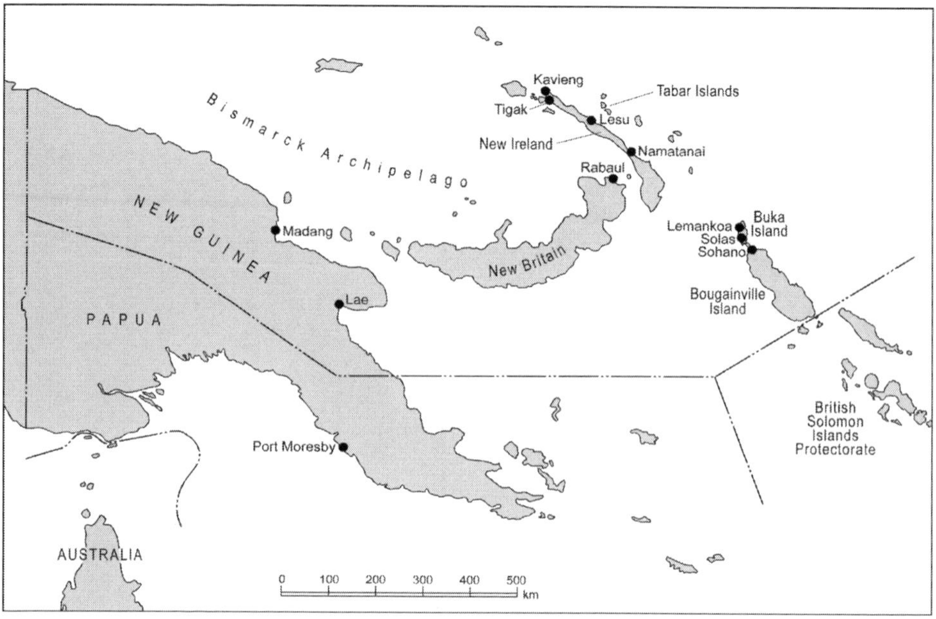

Figure 7.1. Northeast New Guinea and the Bismarck Archipelago, showing the location of Lemankoa and Solas on Buka Island; Tigak and Lesu on New Ireland; and the Tabar Islands. Map drawn by Philip Stickler, Department of Geography, University of Cambridge.

If these had occurred in a medically isolated village, at least two out of three would have died of internal hemorrhage. I also treated several cases of pelvic inflammatory disease, confirming an unusual frequency of conditions often linked to gonorrhea. Adequate penicillin was available to treat these and other infections.

These events are consistent with the progression of a gonorrheal infection from the vagina to the peritoneum. When the ovum is produced it cannot implant in a genital tract infected with gonorrhea. Occasionally it is caught in adhesions in the salpingeal tube, and ectopic pregnancy results. Over time the salpingeal tube is blocked and primary infertility is established. Almost all births occurred unsupervised in the villages, and none of the infants presented with ophthalmia neonatorum.

Tabar Islands

The Tabar Islands are a small group of raised coral and volcanic islands situated twenty-five miles northeast of New Ireland. The islanders speak an Austronesian language and had traditional links with the rest of New Ireland through trade networks, marriage, and ritual connections. In particular, the *malanggan* tradition of Tabar, most of which is thought to have originated there, is shared by six other mainland groups, including the Tigak.[44] In 1929 Powdermaker saw the *malanggan* rituals celebrated in the village of Lesu, on the southern New Ireland coast opposite Tabar, involving "dancing [that] continues throughout the night, and ends with some of the women having intercourse with the men who have been watching them. . . . The taboo against sexual relationship between members of the same moiety holds."[45] At Lesu, even in everyday life, both husbands and wives were free to have extramarital affairs, and there was no social stigma in having lovers.[46] People in Tabar shared many of these beliefs and practices, as revealed in many of the interviews that Ian Downs carried out in 1949.[47] As mentioned earlier the women of Tabar had become well known for their sexual availability.

Direct contact with European whalers and traders did not begin until the mid-nineteenth century. Seven coconut plantations were established by European or Asian planters in the late 1800s. In 1950 there was a European priest at the Catholic mission station on Mapua Island (the very small fourth island of the group), with a small airstrip and a government school with a European teacher on Tatau Island. There were only two resident planters and a few laborers from New Guinea. Each of the three main islands had an aid post, and a trained orderly regularly visited from Kavieng.

The German administration estimated a population of 8,000 in 1908, when the population was already declining.[48] The number enumerated had declined to 5,766 in 1911.[49] I have proposed there were probably 12,000 people living in the Tabar group around 1850.[50] The many vacant village sites confirm there was a much larger population than the 1,462 people counted by me in 1951.[51] It would appear that the total population may have halved every thirty-three years over the ten decades since 1850, representing a persistent yearly decline averaging 3 percent.

The seemingly inevitable extinction of the Tabar people moved the South Pacific Commission to provide a community development grant to support frequent administrative visits, increased medical services, agricultural experiments, a cooperative program, and a resident European teacher. As part of this special attention, in April 1950 Gunther wrote that he had "started something—I doubt whether it will have any significance, but it might give some answers. We are giving every man, woman and child on Tabar 200,000 units of penicillin whether they want it or not."[52] In 1950 all adults of procreative age received a course of penicillin in oil, neoarsphenamine, and sulfamerazine.[53] This use of the antibiotic on the Tabar Islands was possibly the first community penicillin campaign in the world.

Investigation of Infertility

In July 1951 I interviewed men and women in every family in the Tabar group and recorded medical, genealogical, and demographic data to collate and compare with that collected among the Tigak and on Buka. The Tabar villagers were very cooperative, in their hope that the doctor could do something that would bring them children to ensure their survival as a community. The infertility of Tabar women was highest among the twenty-six women still alive who had been born in the nineteenth century, fifty years or more before my census. Nineteen of these twenty-six women were childless (primary infertility), five had one child, one had two children, and only one had the expected eight children. On average women who do not undergo the risk of childbirth live longer. Overall, my survey showed that 30 percent of Tabar unions were childless and another 15 percent had not borne a child for over seven years and were under forty-five years (secondary infertility): a combined childlessness of 45 percent in comparison to the Buka villages, with only 4 percent in Lemankoa and 9 percent in Solas.[54]

In view of these significant differences, I decided to investigate eighty couples drawn from both areas in New Ireland (Tabar Islands and Tigak on the mainland) in the same manner as infertile couples were being investigated in fertility clinics around the world at that time. In due course I examined 120 men to determine the level of their fertility, but it was not practical to bring in the wives of all these men for investigation. The wives of 68 of the 120 men were examined, plus 18 others whose husbands were not seen. The women were aged twenty-three to forty three years. In a sample of 20 women I carried out uterine curettage. A social and medical history was collected and a physical examination was done on all the couples selected. On average husbands were at least five years older than their wives. The men provided semen for microscopy and a testicular biopsy was made on 97. Of the males examined: 56 had normal fertility, 21 were subfertile, and 20 were sterile.[55]

The basal temperature of 39 women was recorded, and of these 30 had an ovulatory peak. Gross adnexal disease was found in 20 percent of the 86 women examined and uterine displacements in 26 percent. A total of seventy-nine lipiodol hysterosalpingograms showed tubal occlusion in 53, the majority of which had fimbrial obstruction with hydrosalpinx. Of the women studied on Tabar, only 7 became pregnant after the investigation. In these women fimbrial adhesions have been broken through by the pressure used in injecting lipiodol. Gonorrheal infection was found in 14 percent of the women from the New Ireland mainland, none of whom had previously received an injection of penicillin.

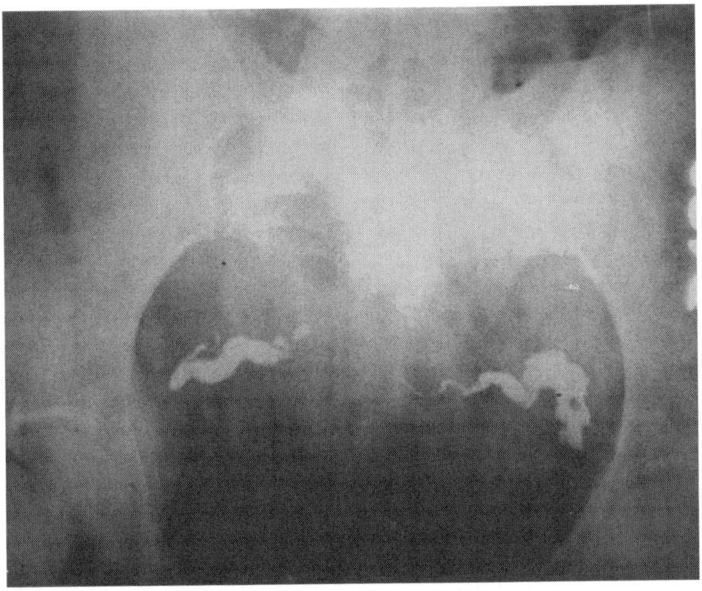

Figure 7.2. X-ray photograph showing bilateral hydrosalpinx due to distally blocked fallopian tubes with retained lipiodol twenty-four hours after injection through the uterine cervix. Lipiodol (Ethiodol in the United States) is an iodized oil used as a radio-opaque contrast agent. This twenty-eight-year-old woman from Tabar had been married ten years and had never been pregnant. Her husband was fertile. Curettage showed secretory endometrium. Gonorrheal infection is the explanation for her childlessness. Photography by the author.

Overall, 80 percent of all the couples investigated had at least one physical reason for their childlessness, and in every case psychological factors could be discounted. No person from Tigak or Tabar had knowledge of an effective contraceptive or abortifacient medicine, contrary to the received wisdom of missionaries, William H. R. Rivers, and others. I found that the main cause of their sterility was tubal occlusion in women as a result of untreated gonorrheal salpingitis and pelvic peritonitis (figure 7.2).[56]

The penicillin injection given to every person on the Tabar Islands in 1950 caused a subsequent resurgence in births, which equaled deaths in 1951 and thereafter exceeded deaths.[57] The evidence became overwhelming that a gonococcal infection, which had first been identified as the principal cause of fallopian tube obstruction in the Western world in 1857, was the main cause of low fertility and depopulation in New Ireland District. In my three-year engagement with the Tigak and Tabar people, it seemed very likely that the frequency of sexual intercourse matched other societies, with comparable symptoms of divorce, extramarital affairs, ectopic pregnancies, and pelvic inflammatory disease. In particular this three-year study indicated that traditional contraceptives and abortifacients were almost certainly nonexistent. It also negated the possibility that either tuberculosis or the yet-to-be-discovered chlamydia was the cause of the infertility, as neither organism would have been eradicated from the community by penicillin.

In 1953 I resurveyed the Buka villages of the Solas people and Lemankoa and collated all the data from the four populations studied from 1948 to 1953. I measured the height, weight, and dental formula of the children in these villages and prepared tables to improve the accuracy of the age data of the New Ireland children. An analysis of the mortality and fertility disclosed four differing demographic patterns. The greatest difference that I found was between Lemankoa and Tabar, which represent the fertility extremes of the communities. Over the initial survey period to 1953, Lemankoa had a crude birthrate of fifty-five and a crude death rate of fifteen, compared to twenty-two and twenty-six in Tabar. In all documented studies of the Tabar people before 1950, only 20 percent of the population was under fifteen years, compared to 50 percent in Lemankoa. Of all communities studied, the six Solas villages in inland Buka had the highest crude birthrate of fifty-seven, generated by the short birth interval after infant deaths attributable to hyperendemic malaria as part of the highest crude death rate of forty. Nowhere were death rates high enough to be a causal factor in depopulation.

The demography of the four communities on Buka (Lemankoa and Solas villages) and New Ireland (Tigak villages and Tabar Islands) were regularly recorded at visits through to 1987. In 1973 the ASFRs for the quinquennial periods from 1947 to 1967 were published. The data showed that after the Tigak people had penicillin in 1952, their fertility rate and that of Tabar had risen to exceed that of the Buka communities.[58]

The age-specific fertility rate (ASFR) in 1953 and 1987 of five-year cohorts of both Lemankoa and Tabar women have been collated for table 7.1. The 1953 ASFR for the thirty-five- to thirty-nine-year-old Tabar women born 1914 to 1918 was only 10 percent of the same cohort in the village of Lemankoa, Buka.[59] The 1987 ASFR for all cohorts younger than thirty-five years in Tabar, who were virgins when they had penicillin in 1950, are not significantly different from that of their contemporaries in Lemankoa. Clearly, gonorrheal infection rates and medical treatments for all cohorts were radically different in these two communities in 1953.

The conundrum was solved, and the doctors working in the community were shown to have been correct. Gonorrhea was proven to be the cause of this severe and widespread infertility in the Tigak and isolated Tabar

Table 7.1. Comparison of age-specific fertility rates for Lemankoa on Buka Island and Tabar Islands east of New Ireland

Age group	Lemankoa 1953	Lemankoa 1987	Tabar Islands 1953	Tabar Islands 1987
15 to 19	133	5	95	139
20 to 24	317	126	144	195
25 to 29	232	251	117	276
30 to 34	446	256	50	262
35 to 39	354	230	35	176
40 to 44	38	100	13	90
45 to 49	0	67	0	38
Total fertility rate	7.594	5.174	2.269	5.880

communities. This previously unrecognized phenomenon is best described as "community infertility." The longitudinal study shows that gonorrhea, introduced early in the history of contact by both Asian and European immigrants, infected both the men and women they employed, who in due course returned to their home villages. Its spread was then facilitated by social customs encouraging relatively high promiscuity and the increasing instability of marriages in New Ireland society.[60] The gonococcus was hidden in the bodies of those who first brought it to the islands, and it triggered an epidemic that continued as an unrecognized endemic disease in the Tabar community for almost a hundred years. Penicillin eradicated gonorrhea from the bodies of those carrying a latent gonorrheal infection and reversed the decline in population.

WHO Scientific Group

In 1974 I was visiting my Papua New Guinea colleagues who had become WHO advisers in Geneva. My visit chanced to coincide with a meeting of the WHO Scientific Group on the Epidemiology of Infertility. I was invited to attend one of their meetings and respond to questions on my studies of the 1950s and the 1973 follow-up. In due course I received a copy of their 1975 report, *The Epidemiology of Infertility*. This report included their opinion that "the most complete epidemiological study of the prevalence of infertility pregnancy wastage is that undertaken by Scragg on the island of New Ireland in the western Pacific."[61]

In 1976 Mark Belsey published his 1974 background paper to this WHO report, which included an ASFR figure he had prepared from data in the 1973 Anne Ring and Scragg paper.[62] Figure 7.3 shows the 1987 collation of the change in ASFR. In a journal article D. G. Muir and Mark Belsey included the same ASFR figure and stated, "The presumed role of gonococcal infection in infertility in Papua New Guinea is supported by the rise in the age-specific fertility rates in women whose reproductive careers benefited from a mass penicillin-therapy program."[63]

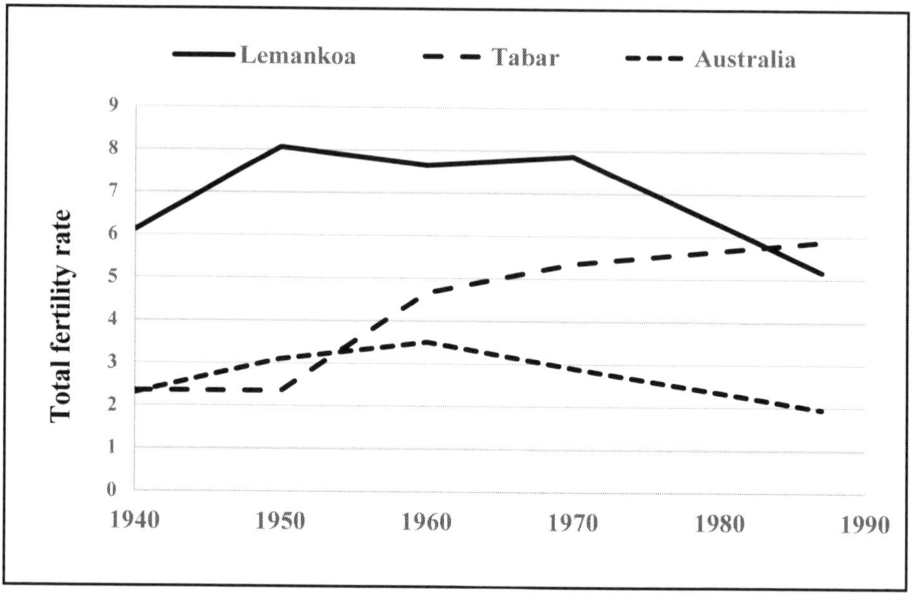

Figure 7.3. Comparison of total fertility rates: Lemankoa, Tabar, and Australia, 1940 to 1987.

Subfecundity

Yet in some quarters the implications of this case study were still not accepted. Joseph and Marguerite McFalls, in their book *Disease and Fertility*, cited malaria, gonorrhea, tuberculosis, and chlamydia as the principal causes of subfecundity. They referred to my 1954 MD thesis and repeatedly challenged my investigations and conclusions, suggesting that my research was a dubious hypothesis. Along with my thesis, the book listed in its bibliography the article by Muir and Besley mentioned earlier but ignored the half-page figure in its text copied from the Ring and Scragg article that proved the role of gonorrhea in the infertility of New Ireland.[64]

The longitudinal studies of four communities on Buka, Tabar, and New Ireland show that, in the Papua New Guinea case, malaria was not the key factor that McFalls and McFalls had asserted. The Solas population on Buka, with the highest level of malaria, also had the highest gross reproductive rate of the four communities.[65] Nor was tuberculosis a potent factor: this disease, spread from infected immigrants, such as the Fijian and Samoan teachers brought to Papua and New Guinea as Methodist missionaries, took years to become a secondary chest infection that could result in a significant prevalence of uterine TB. As for chlamydia, the findings of 1955 trachoma survey suggest that this disease may have arrived in New Guinea with European settlement.[66]

Of the four conditions they list, only gonorrhea can be cured and eradicated by penicillin. In summary, the multifactorial subfecundity concept of McFalls and McFalls was negated in the New Guinea case by the proven role of gonorrhea in infertility. Furthermore, all the multifactorial causes of childlessness resulting from subfecundity would have to be present at the same time in all the populations of the many communities where depopulation occurred. As this multifactorial simultaneity in diverse communities is highly improbable, we should view subfecundity, past and present, as an individual family problem, never a cause of "community infertility." The Tabar study indicates that a high proportion of childlessness in either a social group or in a whole community is pathognomonic of both the existence of promiscuous behavior and a hidden gonorrheal infection.

Innate Reproductive Potential

"Innate reproductive potential" is the capacity of an individual female to reproduce or a population to reproduce itself under optimum natural conditions. Queen Victoria and many of her contemporaries had zero involuntary infertility. In a population the proportion is variable and generally less than 5 percent linked to a base level of physical and hormonal abnormalities.[67]

I have collated the "whole of reproductive life" of all the individual females born before 1950 living in my study communities of Lemankoa, Solas, and Tabar: the urban Tigak community had too much migration to include. These are shown in figures 7.4, 7.5, and 7.6. These graphs show the fertility levels of each designated cohort of all women born prior to 1950 who survived to at least thirty-five years of age. They show a summation of the recorded births to all females aged fifteen and over, based on records of births, deaths, and marriages recorded in mission and village records since 1915, linked with demographic records collected from 1948 to 1987. The cohorts from 1920 on are of five years. The three columns show the percentage of women in each cohort in each fertility category. Primary infertile females have never had a live or a still birth.

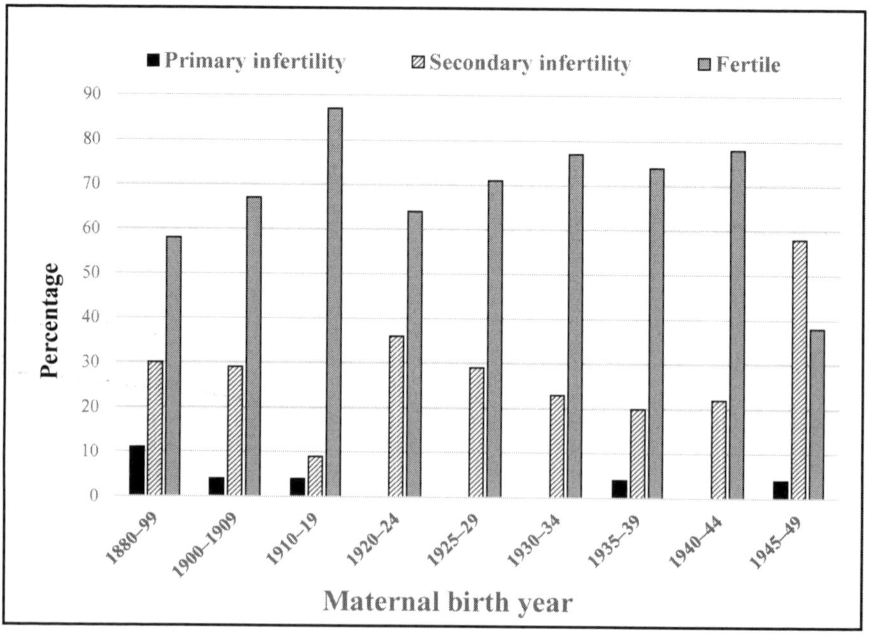

Figure 7.4. Lemankoa. Female reproductive life: fertility pattern of cohorts born 1880 to 1949 and surviving to at least forty years of age (N = 222 women).

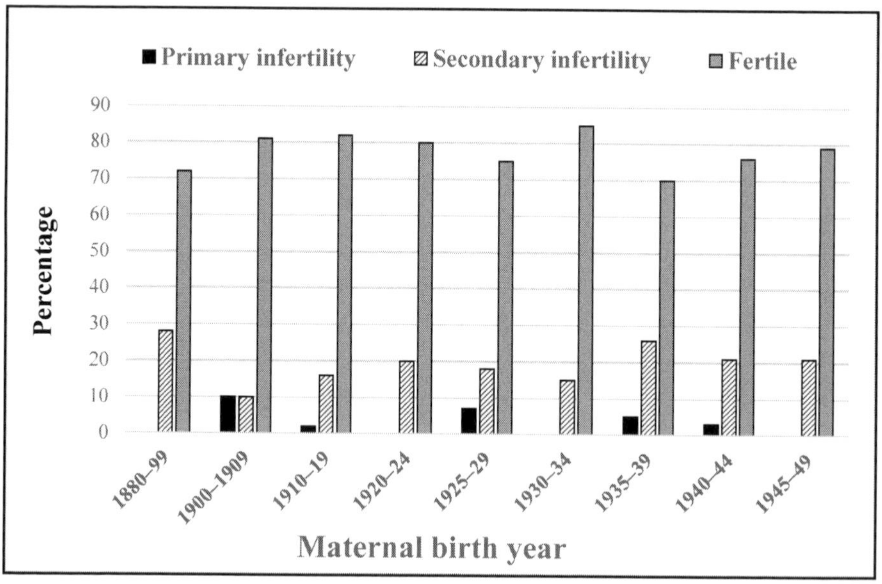

Figure 7.5. Solas. Female reproductive life: fertility pattern of cohorts born 1880 to 1949 and surviving to at least forty years of age (N = 373 women).

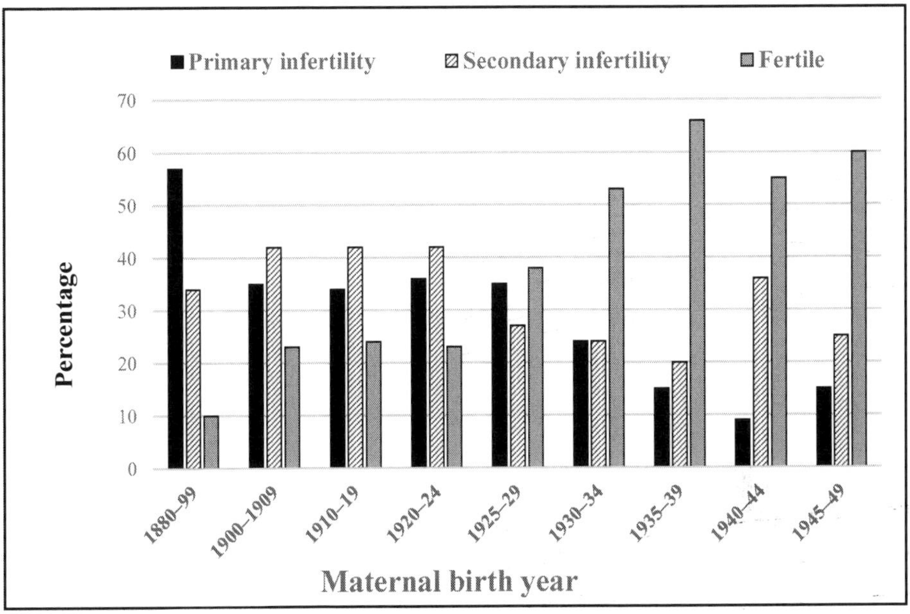

Figure 7.6. Tabar. Female reproductive life: fertility pattern of cohorts born 1880 to 1949 and surviving to at least forty years of age (N = 638 women).

In my 1953 assessment secondary infertility required a woman to have an interval of at least seven years after her last birth to be classified as secondarily infertile. In 1973 the female reproductive span was studied in Buka.[68] The mean age of menarche in 1970 was fifteen years and the age at the birth of the first child was twenty years. Menopause started to occur at forty, and no one over forty-seven was still menstruating. My longitudinal forty-year demographic study indicates that secondary infertility should include all women who had their last child before thirty-five years of age and had not had another child after a lapse of at least three years. If the individual assessment was marginal, the woman was classified as fertile.

In Lemankoa the only significant changes are the higher fertility of women in the 1910 to 1919 cohort and the doubling of secondary infertility in women born after 1945. The Public Health Department's annual reports record that medical stores supplied contraceptives to maternal and child health nurses from 1967. Lemankoa is also the home village of a gynecologist.

The Solas tribal area has a hospital and health services provided at a Catholic mission, and contraceptive medications might be difficult to obtain. The gross reproduction rate was the highest of the three areas, and the infant mortality rate was twice that in Tabar and four times that in Lemankoa. Significantly larger spleens indicated malaria was the main cause of this high mortality.

In Tabar the high proportion of primary infertility in the oldest cohort is consistent with both the lower mortality of barren women and the territory-wide engagement from 1880 to 1925 of pubertal Tabar women by German and other settlers as domestic laborers and concubines. The recruitment of women was prohibited in Australian New Guinea in 1917, but those already employed served out their contracts. The cessation of recruitment of young women and the use of sulfonamides from 1938 triggered the increase in the proportion of fertile women in the 1925 cohort. The availability of penicillin from 1947 and its community-wide use on Tabar in 1950 consolidated the reversal of the fertility picture.[69] The increased secondary infertility in the 1940 cohort is consistent with the availability of contraceptive devices from 1967 and their use by multiparous women in their thirties.

Figure 7.7 compares the lifetime fertility of all women born between 1900 and 1924 with that in Tabar from 1935 to 1949. In the cohorts born before 1924, primary infertility in Tabar was twelve times that in Lemankoa and secondary infertility almost double. The number of fertile women in Lemankoa and Solas was over three times that in Tabar. There was a significant change in both primary and secondary infertility in the Tabar cohorts born after 1935, when many in the 1930 cohort, along with their sexual partners, received penicillin in 1950.

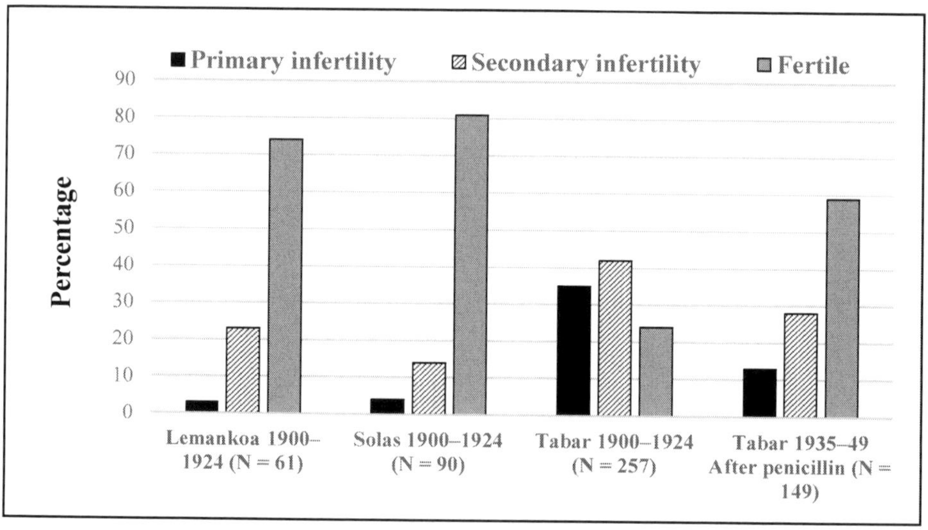

Figure 7.7. Female reproductive life natural fertility from 1900 to 1924 in Lemankoa and Solas compared with the impact of gonorrhea on fertility in the same cohort in Tabar and with the fertility of Tabar women born 1935 to 1949 after community-wide penicillin injections in 1950.

Before 1924 there were no village health services in either Lemankoa or Tabar, and occasional arsenic for yaws was the only effective medication. Adolescents born in 1925 entered puberty after 1938. From 1938 to 1942 sulfonamides were available and may have been used to treat infections involving the generative system. Limited amounts of crystalline penicillin were available from 1947, and ample long acting penicillin from 1949. The Tabar data show that the female cohort, born between 1932 and 1937 and thirty to thirty-four years old in 1967, had an ASFR of 174 and eventually a completed family size of five at menopause. Of these, the twenty-five women born between 1936 and 1937 were prepubertal in 1950. Their average completed family size was eight; two were infertile and the others had from four to thirteen children. It is evident that after 1950 the young women of Tabar entering puberty had sexual partners who no longer had "latent gonorrhea." However, infertility started to reappear in the women born after 1940 due to the use of modern contraceptives and contact with partners from the infected New Ireland mainland, where penicillin administration was given only in response to medical need (figure 7.8). After the community use of penicillin in 1950, the infertile cohorts of women were slowly replaced. The Papua New Guinea national census records that the Tabar population doubled over forty years to reach 3,000 in 1991 and that the restored fertility resulted in it doubling to 6,028 over the twenty years to 2011.

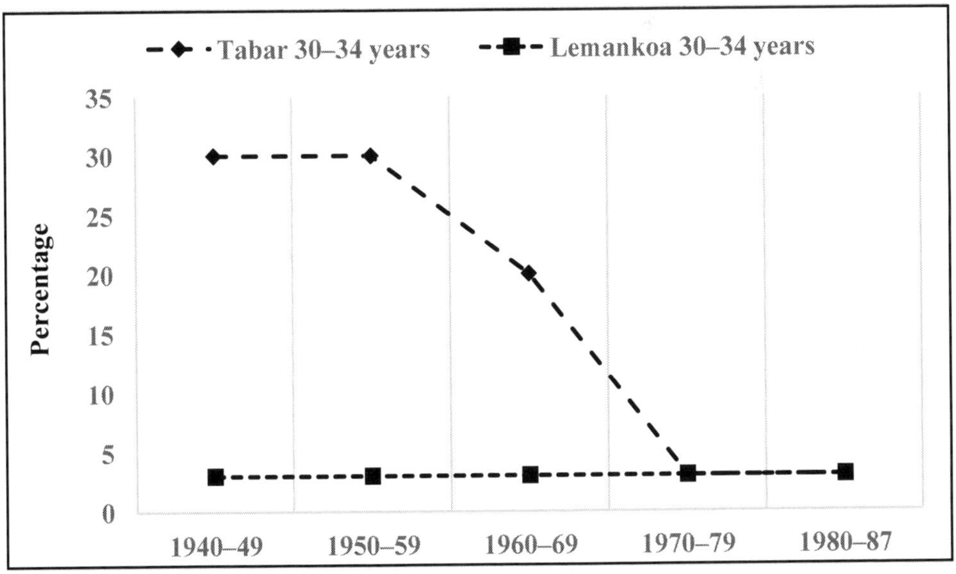

Figure 7.8. Percentage of childless females aged thirty to thirty-four from 1940 to 1987, in Tabar and Lemankoa

Tabar and the World

A sexually transmitted infection in one individual is generally hidden from another individual. In the world at large "community infertility" was also hidden when immigration and invasion concealed the scarcity of progeny within certain socially definable sections of the community or state. For example, it has been estimated that 25 percent of the crews of British sailing ships in the days of Captain James Cook were infected with gonorrhea.[70] Infections transmitted by these men had utterly devastating effects on the societies of the Hawai'ian Islands visited by Cook, but the viability of Britain was not jeopardized by the very high STI levels that prevailed in this particular section of its own society.

Two centuries after Cook the people of Tabar had more than a third of the women of childbearing age childless due to gonorrheal infection. With numbers decreasing at 3 percent per annum, the Tabar population was projected to disappear by 2020. If penicillin had not become available for use in the Tabar Islands, its inhabitants would have now disappeared, as the result of a decision of the New Guinea Company and the German New Guinea government to allow women only from New Ireland and its offshore islands to be exclusively employed to satisfy the domestic and sexual needs of settlers and employers.[71] The New Ireland women were chosen because of their reputation for customary promiscuous behavior. The immediate response of their fertility to penicillin indicates the effectiveness of this antibiotic against gonorrhea: it is the only cause of fallopian tube infection that responds to penicillin.

If the various New Ireland populations had not been subject to a gynecological study in 1950, the opportunity to prove the actual physical cause of population decline would have been slowly lost (figure 7.9). The population growth that followed its nadir would have been ascribed to social initiatives and the amelioration of Rivers's "culture contact." As happened elsewhere in the tropics, the community-wide use of penicillin for yaws and its more selective use on patients for various other problems would, as a side effect, have reduced the incidence of gonorrhea. Its historical role would soon have been hidden by the tidal wave of global antibiotic use.

As World War II ended, the pharmaceutical companies were geared to produce large quantities of penicillin, and it soon became available worldwide. In the armed forces penicillin rapidly became the treatment of choice for both syphilis and gonorrhea. The crystalline form required refrigeration, limiting its use to hospitals and clinics. Long-acting oily penicillin became available in 1949 and quickly replaced arsenicals in the treatment of yaws. In

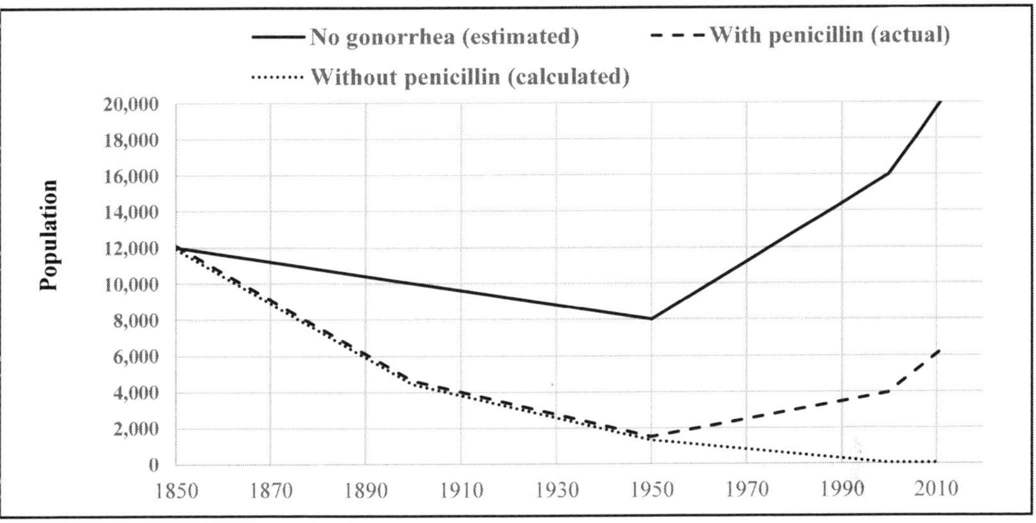

Figure 7.9. Projection of Tabar population, 1850 to 2010, with no gonorrhea (estimated), with penicillin (actual), and without penicillin (calculated).

the mid-1950s community-wide campaigns to eradicate yaws became WHO policy. Penicillin could not open blocked salpingeal tubes, but it was effective in curing pelvic inflammatory disease, epididymitis, and prostatitis and in so doing reduced the amount of involuntary childlessness.

The exponential growth of the Tabar population since the eradication of gonorrhea in the 1950s matched the growth of populations throughout the colonized world. Crude birthrates increased as the innate reproductive potential of populations began to be achieved. The "community infertility" caused by gonorrhea, previously a disease with no effective treatment, had for generations been a damper on fertility in infected communities worldwide. Historically, this hidden affliction was spread to populations within countries of the world as they were being colonized. The study of the isolated population of the Tabar Islands provided a rare opportunity for this hidden process to be revealed.

Promiscuity + Gonorrhea = Childlessness

The equation "Promiscuity + Gonorrhea = Childlessness" aptly summarizes the historical experience of all societies. Gonorrhea spread as empires and nations expanded into what hitherto had been the quarantined spaces of the globe, but the consequences were usually hidden to participants in the process. In these societies childlessness had been a rare event, one linked in the minds of people to either the consumption of plant materials reputed to be known only to certain older women or to a spell placed by a sorcerer preventing conception in an otherwise healthy woman. The link between the strange invaders and the respiratory and gastrointestinal infections that they brought was generally recognized, but not the link between the strangers and the increasing prevalence of childlessness.

Searching for references on childlessness, I first came on the concern of the Emperor Augustus at the failure of the Roman patriarchy to generate the required number of births to match the number of deaths in their section of Roman society and the special laws he promulgated to encourage the Romans to reproduce in the same manner as the Christians.[72] My next discovery was the story of Spartan women around four hundred years earlier.[73] The Greeks had coined the word *oliganthropia* to describe sparse population, and Pomeroy considers every social, psychological, and economic aspect of the Spartan decline that had commenced about 480 BCE. However, there is no mention of a high mortality epidemic or venereal disease. In October 2017 I chanced on the PhD thesis by Timothy Doran on the same subject.[74] As it is a demographic thesis, it is more precise and specifies that eight thousand Spartiates in 480 BCE declined to one thousand by 330 BCE. Fortunately, true Spartans maintained records and a census to prove their identity. Again, the discourse covers all aspects of the society, including promiscuity, but epidemics and venereal disease are not mentioned. Centuries before this decline hordes of Greeks and Phoenicians invaded the western Mediterranean and established colonies as far as the Atlantic coast. The question is, why did societies that could produce hordes become societies that needed miscegenation to maintain their population?

Human Petri Dish

Unknowingly, the recruitment from 1880 to 1925 of pubertal Tabar women by German and other settlers for use as concubines created a unique biological experiment in which the women were infected with all the venereal diseases transmitted by their partners, randomly drawn from many countries. The 35 percent primary infertility is indicative of the efficiency of *Neisseria gonorrhoeae* in establishing a hostile uterine environment and in due course blocking the fallopian tubes and acting as a permanent contraceptive. Promiscuous social behavior, matched with the high prevalence of gonorrhea in the settler community, resulted in a combined primary and secondary infertility of 77 percent of the Tabar women.

Their male partners would have also brought syphilis with them, but frambesia (yaws), which was endemic in tropical New Ireland, gave the women immunity. However, the original inhabitants of southern Australia and New Zealand had no such immunity and were infected with epidemic syphilis with symptoms matching those that occurred in Europe in the sixteenth century.[75] The residual secondary infertility in Tabar was not significantly less than that in Lemankoa, indicating that if genital *Chlamydia trachomatis* was transmitted by the settlers, it had little perceptible effect on fertility.

Antiquity of Gonorrhea

My thesis is that gonorrhea is the only organism that will produce population decline in a promiscuous society or in a section of a society that is promiscuous. The written history of the world in antiquity is centered around the Mediterranean. Century after century distant northern and northeastern societies without gonorrhea invaded southern Europe and the Mediterranean littoral with its declining populations due to gonorrhea. After Bartolomeo Diaz rounded the Cape of Good Hope in 1482, gonorrhea slowly became a hidden pandemic, doing its part to keep global population growth under 1 percent per annum.

Only gonorrhea can cause a significant level of primary infertility. Pelvic inflammatory disease and orchitis were described by Greek physicians.[76] Gonorrhea is a silent disease, and many of the women of Tabar would have thought their pelvic pain was just a bad period. Childlessness ascribed by Rivers in the Southwest Pacific to psychic causes and ascribed by Cicero and Polybius in Greek and Roman societies to socioeconomic causes is the most evident symptom of hidden gonorrhea.

The earliest common recent ancestor of the current gonorrhea serovars has been identified as appearing no later than 1544.[77] I postulate that missing genetic links could have been destroyed by the Black Death in the fourteenth century. The highest incidence of the plague was in the towns and settlements where gonorrhea was most prevalent. Gonorrhea occurred only in Eurasia. The plague would have eliminated the serovars needed to provide a projection back to a tMRCA of the tissue invading gonococcus in Egypt around the year 600 BCE.

For how long in the twenty-first century will our current control of this hidden affliction continue? Over the past eighty years, the gonococcus has repeatedly rearranged its genetic biochemistry to neuter antibiotics—sulfonamides from the 1940s, penicillins from 1955, tetracyclines from 1975, cephalosporins from 1985, fluoroquinolones from 1990, and azythromycins from 2015. Slowly but surely the gonococcus has ensured its survival as an obligate parasite, limiting human reproduction with great effectiveness. The exponential growth in human population that followed the conquest of gonorrhea by penicillin has contributed to the population crisis that we now recognize to be unsustainable. Perhaps this biological community contraceptive will continue to mutate, thus protecting humans from their innate propensity to overpopulate?

Notes

1. John T. Gunther to Roy Scragg, June 20, 1950, Sir John Gunther Papers, 1947–1984, ANAU 321, Australian National University Archives, Canberra.

2. Edwin Holland, *Depopulation East Coast, New Ireland: Official Report* (Kavieng: Public Health Department, 1931); Ernest W. P. Chinnery, "Demographic Study of Native Populations, East Coast of New Ireland, 1911–1950," in *Anthropological Report, New Guinea, No. 6* (Canberra: Green/Government Printer, 1931).

3. Holland, *Depopulation*, 6.

4. Margrit Davies, *Public Health and Colonialism: The Case of German New Guinea, 1884–1914* (Wiesbaden: Harrassowitz, 2002), app. 5, tabulated from the *Medizinal-Berichte uber die Deutschen Schutzgebiete*, 1903–13.

5. Stewart Firth, *New Guinea under the Germans* (Carlton, Victoria: Melbourne University Press, 1983), 125–26.

6. Davies, *Public Health and Colonialism*, 217, tabulated from the *Medizinal-Berichte*, 1903–13.

7. Peter Sack and Dymphna Clark, eds., *German New Guinea: The Annual Reports* (Canberra: Australian National University Press, 1979), 160.

8. The statistics published in Berlin from 1905 onward in *Medizinal-Berichte* are analyzed by Daniel J. Walther, *Sex and Control: Venereal Disease, Colonial Physicians, and Indigenous Agency in German Colonialism, 1884–1914* (New York: Berghahn, 2015), 66–67, 152–55.

9. Several other venereal diseases were also diagnosed and treated in the German colony over this period: bubo (87 cases), epididymitis (84), genital warts (119), ulcus molle (239), venereal granulum (106), and "other" (78); see Walther, *Sex and Control*, 152–55. Bubo and epididymitis could have been symptoms of gonorrhea.

10. Roy F. R. Scragg, "Depopulation in New Ireland: A Study of Demography and Fertility" (MD thesis, University of Adelaide), 1954, 93.

11. Willi Hoffman, "Nichamtlichen Teil: Über die Gesundheitsverhältnisse der Eingeborenen im Nordöstlichen Neumecklenburg," *Amtsblatt für das Schutzgebiet Neu-Guinea*, no. 11 (June 1, 1913): 120–21.

12. Sack and Clark, *German New Guinea*, 341.

13. Davies, *Public Health and Colonialism*, 154, quoting from the 1912–13 quarterly report, 1.7.1912–31.12.1912, Reichskolonialamt Records, Berlin, 5772, 196/7.

14. Davies, *Public Health and Colonialism*, 167, 204.

15. Sack and Clark, *German New Guinea*, 311.

16. Sack and Clark, *German New Guinea*, 324.

17. Dr. Willy Wick, "Arbieterfürsorge in Deutsch-Neuguinea, 1914," BArch R1001/5773, Budesarchiv, Lichterfelde, German Federal Archive, Berlin, 38, cited and translated by Walther, *Sex and Control*, 97.

18. Charles Rowley, *The Australians in German New Guinea, 1914–1921* (Carlton, Victoria: Melbourne University Press, 1958), 127, 128, 130.

19. Rowley, *Australians*, 120, 127.

20. Hortense Powdermaker, "Vital Statistics of New Ireland (Bismarck Archipelago) as Revealed in Genealogies," *Human Biology* 3, no. 3 (1931): 351–75.

21. Phyllis Cilento, pers. comm. describing her Western Islands investigations, 1982. Reported in Raphael W. Cilento, *The Causes of the Depopulation of the Western Islands of the Territory of New Guinea* (Melbourne: Australian Government Printer, 1928), 19–20.

22. Ernest W. P. Chinnery, *Repeat Study of the Native Population of the East Coast of New Ireland*, report to the Department of External Territories (Canberra: Government Printer, 1950).

23. Stephen H. Roberts, *Population Problems of the Pacific* (London: Routledge, 1927), 389–90.

24. Bolton G. Corney, J. Stewart, and B. Thomson, *Report of the Commission Appointed to Inquire into the Decrease of the Native Population* (Suva, Fiji: Government Printer, 1893).

25. Ian F. G. Downs, "District of New Ireland: Patrol Report No 5, Tabar Island Group; 15 February 1949," UC San Diego Digital Collections, accessed September 2017, www. http://library.ucsd.edu/.

26. Anita Herle and Sandra Rouse, eds., *Cambridge and the Torres Strait: Centenary Essays on the 1898 Anthropological Expedition* (Cambridge: Cambridge University Press, 1998).

27. Ben Shephard, *A War of Nerves: Soldiers and Psychiatrists, 1914–1974* (London: Cape, 2000), 89–90; Tim Bayliss-Smith, "Colonialism as Shell Shock: W. H. R. Rivers's Explanations for Depopulation in Melanesia," in *The Ethnographic Experiment: A. M. Hocart and W. H. R. Rivers in Island Melanesia, 1908*, ed. Edvard Hviding and Cato Berg (New York: Berghahn, 2014), 179–82; and, more generally, see also Tracey Loughran, *Shell-Shock and Medical Culture in First World War Britain* (Cambridge: Cambridge University Press, 2017).

28. John Forrester, "The English Freud: W. H. R. Rivers, Dreaming and the Making of Early Twentieth-Century Human Sciences," in *History and the Psyche*, ed. Sally Alexander and Barbara Taylor (New York: Palgrave Macmillan, 2012), 71–104.

29. William H. R. Rivers, "The Dying Out of Native Races," *Lancet* 98 (1920): 42–44; Rivers, *Instinct and the Unconscious: A Contribution to a Biological Theory of the Psycho-Neuroses* (Cambridge: Cambridge University Press, 1920); Rivers, "The Psychological Factor," chap. 8 in *Essays on the Depopulation of Melanesia* (Cambridge: Cambridge University Press, 1922), 84–113.

30. Philippe Ricord, *A Practical Treatise on Venereal Disease* (London: Longman, Brown, 1842).

31. Gustave Bernutz and Ernest Goupil, "Cliniques memoires sur le maladies de femmes," *Archives générales de médecine*, 5 series t (March 1857): IX.

32. Emil Jacob Noeggerath, "Latent Gonorrhea, Especially with Regard to Its Influence on Fertility in Women," *Transactions of the American Gynaecologic Society* 1 (1876): 268–300; Albert Neisser, "Über eine der Gonorrhoe eigentümliche Micrococcusform," *Zentralblatt für die Medizinischen Wissenschaften* 17 (July 12, 1879): 497–500.

33. Elliott Bowen, "Limits of the Lab: Diagnosing 'Latent Gonorrhea,' 1872–1910," *Bulletin History of Medicine* 87 (2013): 63–85. See also Christina Benninghaus, chap. 10; Fabrice Cahen and Adrien Minard, chap, 11; and Simon Szreter and Kevin Schürer, chap. 12, all in this volume.

34. See also Tim Bayliss-Smith, chap. 6, in this volume.

35. Rivers, *Essays on the Depopulation.*

36. Rivers, "Psychological Factor," in *Essays on the Depopulation of Melanesia*, 104.

37. Roberts, *Population Problems*, 85.

38. George H. F. L. Pitt-Rivers, *The Clash of Cultures: An Anthropological and Psychological Study of the Laws of Racial Adaptability, with Special Reference to the Depopulation of the Pacific and the Government of Subject Races* (London: Routledge, 1927), 142–48.

39. Bayliss-Smith, "Colonialism as Shell Shock," in Hviding and Berg, *Ethnographic Experiment*, 189–92.

40. Judith Bennett, "A Vanishing People of a Vanishing Discourse? W. H. R. Rivers's 'Psychological Factor' and Depopulation in the Solomon Islands and New Hebrides," in Hviding and Berg, *Ethnographic Experiment*, 214–51.

41. Hoffman, "Nichamtlichen Teil," 114–31, 115, 120–21, 119.

42. Chinnery, "Demographic Study of Native Population, East Coast of New Ireland, 1950," October 19, 1950, Department of External Territories, A.806/1/3, pp. 1–17.

43. Roy F. R. Scragg, "Report on Two Cases of Ectopic Pregnancy in New Guinea Natives," *Medical Journal of Australia* 2 (1951): 53.

44. Michael J. Gunn, "Rock Art on Tabar, New Ireland Province, Papua New Guinea," *Anthropos* 81, no. 4 (1986): 455.

45. Hortense Powdermaker, *Life in Lesu: The Study of a Melanesian Society in New Ireland* (New York: Norton, 1933), 144.

46. Powdermaker, *Life in Lesu*, 244–46.

47. Downs, "District of New Ireland," includes a fifteen-page appendix, titled "Vital Statistics and Causes of Depopulation in Tabar Island Group and the East Coast of New Ireland," in which Downs presents the results of interviews he carried out with seventy-nine senior men. They were all asked, "Why do your modern women fail to produce children?" A frequent response was regret that the periodic *malanggan* feasts and dances had declined in popularity, so now there was less sexual intercourse and more feelings of shame induced by church-led sanctions.

48. Downs, "District of New Ireland," app. "Vital Statistics," which includes five population figures for Tabar, as counted in 1908, 1928, 1941, 1947, and 1949. He notes, "In 1908 the count was made by Kramer, Sapper, Behrmann and Hoffman, and Father Krumpel at Mapua Mission states that the figure was counted up to 8,000 (but was not complete)."

49. Amtsblatt, "Engebnis der Eingeborenenen Kopfstener des Bezirks Neu-Mecklenburg-Nord," *Amtsblatt für das Schutzgebiet Deutsch-Neuguinea*, 3, no. 11 (1911): 141.

50. Roy Scragg, "Science and Survival in Paradise," *Health and History* 12, no. 2 (2010): 57–78, 58.

51. Scragg, "Depopulation in New Ireland," table 3.

52. John T. Gunther to Robert Melrose, April 13, 1950, ANAU 321.

53. Scragg, "Depopulation in New Ireland," 75.

54. Scragg, "Depopulation in New Ireland," 51, tables 29, 31.

55. Scragg, "Depopulation in New Ireland," 100, table 35.

56. Scragg, "Depopulation in New Ireland," 90.

57. Scragg, "Depopulation in New Ireland," table 11.

58. Anne Ring and Roy Scragg, "A Demographic and Social Study of Fertility in Rural New Guinea," *Journal of Biosocial Science* 5 (1973): 92–94.

59. Scragg, "Depopulation in New Ireland," table 20.

60. Ring and Scragg, "Demographic and Social Study," 113.

61. WHO Scientific Group on the Epidemiology of Infertility, "The Epidemiology of Infertility," *WHO Technical Report Series, No. 582* (World Health Organization: Geneva, 1975), 10.

62. Mark A. Belsey, "The Epidemiology of Infertility: A Review with Particular Reference to Sub-Saharan Africa," *Bulletin of the World Health Organization* 54, no. 3 (1976): 319.

63. D. G. Muir and Mark A. Belsey, "Pelvic Inflammatory Disease and Its Consequences in the Developing World," *American Journal of Obstetrics and Gynaecology* 138 (1980): 913–28.

64. Joseph A. McFalls and Marguerite H. McFalls, *Disease and Fertility* (Orlando: Academic Press, 1984), 295.

65. Scragg, "Depopulation in New Ireland," 39, table 21.

66. Ida Mann and Janos Lorschdorfer, *Ophthalmic Survey of the Territories of Papua and New Guinea* (Port Moresby: Government Printer, 1955).

67. WHO Scientific Group, "Epidemiology of Infertility," 5.

68. Roy F. Scragg, "Menopause and Reproductive Span in Rural Papua New Guinea" (paper presented at the Medical Society of Papua New Guinea, Ninth Annual Symposium, 1973), 126–44.

69. Ring and Scragg, "Demographic and Social Study," 89–121.

70. Charles C. Norris, *Gonorrhea in Women* (London: Saunders, 1913), 176.

71. Walther, *Sex and Control*, 24–30.

72. John Percy Vyvian Dacre Balsdon, *Roman Women: Their History and Habits* (London: Bodley Head, 1962) 194ff.

73. Sarah B. Pomeroy, *Spartan Women* (Oxford: Oxford University Press, 2002).

74. Timothy D. Doran, "Demographic Fluctuation and Institutional Response in Sparta: Ancient History and Mediterranean Archaeology" (PhD diss., University of California Berkeley, 2011), 61.

75. Peter J. Dowling, "A Great Deal of Sickness: Introduced Diseases among the Aboriginal People of Colonial South East Australia, 1788–1900" (PhD diss., Australian National University, 1997); D. E. Hanham, "The Impact of Introduced Diseases in the Pre-treaty Period, 1790–1840" (master's thesis, University of Canterbury, New Zealand 2003).

76. William J. Stewart McKay, *The History of Ancient Gynaecology* (London: Tindall and Cox, 1901).

77. See Simon Szreter's introduction to this volume, p. 24.

Chapter Eight

Fertility, STIs, and Sexual Behavior in Early and Mid-Twentieth-Century East Africa

Shane Doyle

Problematic Generalizations: Fertility and STIs in African History

Narratives around fertility and sexually transmitted infections in Africa have commonly been characterized by assumptions of universality. Influential theories promoted by Jack Goody and Jack Caldwell identified African cultures as profoundly pronatalist, with the prioritization of the expansion of the lineage causing infidelity to be tolerated and polygamy encouraged. Caldwell and colleagues expanded on this thesis in light of Africa's HIV pandemic, to suggest that pronatalism exposed Africans to a high risk of STI infection.[1] Explanations for the delay in population growth until the 1950s across much of Africa similarly typically focused on gonorrhea and syphilis as the primary cause of subfertility.[2] Moreover, historical analyses of medical interventions against STIs have been consistently negative, owing to a focus on the early colonial experience.[3]

This chapter addresses this tendency toward an assumed homogeneity in depictions of the history of fertility and STIs in Africa. It compares the history of two neighboring societies, Buganda in modern-day Uganda and Buhaya in Tanzania (formerly Tanganyika). It shows that although commonalities in these societies' experience of fertility change, gonorrhea, and syphilis can be identified, fundamental differences existed in both causation and response. The importance of these findings is threefold. Most obviously, this comparison suggests that if significant levels of variation in local experience over time and space existed, despite Buganda's and Buhaya's core similarities, then assumptions of continent-wide patterns of change should be reconsidered. Second, the analysis of the growing liberalism of STI interventions in Buganda from the 1920s illustrates the capacity of colonial medicine to adapt to both local and metropolitan pressures. The third aspect of this study, which has broader significance, is that, while STI campaigns were most effective where local populations accepted external assertions that subfertility resulted from gonorrhea and syphilis, overall STI interventions' impact was so great because they provided a vehicle for a broader transformation in reproductive health care.

Buganda and Buhaya: Subfertility and STIs

Buganda and Buhaya, though separated today by an international border (see figure 8.1), share fundamental geographic and cultural characteristics. Their languages are to a large degree mutually intelligible; their social relationships have been shaped by a history of monarchical government; their indigenous religions drew on similar core beliefs and structures; and neither society was especially pronatalist.[4] Haya families lost their land if they lacked a legitimate heir but, because cultivable land was relatively limited, did not particularly value extremely large families. Girls who became pregnant before marriage were encouraged to abort or, it is claimed, were murdered. Mothers were pressured to breastfeed for up to four years, which was (correctly) believed to suppress the chances of a further conception. Women who conceived soon after giving birth were sent away to their parents when their next child was born to avoid another short birth interval. This was a culture that encouraged caution in childbearing.[5] Similarly, in Buganda, while having several children was highly valued, women who had extremely large families were socially defined as lacking self-control. Proverbs described such women as reproducing "like a dog" and referred to giving birth as a "deadly thing." Some sources suggest it was common for inconvenient pregnancies to be terminated, and social norms did not expect a widow with children to remarry. As in Buhaya, women aimed for very long birth intervals.[6]

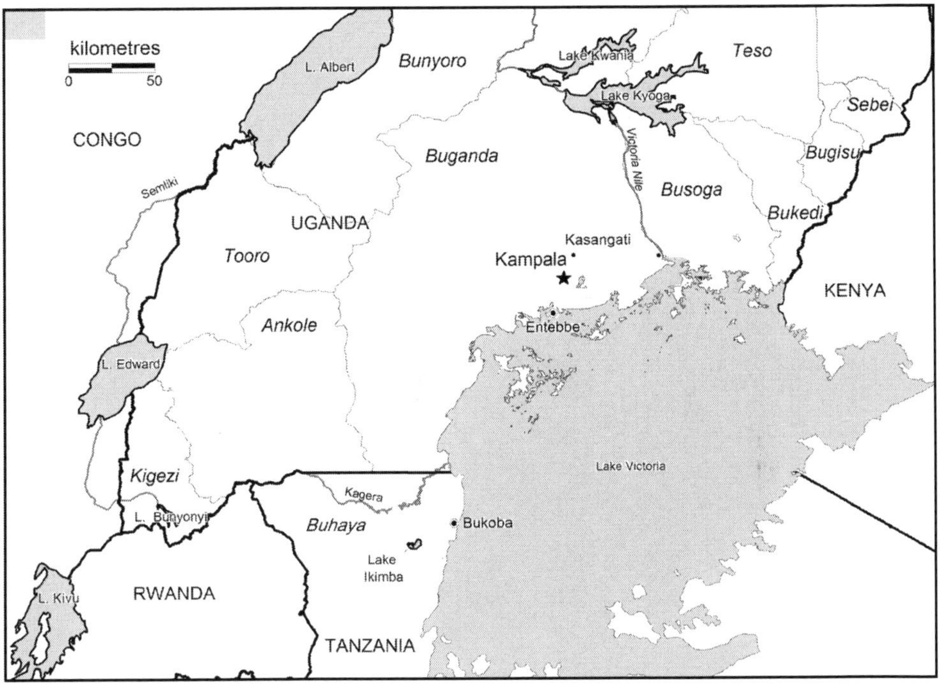

Figure 8.1. Map of Buganda, Buhaya, and the Great Lakes region. Map created by Vincent Hiribarren.

The experience of colonial rule within Buganda and Buhaya, moreover, was also directly comparable. Both were characterized by early, successful missionization, and each possessed highly developed educational and medical systems and enjoyed unusual prosperity through cash cropping. Strikingly, both societies also followed similar trajectories of demographic and medical change. During the first half of the twentieth century, Buganda and Buhaya were notorious for high reported STI rates, and very low recorded fertility. Then, from the 1950s, STI incidence in both societies fell sharply, and total fertility rates doubled within a generation.

While the underlying similarities in socioeconomic characteristics and demographic trends are undeniable, the causation of fertility change varied significantly across the two case study areas. Moreover, the apparent homogeneity in STI patterns was in large part a product of a shared moral discourse and common principles of (mis)diagnosis that drew on, and reinforced, a sense of regional crisis. In the late nineteenth and early twentieth centuries, a series of famines and epidemics, from sleeping sickness to smallpox, created a sense of unease among European administrators of the new colonial dependencies of Tanganyika and Uganda. Population decline seemed to undermine the legitimacy of an enterprise self-justified by Rudyard Kipling's promise to "Fill full the mouth of famine / And bid the sickness cease."[7] More immediately, it threatened the career progression of those tasked with bringing these initially unpromising territories to financial self-sufficiency, given that a falling population limited both the tax base and the potential for a rapid expansion of exports. As one official put it in 1911, a "declining birth-rate which under present conditions appears to be inevitable means in years to come declining revenue. . . . Therefore from a financial point of view apart from a higher motive these people must be prevented from allowing themselves to commit race suicide."[8] It was this context that explains colonial governments' willingness to both consider medical interventions of remarkable coerciveness and accept missionary claims that the primary cause of demographic decline was an epidemic of STIs, and in particular of syphilis.

Buganda: From Coercion to Liberalism

Missionary influence rested above all on the shoulders of Albert Cook, a Cambridge-trained doctor who founded Uganda's first hospital in 1897 and was the consultant of choice for East Africa's colonial elite until his retirement in 1934. Cook's ability to shape secular policy drew not only on his reputation for medical expertise but also on his undoubted skills as a propagandist and his initial monopoly of medical data. Before World War I, the region's only apparently credible source of information on epidemiological trends was Cook's carefully maintained, but problematically analyzed, register of in- and outpatients at Mengo Hospital (the oldest hospital in Kampala, founded by missionaries in 1897). This statistical authority provided the leverage that enabled missionary anxieties about the moral decline of Uganda's first generation of converts to be salved through secular legislation of unique severity.[9] In 1913, for example, Cook claimed that "70 percent of the children in Uganda either die from premature birth, or are still-born, or die in the first week after birth. In England the corresponding infant mortality is 14 percent. . . . This heavy infant mortality is accounted for by (1) the virulent epidemic of venereal disease in the country (2) native ignorance and neglect."[10] Reports of this kind reached a crescendo as World War I drew to a close, ultimately causing Uganda's governor Robert Coryndon to fund a national Social Purity campaign, led by Cook and his wife, and to support the establishment of a network of Anglican maternity centers, which sought to address the "twin evils" of STIs and infertility by establishing a new culture of Christian familyhood and hygienic maternity care.[11]

Missionaries then gave Uganda's early response to STIs its strong weighting toward moralistic admonition and pronatalist interventionism. Indirectly, mission influence also resulted in the remarkably coercive intrusiveness that would make the country notorious among liberal observers in the metropole. Cook's apocalyptic predictions of demographic collapse due to STIs resonated with the local chiefly elite, who saw that STI control could provide a mechanism for the restoration of their authority over an increasingly mobile and assertive population. Chiefs' anxieties, backed up by Cook's claim "that between 1897 and 1907 . . . the incidence of syphilis [had] increased rapidly" at Mengo Hospital, prompted Uganda's governor to ask the Colonial Office to send an STI specialist to set up a syphilis-control program in the protectorate.[12] That the expert appointed was one of the Royal Army Medical Corps' leading syphilologists, Col. Francis Lambkin, was indicative of colonial preconceptions and would ensure that Uganda's program would be run on military lines from the beginning. Lambkin claimed that due to moral and social disintegration the majority of the population were infected with syphilis and that the epidemic, if unchecked, would "decimate some of [Uganda's] tribes, and the remainder will become so degenerate as to be practically useless." This cataclysmic analysis brought three further RAMC specialists to establish an STI-control program, focusing on Uganda's central kingdom of Buganda, whose chiefly elite were particularly vociferous in their demands for radical intervention.[13]

Buganda's leading chiefs had seen their power constrained by the imperial takeover but found that the colonial administration would legitimize their exertion of authority when the state's fundamental interests were threatened. Public health was a sphere where senior chiefs could display their dedication to Britain's civilizing mission and so secure official endorsement for coercive interventions that would not have been accepted in most other policy domains.[14] Thus county chiefs' proposal that a new law be passed to compel the treatment of the sick was greeted with enthusiasm. Lt. George Keane, the RAMC officer tasked with drafting the legislation, recognized that compulsory treatment could resolve declining revenue as well as authority and morality, anticipating that compulsion would enlarge the labor supply by up to 20 percent.[15] The simultaneous publication in 1913 of the protectorate government's "Townships (Venereal Diseases) Rules" and the Buganda kingdom government's "Law for Preventing Venereal Disease" symbolized this coercive alliance. Syphilis was declared a dangerous disease, and those suspected of being infected faced compulsory examination, while the infected would submit to a full course of treatment, during which they could not trade, marry, or have sex. Heavy fines or imprisonment would penalize non-compliance. Sex workers were particularly targeted for intense supervision by chiefs and police, but it was the remarkable degree to which the entire Ganda population would be monitored by the chiefly hierarchy that is so striking. Local landlords and chiefs were required to check every fortnight whether any new infections had occurred among their tenants and subjects and to force new cases to accept treatment.[16] Uganda's legislators were clearly influenced by previous metropolitan and imperial interventions, but the universality of compulsion set Uganda apart from India, for example, whose Contagious Diseases Acts explicitly focused attention on women.[17]

While limited funds narrowed the geographic focus within Buganda, the campaign's impact was intense. STI specialist officers, energetically supported by chiefs, organized regular mass examinations of entire communities. In addition to systematic village-level investigations, during which inhabitants were required to submit to a cursory, public inspection of their genitalia, chiefs were paid for reporting suspected victims of syphilis to a treatment center. The presence of potentially syphilitic sores resulted in an order to complete a course of treatment, with defaulters tracked down by the local police. RAMC officers understood syphilis treatment as essentially a form of inoculation, designed to limit further disease transmission, with the greater good of the community outweighing the liberty of the individual. Compulsory injections suited the overstretched early colonial health system, as they freed the "patient of all participation in his treatment and the medical officer is independent of his assistance and makes no demands on him."[18]

Uganda's program ended not because of its lack of interest in behavioral change but because of the fallout following an incident in which a recently arrived female venereologist, Dr. Margaret Lamont, was dismissed from the colonial medical service in 1922 for complaining about oppressive and degrading mass examinations. This prompted the United Kingdom's Association for Moral and Social Hygiene (AMSH), a pressure group that had long campaigned against STI policies that unfairly victimized women, to take up her case, forcing the Colonial Office to launch an inquiry. For Keane, the head of Uganda's program, that "the compulsory measures of Uganda are the most rigorous and far-reaching" in the world was justified by the scale of the crisis, as, he claimed, the protectorate's population suffered 90 percent STI prevalence, infant mortality of up to nine hundred per thousand, and a stillbirth rate of 12 percent.[19] Cook also endorsed the colonial system by referring to case records that showed that 22 percent of recent outpatients were diagnosed with an STI, while two-thirds of maternity cases had a current or previous syphilis infection.[20] Policy in Uganda had been driven for fifteen years by such estimates, but only now were they examined skeptically. The AMSH dismissed prevalence rates derived from the examination of individuals suspected by their chiefs of suffering from STIs or from people seeking hospital treatment. The assumption that all stillbirths were caused by syphilis was equally indefensible. That the reported stillbirth rate among mission maternity cases was almost three times higher than in the general population indicated to AMSH specialists that they had an atypical experience of STIs. Lamont complained that laboratory testing was restricted purely on the grounds of expense but reported that her own inspection of the general female population found evidence of active infection in only 5 percent of women. The AMSH considered that the data, taken together, indicated that the STI situation in Uganda, with perhaps 10 to 20 percent prevalence, was probably similar to that in the United Kingdom, "but we don't adopt Ugandan measures." The UK government, embarrassed by these revelations of how the excessive power of the colonial state could be abused, ordered the abandonment of Uganda's RAMC model of STI control.[21]

While this story is well known, the transformation in Ugandan policy after 1922 has not been fully recognized in previous scholarship, despite the similarities with metropolitan trends.[22] The protectorate drew back from comprehensive compulsion, shifting toward a model based on persuasion supported by mass availability of treatment. Interventions were not entirely free of coercion, but this was no longer policy's defining characteristic. In 1941 the colonial state did quietly approve legislation that granted new powers to detain and examine sex workers, who were defined rather loosely. This was justified as a wartime measure because of the fear that STIs would lower troops' efficiency and, it seems, was largely forgotten until the 1950s, when male fears about the increase in female industrial employment and growing ethnic neoconservatism resulted in sporadic assaults on independent women in Buganda. At this point the 1941 law came back into sporadic use, as women traveling alone to Kampala were removed from buses and forced to return to the countryside, others were randomly arrested on city streets and carried off to be tested for STIs, and schools had to close due to unmarried teachers being charged with prostitution. Each outbreak of gender repression proved short-lived, in part because of pressure in response exerted by metropolitan groups, such as the Mothers' Union and AMSH, on the Colonial Office, and so there was overall no discernible impact on the number of autonomous women in the city, prostitution, or STI prevalence.[23]

The tone of health education meanwhile also grew more positive as colonial rule matured, focusing less on fear and morality and more on modernity and familial development. STI propaganda increasingly focused on the male household head, encouraging sexual restraint so that he could concentrate his expenditure within the bounds of the nuclear family and so raise its health and living standards. The most obvious attempt to Africanize this improving vision of modernity was the emphasis placed on the need to avoid STIs to satisfy the assumed desire for high levels of fertility.[24] By the 1960s, as radical nationalism and decolonization reframed the state-subject relationship, STI strategies drew back from an explicit attempt to critique and transform indigenous culture. Instead, they refocused on the pragmatic goal of understanding how sexual behavioral patterns had changed so that public health information on how to minimize infection risk could be best targeted.[25] Attention shifted from the moral to the social context of STI infection, such as the role played by alcohol usage and Buganda's changing age structure. The fixation with prostitutes and barmaids, and the desire to redefine marriage, was dropped, as studies showed that 70 percent of Kampala's STI cases were unmarried, 15 percent were schoolchildren, and police, army, truck and bus drivers, and university students were all identified as having particularly high levels of infection.[26]

This redirection of focus in relation to STI policy was to a large degree shaped by the legacy of the 1922 scandal. The records of the AMSH indicate that Uganda's treatment of women in general, and sex workers in particular, was particularly closely monitored by metropolitan pressure groups throughout the remainder of the colonial period. Criticism of Uganda's misuse of data and systematic misdiagnosis prompted a shift toward an unusually empirical, cautious interpretation of signs and symptoms. Diagnostic practice was increasingly modeled on norms established at Mulago Hospital (founded in Kampala in 1913), whose role as East Africa's center of medical research between the 1920s and 1960s permitted sustained consideration of STI trends. Analysis of postmortems between 1931 and 1946, for example, revealed evidence of previous syphilitic infection in only 11.8 percent of cases, much lower than estimates produced through serology or clinical signs and very similar to rates recorded in contemporary US autopsies. Pathological examination revealed that most neonatal deaths were in fact due to birth-related infection, while infant deaths were mainly the result of pneumonia, malaria, meningitis, and malnutrition. That syphilis, which had previously been blamed for most child mortality, was found to be of marginal significance prompted a revision of protocols around the interpretation of Kahn tests so that only strongly positive results would be taken as an indicator of syphilitic infection among all age groups.[27]

A gradual shift toward diagnostic caution had begun almost immediately in Uganda's secular hospitals following the Lamont scandal, but it was delayed in rural dispensaries and mission units, where assumptions of sinfulness proved particularly entrenched. Thus, the proportion of maternity patients at Mengo Hospital who were recorded as having a history of syphilis fell from 44 percent in 1929 to 33 percent, still a very high level, a decade later. That this decline was a consequence of growing diagnostic accuracy is suggested by the strengthening relationship between a history of syphilis and neonatal mortality over this period. Rates of neonatal mortality varied by only 0.6 percent in 1929, depending on whether a history of syphilis was recorded or not. By 1939 the incidence of neonatal mortality was 7.3 percent among patients with a history of syphilis and 4 percent for those without.[28] As late as 1953, while only 1 percent of infants attending secular child welfare clinics around Kampala were found to be syphilitic, the proportion of all cases diagnosed in the children's clinic at Nsambya Catholic Hospital between 1952 and 1954 identified as syphilis was 13 percent. Although these figures may appear to be a comparison of prevalence and incidence data, as child welfare clinics were aimed at preventing rather than curing disease, in fact child welfare specialists frequently complained that many women brought their children only when they were ill. The doctor who led the child welfare program in Kampala had in fact initially come to Uganda as a medical missionary but quickly moved to the state sector, partly because of what she considered gross overdiagnosis of STIs: "When I went out in '46 the first thing I was told was that c. 80 percent of the population were syphilitic."[29]

Buhaya: The Vernacularization of Colonial Discourse

Discourse and policy around STIs and fertility in Buhaya mimicked Buganda's in many ways. In part, this reflected pressures and preconceptions that were common across early colonial contexts in Africa. But beyond racial assumptions around the oversexed African, and underfunded imperial peripheries, there existed a conscious imitation of Buganda across much of British Africa in the early decades of the twentieth century. Buganda had negotiated a unique constitutional relationship with its British overrulers; it was perhaps the continent's most famous site of mission activity, and its long-standing unusual wealth and highly educated society, predating colonialism, permitted it to exert influence across the entire region. Administrators and clergy deliberately observed and learned from the Buganda model, but their fixation with low fertility and high STI rates derived from their observation of local conditions as well as external influences. European descriptions of Haya villages repeatedly noted the jarring paucity of children. The seeming tolerance by Haya of extramarital affairs in specific circumstances unsurprisingly encouraged assumptions among both missionaries and administrators that subfertility and high infant mortality were the consequences of "diseases of immorality," a process of logic that Haya themselves would absorb, as decades of condemnatory sermons and public health campaigns were reinforced by a comparative ethnography driven in part, as Derek Peterson has shown, by a competitive ethnic patriotism.[30]

In Buhaya, as in Buganda, fertility and STIs were frequently discussed in apocalyptic terms during the first quarter of the twentieth century. In 1913 one of many missionary jeremiads stated, "We live among a dying people. We always return from the clinic with this impression: sick from top to bottom. Unclean diseases have penetrated the people to a terrifying degree."[31] Successive administrative reports associated population decline with promiscuity and STIs and, worried about declining tax revenues, defined the apparent decline in the birthrate as being "of the utmost importance."[32] Where Buhaya diverged from its northern neighbor was that such predictions of imminent disaster persisted far beyond the early 1920s, almost until the end of the colonial era. In 1938 a missionary doctor preached that "'venereal disease has become rampant. We try to heal but it does not seem to help. . . . The Haya are a dying people. Your country will be eaten up by another people. Hayaland stands at the door of death.'"[33] That year steadily declining tax receipts caused Tanganyika's colonial government to dispatch Arthur and Geraldine Culwick, regarded as demographic specialists, to propose solutions to what was regarded as a population crisis. The Culwicks' report mimicked the missionaries' millenarian warnings: "The Bahaya are threatened with extinction as the result of venereal disease."[34] When census returns showed that Buhaya was an exception to the accelerating demographic growth that characterized East Africa, the colonial administration interpreted a fractional fall in the number of Haya from 259,931 in 1931 to 259,338 in 1948 as confirming "the trend foretold by Culwick. . . . The population is rapidly disappearing due to VD, prostitution and the general break-up of family life."[35] As late as 1952, a medical report reaffirmed that "the tribe is dying."[36]

Buganda's and Buhaya's rates of natural increase, or lack thereof, were in fact rather similar in the mid-twentieth century, but Buganda's perceived crisis was largely forgotten because of the enormous immigration of particularly fecund ethnic groups from the 1920s. Just as visible population expansion provides one explanation for the growing liberalism of Buganda's STI policy, so the enduring, if misguided, sense of imminent demographic collapse in

Buhaya helps account for the sustained extremism of its interventions over the colonial period. Energy and anxiety also stemmed from repeated medical reports that STIs were more common in Buhaya than anywhere else in Tanganyika. In 1925, for example, syphilis and gonorrhea accounted for 31 and 7 percent, respectively, of all outpatient diagnoses at Bukoba Hospital. Three years later 42 percent of cases treated in Buhaya's many rural medical units were diagnosed as syphilis, three and a half times the Tanganyikan average. In the early 1940s a quarter of antenatal cases had strongly positive Kahn tests, and a fifth of military recruits were diagnosed as suffering from gonorrhea. A third of all operations at Bukoba Hospital were believed to be related to gonorrhea.[37] That Haya dominated East Africa's sex trade added credibility to such figures, while the cyclical movement of large numbers of sex workers in and out of the district provided a convenient target on which to focus. Decade after decade proposals aimed at preventing suspected prostitutes from boarding ferries and buses, confining their operations to licensed brothels, or simply incarcerating them were repeatedly proposed.[38]

Buhaya's assimilation into the British Empire during World War I involved the transfer of administrative models and colonial and missionary personnel from Uganda. Albert Cook himself journeyed to Bukoba in 1919 to advocate for the adoption of Ugandan models of STI control. Struck by the coalescence of demographic, medical, and moral crises, Bukoba's administrators immediately requested permission from the colonial office to enforce compulsory inspection and treatment. It is particularly striking that less than a year after Uganda formally abandoned its coercive STI program, Buhaya's administration's requests for its replication within Tanganyika reached a crescendo: "Otherwise this rich and fertile district will . . . become depopulated and revert to bush."[39] Permission to replicate the Ugandan model was refused. Instead, in 1924 Buhaya instituted an intensive if toned-down program of mass semi-voluntary inspection and treatment, delivered through a new network of dispensaries run by tribal dressers. This approach was utterly unsuccessful, largely because the reliance on bismuth as the treatment for syphilis required numerous painful injections over so many months that defaulting was universal. In 1948 3,881 bismuth injections for syphilis given in nine dispensaries had achieved not one single cure because no patient had completed the course.[40]

As it became obvious that mass treatment offered little hope of controlling STIs, the sense grew between the wars that only a change of attitudes and behavior could save the Haya. STIs featured prominently in missionaries' sermons, official speeches, and school visits. Both the chiefly council and the Lutheran Church ruled that infections with gonorrhea or syphilis were grounds for divorce. And colonial experts recommended that the infected should wear a special badge, be separated from society, and undergo compulsory treatment, largely as an example to the uninfected.[41] After World War II popular discourse began to reflect external anxieties about demographic extinction and moral degradation. As indigenous politics in East Africa became restructured around a competitive patriotism that sought to control or reject emergent nationalist movements, populist demands for extreme measures against suspected prostitutes escalated beyond what was considered tolerable even by the illiberal standards of Tanganyika's colonial administration.[42] In 1951 anger turned against the imperial system: Europeans' repeated linkage of immorality, STIs, and demographic collapse was turned against them. With colonial inaction being interpreted as a "deliberate policy designed to reduce the population of the District," administrators cast around for radical new interventions. The development of regional research organizations such as the East African Medical Survey (EAMS) offered officials external solutions to local impasses. When the EAMS's pilot study indicated that the mass use of penicillin could eradicate syphilis and gonorrhea, the district commissioner convinced the Haya to pay for such a program through a special tax on coffee exports. Accepting the failure of moral admonition, it was now hoped that the assumption of financial responsibility would encourage the Haya to accept liability for their own health and so reform their sexual practices. "If not, the Haya would learn at their own expense that a purely medical approach will not work, and they would in future have only themselves, instead of government, to blame."[43]

That EAMS staff gave implicit support to the concept of mass compulsory treatment might seem an example of researchers being captured by the concerns of their subjects. But in fact their acceptance of compulsion followed their rejection of the local fixation with female immorality. While the EAMS accepted that prostitution had to be controlled, women were depicted as the victims of Buhaya's STI problem. Researchers believed that "men spent most of their time womanizing and drinking," that most female infections resulted from their husbands' infidelity, and that owing to social embarrassment and physiological obstacles to self-diagnosis, the female reproductive system had typically already been damaged by gonorrhea by the time women sought treatment.[44] A voluntarist campaign therefore would leave most female victims of STIs untreated.

The success of Buhaya's STI control program followed the decision to use a single-shot high-dosage injection of procaine penicillin as treatment for both gonorrhea and syphilis. The initial strategy prioritized speed, treating everyone with a history of STI infection or low fertility and rejecting the time-consuming niceties of testing. Medical teams depended on forceful persuasion, relying on missionaries and local chiefs to ensure attendance. As one participant in the program recalled, "They brought the medicine there, and people were being injected compulsorily. . . . There was really meaningful propaganda going on, and the force behind it in the villages was kind of hand in glove." Only as the campaign matured in the mid-1950s did testing begin to take on more prominence. This followed the decision to shift from a targeted peripatetic program that sought to radically reduce STIs within a locality to a mass campaign of easily accessible treatment, with injections being made available in each of Buhaya's twenty-three dispensaries. This reflected a new strategy, shaped by a new generation of Tanganyikan doctors, which sought to integrate STI control within a wider push to improve public health, from antimalarial measures to water sanitation and nutritional health education.[45]

Discussion: Fertility Change and STIs in a Sociomedical Context

In both societies impressive investments in fundamentally different control programs after 1950 were associated with rapid declines in STI prevalence and coincided with some of the sharpest increases in fertility rates in recorded history. As demonstrated earlier in the chapter, misdiagnosis of primary and secondary syphilis was so commonplace before the 1950s that longitudinal data relating to these conditions are of limited value. Tertiary syphilis, however, was less affected by difficulties in differential diagnosis, and so data relating to its impact on the nervous and cardiovascular systems can be regarded as reasonably reliable. Studies at Mulago Hospital in Kampala found that the incidence of neurosyphilis declined from 0.30 percent in 1937–41 to 0.04 percent in 1960–64, while conditions linked to syphilis accounted for 27 percent of cardiac admissions in 1952, 12 percent in 1957, 6 percent in 1965, and 4 percent in 1970.[46] Surveys, censuses, and Demographic Health Surveys estimated that Buganda's total fertility rate rose sharply from 3.0 in 1952 to 4.9 in 1959, 5.3 in 1969, and 8.0 in 1982–84. Rates of female sterility in Buganda meanwhile fell from 25 percent in 1948 to 18 percent in 1969 and 5 percent in 1994.[47] Buhaya's transformation was even more sudden. Here the total fertility rate rose from 3.0 in 1952 to 7.2 in 1967. Buhaya seems to have suffered less severely from primary sterility than Buganda. From a peak in 1938 at 18.5 percent, rates fell rapidly from the 1960s so that by 1984 southern Buhaya had the lowest levels of female infertility of seven districts surveyed in Tanzania, and in 1991 only 2 percent of ever-married women in Kagera region, within which Haya were the largest population group, were childless.[48] Buhaya's major problem had been secondary sterility. The proportion of ever-pregnant women in their twenties who had not conceived in the past five years fell from 51 to 8 percent between 1951 and 1973, while for women in their thirties the proportion fell from a remarkable 88 to 36 percent.[49] The relationship between STIs and fertility, however, was complex.

That STIs could provide only a partial explanation for subfertility was recognized even by researchers commissioned to analyze the demographic consequences of syphilis and gonorrhea. The EAMS noted in 1953 that STI rates were almost identical in Buhaya and the nearby region of Ukara, yet Ukara's fertility rates were 75 percent higher. Its report observed that in Buhaya it was necessary also to consider the "growing breakup of family life at an early stage with a consequent low birth rate in the later years of the female's reproductive life."[50] This comparative perspective highlighted that the reproductive impact of STIs depended not just on medical interventions but on social responses. In some African societies, typically those such as Buhaya, where childlessness threatened the loss of landed property, or regions where the slave trade and a particularly disruptive colonialism destabilized familial relationships, subfertility engendered a cycle of self-defeating behaviors.[51]

Among the Haya intense pressure to produce an heir accelerated partner exchange and divorce. A survey in the 1950s found that 22 percent of ever-married women in their twenties were divorced or separated, and another 24 percent were on their second or third marriage.[52] Infertility, as in many societies, implied a moral failure that legitimized divorce: "The parents of the husband would argue that it was justifiable for him to divorce because the wife had produced no children and so she was like a prostitute to him."[53] What was remarkable in Buhaya was how little time a couple was granted before alternative avenues to conception were proposed. A female interviewee remembered how "old women advised you to go with other, potent men" if, like her, pregnancy did not quickly follow a wedding. The alternative was bleak: "They hated [a childless woman], especially in the husband's family." Several women stated that they were divorced within a year of marriage, accused of being barren. Men were also pressured to seek children outside marriage, according to informants: "Very few men can tolerate to live with a barren woman and be faithful to her." Those who tried repeatedly to secure a child in new relationships were regarded as particularly likely to transmit STIs, saboteurs of Haya fertility. As one interviewee put it, "Old, infertile men would take girls of fifteen or sixteen and start trying to have children with them, so they spoiled the factory." Other men abandoned their Haya wives to marry women from ethnic groups known to be particularly prolific, such as Bahangaza: "Those are the women who had many children" in colonial Tanganyika. Less problematic, given the relative infrequency of church marriage, but significant nonetheless, was the insistence of missions during the mid-twentieth century that a wedding could be permitted only when both partners had a negative Kahn test. Given the retrospective realization that such tests produced frequent false positives before the technical improvements of the mid-1950s, many couples must have been wrongly denied the opportunity to form a reproductive union.[54]

The attempt by East African secular and religious authorities to convince local populations of sexually transmitted diseases' severity and ubiquity, and their dominant role in causing infertility, was remarkable in its intensity and longevity. Although authorities' understanding had become more nuanced by the 1950s, the success of penicillin-based STI campaigns between 1950 and 1970 was in part due to earlier propaganda forcing a revision in indigenous thinking about the nature of syphilis and about the connection between STIs and subfertility. In Buganda, as in much of the region, precolonial characterizations of syphilis, in contrast to gonorrhea, did not automatically define it as a sexually transmitted disease. Proverbs referring to gonorrhea emphasized its association with immorality and sexual means of transmission; those relating to syphilis did not. Oral accounts and local practices indicated that the disease was thought to spread usually by nonsexual contact or through in utero transmission. The broad consensus in the scholarship is that early European observers mistakenly assumed that all symptoms of treponemal disease they encountered were due to sexually transmitted syphilis, whereas most cases would in fact have been endemic syphilis or yaws. The lack of shame that so outraged missionaries and medics was sincere and appropriate, in the early colonial period at least. It is hypothesized that over time improved hygiene and increased use of clothing among children reduced the prevalence of nonsexual treponemal diseases, facilitating their displacement by sexually transmitted syphilis. Certainly, this displacement occurred to a large degree within local popular conceptualizations of syphilis. Even in the early 1940s newly arrived doctors were still shocked and amused by the frequency with which their medical encounters with patients went as follows: "What's the matter? 'Oh, I've got syphilis,' with a beaming smile." In the decades that followed, such reports gradually disappeared from the repertoire of medical anecdotes.[55]

In Buhaya in particular there developed an extremely powerful association in vernacular discourse between promiscuity, sexually transmitted disease, and infertility. Deepening anxiety about reproductive failure prompted internal debates where consensus was achieved that STIs were the primary, though not sole, agent, and immorality was the underlying cause of STIs. Agreement about exactly whose morality was most problematic was of course harder to come by, but the broad linkage was dominant in both contemporary sources and oral memory relating to the 1950s and 1960s. According to one group of male students writing in 1961, "Prostitutes are disseminators of disease. . . . Because of these diseases many women do not give birth."[56] Oral informants tended to be less accusatory, emphasizing recognition of the value of openness about the risks of promiscuity. "They used to tell young boys and girls not to do sexual intercourse; otherwise they would get diseases such as syphilis and gonorrhea. They said that those diseases could destroy the reproductive system. . . . The increase in fertility . . . coincided with . . . syphilis being reduced, by antibiotics."[57] "Fertility increased because people learnt not to keep STIs a secret, but to go to the doctor because they were an obstacle to reproduction."[58]

The extent to which mission-led theories of causality had been absorbed is indicated by the acceptance of their reverse logic. In the early 1950s an anthropologist working with the East African Medical Survey found that "if women had living children, they replied negatively to questions about having noticed symptoms of one of the venereal diseases even though when tested they had a strong positive reaction to the Kahn test. If women had no children or if one or more of their children had died, they replied affirmatively to the same question, even though when tested they had double negative Kahn reactions. Haya women held venereal disease to be responsible . . . for the fate of their [childless] condition apparently irrespective of their actual medical condition."[59] A decade earlier another medical researcher had made a similar observation: "If you believe . . . all who confessed to VD you would be led to assume that the disease was universal in the strictest sense of the word, yet many women who confessed to syphilis, the all-powerful, mysterious and ubiquitous disease, had a negative laboratory result."[60] One striking feature of my interviews with elderly Haya was the revelation that every single woman had used traditional herbs in an attempt to prevent STI infection, an indication of the actual or assumed frequency of extramarital affairs, and STIs, within the society. "If a woman conceived she had to put inside local herbs for the treatment of diseases liable to cause miscarriage." That this practice largely died out was due partly to recognition of the superior curative power of penicillin and partly to public health advice that "these herbs could cause infertility, because they block the cervix."[61]

This willingness to believe in their own immorality and infected status contributed to the particular enthusiasm with which Haya participated in the penicillin campaign of the 1950s and 1960s. Reports of the miraculous cure—its efficacy, immediacy, and painlessness contrasting so sharply with earlier treatments—created a sense of reproductive urgency, according to informants' accounts. The older generation, convinced that penicillin had removed the brake on population growth, pressured those of reproductive age to maximize their family size, to compensate for their own subfertility. As one man who came to maturity in the 1960s remembered, "My parents, they said that because we did not have enough children, for example, I was born alone, my mother she is the only daughter of her parents, when I said that I would like to have not more than six children, they said, 'you will be blessed to have as many children as possible.' . . . I should have children who would replace those they would have borne."[62] This shift in thinking was reflected in a remarkable change in reported ideal family size. In 1952 most answers fell between two and six, far lower than the norm elsewhere in colonial Africa. Yet in the context of early 1950s Buhaya, hoping for six children would have seemed wildly ambitious. By 2000 typical answers were ten or twelve, even though Buhaya's population had quadrupled, and population pressure on the land was high.[63] Haya reproductive optimism was also reflected in a stabilization of marriage, with the proportion of ever-married women who had been divorced by the age of thirty falling from a half to a third in two decades.[64]

The late colonial STI campaigns do seem to have contributed to a rapid increase in fertility and to a change in marriage patterns in Buhaya. That neurosyphilis, cardiovascular syphilis, and rates of primary and secondary sterility declined so sharply in the third quarter of the twentieth century indicates that penicillin markedly reduced the destructive consequences of ineffectively treated STIs. The penicillin-based campaigns' impact on sexual behavior and overall STI incidence and prevalence, however, should not be exaggerated. While Uganda's data from the 1950s and 1960s tell a story of steady declining incidence of some STIs (see figure 8.2), these figures should not be taken at face value. They were affected by greater accuracy and caution in diagnosis, as discussed earlier. Moreover, the treatment itself altered the behavior of the sick and created a selection effect that altered the relative frequency of the various STIs. One of the most striking consequences of penicillin's emergence was that it radically changed STI patients' gender profile. Before the 1950s men had made up the great majority of patients diagnosed with STIs in local clinics across the region. This was explained by the EAMS in both cultural and physiological terms: "Firstly the symptoms of gonorrhoea among women were often not severe enough either to warrant a trip to a clinic or to be detectable by a doctor, and secondly women in the lakes region were generally unwilling to come forward for gynaecological examination for whatever reason." This was immediately transformed by penicillin. By 1952 women made up 73 percent of STI patients attending Bukoba Hospital. It seems that it was awareness of a rapid, effective cure that encouraged women to accept the elevated risk of social embarrassment they faced and to seek testing and treatment. Penicillin also drew out sufferers of gonorrhea, which constituted 42 percent of all STI cases in that year, compared to syphilis's 49 percent, highlighting the misguided fixation with syphilis alone that had characterized the previous half century.[65]

In Uganda the incidence of syphilis fell steadily through the 1950s, whereas that of gonorrhea remained relatively steady. It is likely that this was partly due to individuals with long-standing gonococcal infections coming forward for treatment. It may also reflect misidentification of nongonococcal urethritis, including chlamydia, as well as new infections of penicillin-resistant gonorrhea, which was reported to be common around Kampala by the 1960s.[66] That penicillin seems to have provided a competitive advantage for STIs other than gonorrhea and syphilis is suggested by the much higher incidence of conditions such as chancroid around Kampala, by far the most intensively medicated community in East Africa, compared to the rest of Uganda. Thus in 1966 gonorrhea and syphilis accounted for 81 percent of all STI diagnoses nationally, but only 53 percent in the urban university clinic of Makerere.[67]

STI campaigns then were generally sufficiently effective to avert fertility-affecting sequelae by the 1960s, but new STI infections remained common and would of course facilitate the rapid spread of HIV in Buganda and Buhaya through the 1970s and 1980s. When penicillin was first introduced as an STI treatment in the region, it was feared that it would not "overcome the propensity to reinfection so frequently revealed. . . . The social attitude towards promiscuity, which is the basic predisposing cause of venereal disease, will need radical alteration if there is to a substantial reduction in the reservoir of infection."[68] The stabilization of marriage seen in Buhaya was not matched in Buganda, where instead fertility rose in part due to a growing tolerance of pre- and postmarital reproduction in the 1950s and 1960s.[69] While tales of the agony suffered by men affected by urethral stricture were common during discussions of the prepenicillin era, most informants felt that fear of STIs disappeared with penicillin. "Male promiscuity even increased because after whites came, the STIs could be healed." "People didn't fear gonorrhea very much because they could be treated and go back home, get infected again and go back for more treatment."[70] A 1966 study found that 28 percent of all

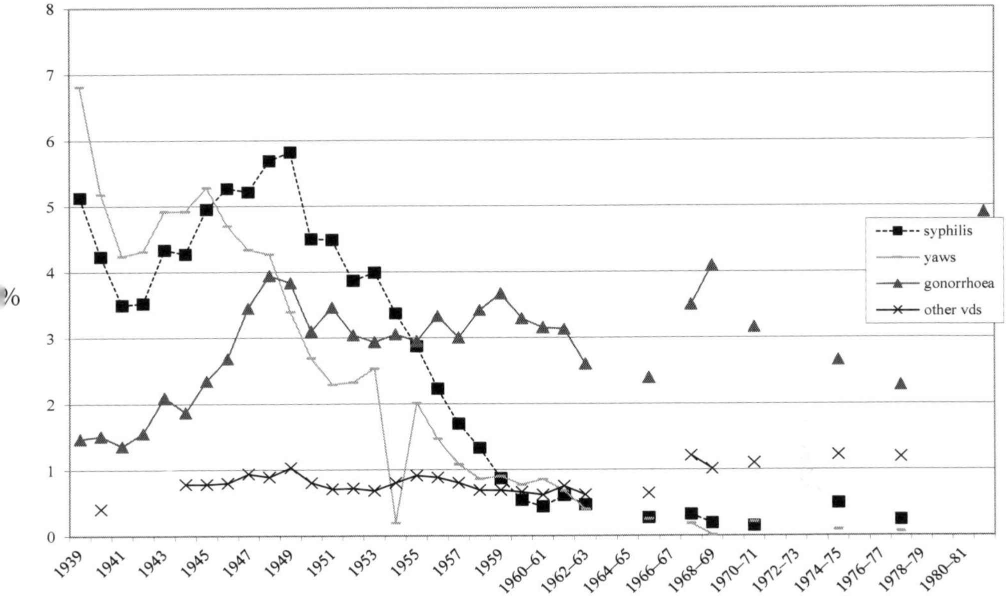

Figure 8.2. STDs and yaws as a percentage of all new outpatient cases at government hospitals in Uganda, for years with data (1939–82). Uganda Annual Reports, TNA, CO/685.

male undergraduates at Makerere University had had at least one STI within the previous year; half of the cases effected no behavioral change, and of these two-thirds suffered a reinfection. A few students felt anxiety around STI risk, but crucially, in terms of fertility, concealing infection or avoiding treatment was thought to be exceptionally unusual.[71]

Legacies

The case studies of Buganda and Buhaya are so significant because so many people for so long believed that eradicating STIs would resolve these societies' fertility crises. The intensity of this association was particularly mobilizing in Buhaya, because there, more so than in Buganda, public opinion in the 1950s and 1960s absorbed the unilinear argument that subfertility was due to STIs, which were due to promiscuity. Decades later elderly Haya informants displayed a much more nuanced and reflective understanding of fertility problems than was evident within popular discourse during the period of their young adulthood. While their memories of the late colonial period sometimes conjured up the narrow logic and moral anger that provided an appealing clarity and immediacy to the narratives necessary to the letter writers and speech makers of the mid-twentieth century, their individual fertility histories indicate that Buhaya's crisis ended because of a general improvement in the quality and range of reproductive health interventions.[72] While some women reported that penicillin enabled them to conceive or carry pregnancies to term, more stated that their ability to have children depended on careful antenatal monitoring, malaria treatment during pregnancy, various surgical procedures, and hospital delivery involving the use of forceps, vacuum extraction, or caesarean section. Institutionalized delivery had become so popular by 1959 that government clinics discussed introducing charges to deter nonemergency cases. Others reported that they received tetanus inoculations and that traditional birth attendants were trained to adopt more hygienic procedures, such as using new razor blades to cut the cord. Such innovations must have reduced maternal (and neonatal) mortality and prevented potentially sterilizing postpartum infections.[73]

STI campaigns in colonial Africa might appear to be typical, problematic examples of vertical interventions, treating one health condition in isolation. In fact, their significance is their longevity and their role in delivering mass preventive and curative health care provision.[74] Uganda's national referral hospital, Mulago, came into existence as a specialist VD unit. Buganda's remarkable improvements in reproductive health in the 1950s were based in large part on antenatal coverage reaching a staggering (for the time) 90 percent of pregnant women. The foundation for this achievement was the creation of dozens of mission maternity centers in the 1920s, designed to combat immorality. Buhaya's STI campaign of the 1950s similarly was so broad in its impact because it could utilize an exceptionally dense network of rural medical units that had been set up to deliver bismuth to the Haya masses. Penicillin, moreover, was rapidly made part of a regeneration of Buhaya's health care system, being tied to new interventions in malaria prevention and treatment, nutrition, and maternity care (all of which would have increased birthrates). STIs' emotive power energized colonial biomedicine. They proved particularly effective at leveraging extra funding from the notoriously parsimonious British Colonial Office. The message that individual behaviors increased the risk of infection and could lower fertility ultimately resonated simply because it was repeated decade after decade.

Yet it is necessary to end with some notes of caution. The success of penicillin-based STI campaigns in the 1950s and 1960s was in part due to changes in indigenous understandings of the nature of syphilis and the relationship between STIs and subfertility. But both of these conceptual shifts were based on partial misapprehensions. It is unlikely that non–sexually transmitted treponemal diseases had disappeared completely by 1950, while iatrogenic transmission of gonorrhea and syphilis must have been common, given the frequency of injections and blood transfusions in Kampala in particular. In addition, the role of STIs in limiting population growth, while important, was exaggerated. With hindsight some informants believed that they had been manipulated by the authorities in the 1950s and expressed skepticism about the sincerity of the motivations underlying medical interventions.[75] Health information campaigns did change popular opinion, but not completely, nor irreversibly. STI campaigns' tendency toward exaggeration and moral condemnation may have proven effective in some contexts in the past, but these tendencies are also likely to have contributed to the skepticism that has so often characterized many East Africans' responses to STI interventions over the past century, most notably during the subsequent era of AIDS.

Notes

1. Jack Goody, *Production and Reproduction: A Comparative Study of the Domestic Domain* (Cambridge: Cambridge University Press, 1976); Jack Caldwell, "The Social Repercussions of Colonial Rule: Demographic Aspects," in *UNESCO General History of Africa*, ed. Albert Adu Boahen, 7th ed. (London: Heinemann, 1985), 458–80; Jack Caldwell, Pat Caldwell, and Pat Quiggin, "The Social Context of AIDS in Sub-Saharan Africa," *Population and Development Review* 15, no. 2 (1989): 185–234.

2. Anne Retel-Laurentin, "Sub-fertility in Black Africa: The Case of the Nzakara in Central African Republic," in *Subfertility and Infertility in Africa*, ed. Babatunde Adadevoh (Ibadan: Caxton, 1974), 69–80; Anatole Romaniuk, "Increase in Natural Fertility during the Early Stages of Modernization: Evidence from an African Case Study, Zaire," *Population Studies* 34 (1980): 293–310; Gilles Sautter, *De l'Atlantique au fleuve Congo: Une géographie du sous-peuplement* (Paris: Mouton, 1966). Note, though, that these scholars acknowledged that STIs were the most important, but not the sole, cause of low fertility.

3. Michael Tuck, "Syphilis, Sexuality, and Social Control: A History of Venereal Disease in Colonial Uganda" (PhD diss., Northwestern University, 1997); Megan Vaughan, *Curing Their Ills: Colonial Power and African Illness* (Cambridge: Polity, 1991). While the focus is wider within Maryinez Lyons, "Sexually-Transmitted Diseases in the History of Uganda," *Genitourinary Medicine* 79 (1994): 138–45, the period of 1922–60 is dealt with in less than a page.

4. Jean-Pierre Chrétien, *The Great Lakes of Africa: Two Thousand Years of History*, trans. Scott Strauss (New York: Zone, 2003). For further cultural, demographic, and

medical context, see Shane Doyle, *Before HIV: Sexuality, Fertility and Mortality in East Africa* (Oxford: Oxford University Press, 2013).

5. Interview with the author (Int.) SK, Rubya, June, 21 2000; Priscilla Reining, "The Haya of North-Western Tanzania," in *Cultural Source Materials for Population Planning in East Africa*, vol. 3, *Beliefs and Practices*, ed. Angela Molnos (Nairobi: EAPH, 1973), 217–20; James Cunningham, *Uganda and Its Peoples: Notes on the Protectorate of Uganda, Especially the Anthropology and Ethnology of Its Indigenous Races* (London: Hutchinson, 1905), 284–93; G. Rwegelera, "Tribal Customs in Infant Feeding I: Among the Haya," *East Africa Medical Journal* 40 (1963): 366–69.

6. Mere Kisekka, "The Baganda of Central Uganda," in *Cultural Source Materials for Population Planning in East Africa*, vol. 2, *Innovations and Communication*, ed. Angela Molnos (Nairobi: EAPH, 1972), 167; Birth customs, October 20, 1954, Maryamu, Kisozi, Audrey Richards Papers, London, London School of Economics, 7/16; John Roscoe, *The Baganda: An Account of Their Native Customs and Beliefs* (London: Macmillan, 1911), 96, 237, 270; Albert Cook, *A Medical Vocabulary and Phrase Book in Luganda* (1903; repr., Kampala, 1921); Edwin Haydon, *Law and Justice in Buganda* (London: Butterworths, 1960), 217.

7. Rudyard Kipling, *100 Poems Old and New*, ed. Thomas Pinney (Cambridge: Cambridge University Press, 2013), 111–13.

8. Franz Stuhlmann, *Mit Emin Pascha ins Herz von Afrika* (Berlin: Reimer, 1894), 712, 726; Hermann Rehse, *Kiziba: Land und Leute* (Stuttgart: Strecker und Schröder, 1910), 1–30; Robert Moffat to Captain Greig, May 16, 1905, Bruce Papers, Albert Cook Library, Kampala; Henry Bell, "Uganda Diary, 1906–09," May 3, 1906; June 24, 1906, MSS 1975, Royal Commonwealth Society Archive, Cambridge; Hesketh Bell to Robert Crewe, January 6, 1909, National Archives (NA), CO/536/25; Lt. George Keane, Medical Officer, Venereal Disease Investigations, to the Provincial Commissioner, Buganda, May 19, 1911, in Buganda Annual Report, 1910–11, Entebbe Secretariat Archives, A46/420.

9. Albert Cook, "An Urgent Need in Uganda," *Mercy and Truth* 12 (1908): 44–50; Albert Cook, "Syphilis in the Uganda Protectorate," *British Medical Journal* 2, no. 2502 (1908): 1780–81; William Foster, *The Early History of Scientific Medicine in Uganda* (Nairobi: East African Literature Bureau, 1970), 70.

10. CMS Mengo Hospital Annual Report, 1912–13, Albert Cook Archive, Mulago Hospital, Kampala. As this quotation demonstrates, Cook's statistical authority reflected the absence not only of alternative sources of data within the Ugandan health care system but of significant critical analysis of numerical claims. Cook not only miscategorized miscarriage, stillbirth, and neonatal mortality as infant mortality; he also seems to have plucked figures from the air. The government had begun compiling stillbirth data in 1911, recording a Ugandan average of 13.7 percent, based on a limited sample, but gathered no data on miscarriage or neonatal mortality. Cook's figures exceeded even those recorded in his own hospital during this period, with only 26 percent of Mengo Hospital's maternity cases resulting in miscarriage, stillbirth, or neonatal death.

11. Robert Coryndon to Secretary of State, May 30, 1918, NA, CO/536/89; George Keane, report on venereal disease measures, Medical Report 1921, NA, CO/536/119; Coryndon to Secretary of State, November 11, 1920, NA, CO/536/101; Holger Hansen, *Mission, Church and State in a Colonial Setting: Uganda, 1890–1925* (New York: St. Martin's, 1984), 294; Albert Cook, *Uganda Memories, 1897–1940* (Kampala: Uganda Society, 1945), 342; Vaughan, *Curing Their Ills*, 130–36; Maryinez Lyons, "Medicine and Morality: A Review of Responses to Sexually Transmitted Diseases in Uganda in the Twentieth Century," in *Histories of Sexually Transmitted Diseases and HIV/AIDS in Sub-Saharan Africa*, ed. Philip Setel, Milton Lewis, and Maryinez Lyons (London: Greenwood, 1999), 97–117; Michael Tuck, "Venereal Disease, Sexuality, and Society in Uganda," in *Sex, Sin and Suffering: Venereal Disease and European Society since* 1870, ed. Roger Davidson and Lesley Hall (London: Routledge, 2001), 191–204.

12. Cook, "Urgent Need in Uganda"; Cook, "Syphilis"; Foster, *Early History*, 70.

13. Francis Lambkin, "An Outbreak of Syphilis on Virgin Soil," *Lancet* (1908): 1022; Francis Lambkin, Mission, to the Uganda Protectorate, report on the prevalence of venereal diseases, summary of evidence, December 1907, NA, CO/536/15; Vaughan, *Curing Their Ills*, 132–34; Lambkin, report on the prevalence of venereal disease in the Uganda Protectorate, December 1907, NA, CO/879/99; Carol Summers, "Intimate Colonialism: The Imperial Production of Reproduction in Uganda, 1907–1925," *Signs* 16, no. 4 (1991): 800; Hesketh Bell to E. E. K., January 20, 1908, NA, CO/536/18; Aubrey Hodges to Deputy Commissioner, April 1908, NA, CO/536/19. Lambkin's reference to degeneracy was a relatively rare example of eugenicist discourse within colonial Uganda. Eugenics' popularity was greatest in Britain's settler colonies, where whites' uneasy preeminence promoted assertions of African racial deterioration and colonists' tropical vigor. See Chloe Campbell, *Race and Empire: Eugenics in Colonial Kenya* (Manchester: Manchester University Press, 2007).

14. Diane Zeller, "The Establishment of Western Medicine in Buganda' (PhD diss., Columbia University, 1972), 195–99.

15. Keane to Provincial Commissioner, May 19, 1911, Entebbe Secretariat Archives.

16. Uganda Protectorate, "Annual Medical and Sanitary Report for 1913," NA, CO/685/2; Zeller, "Establishment," 197–201. The standard treatment provided in the program's early years was mercury or calomel, which would hardly have added to its popularity or efficacy. The effectiveness of Salvarsan was recognized, but it was made available only to patients who could pay for its application. Uganda Protectorate, *Annual Medical and Sanitary Report for the Year Ended 31st December 1921* (Entebbe: Government Printer, 1922).

17. Philippa Levine, "Venereal Disease, Prostitution, and the Politics of Empire: The Case of British India," *Journal of the History of Sexuality* 4, no. 4 (1994): 579–602. Admittedly, in practice Ugandan women suffered more than men from compulsory medical interventions.

18. Uganda Protectorate, "Annual Medical and Sanitary Report for 1919," NA, CO/685/3, p. 8; Uganda Protectorate, "Annual Medical and Sanitary Report for 1920," NA, CO/685/4, p. 9; Dr. Margaret Lamont to Dr. J. Walker, January 1, 1922, Uganda 1908–54, Women's Library, London, 3AMS/D/49; Lyons, "Sexually-Transmitted Diseases," 140; Reports on the treatment of venereal diseases from January 27, 1909, to March 31, 1910, NA, CO/536/33.

19. Lyons, "Sexually-Transmitted Diseases," 140; George Keane, report, in J. Hope Reford, Ag PMO, to National Council for Combating Venereal Diseases, August 22, 1922, Uganda 1908–54, Women's Library, 3AMS/D/49.

20. Jack Cook to Mrs. Smithett, YMCA, April 3, 1922, Uganda 1908–54, Women's Library, 3AMS/D/49.

21. Visit of Mrs. Smithett and A. Neilan to Albert Cook and Katherine Cook, [1922?], Uganda 1908–54, Women's Library, 3AMS/D/49; A. Neilans, AMSH, some notes on the memorandum issued by the CO concerning antivenereal measures in Uganda, Uganda 1908–54, Women's Library, 3AMS/D/49; Dr. Margaret Lamont to Dr. J. Walker, January 1, 1922, Uganda 1908–54, Women's Library, 3AMS/D/49; Webb, interview, April 20, 1922, NA, CO/536/120; George Keane, venereal diseases in Uganda, 1922, NA, CO/536/120; Notes of a conference on venereal measures, April 6, 1922, NA, CO/536/123.

22. As in Buganda, the shift toward voluntarism in England was not absolute. See Pamela Cox, "Compulsion, Voluntarism, and Venereal Disease: Governing Sexual Health in England after the Contagious Diseases Acts," *Journal of British Studies* 46, no. 1 (2007): 91–115.

23. Anonymous to M. Billson, AMSH, February 1, 1951; F. Webber, CO, to General Secretary, AMSH, October 30, 1951; Mary Stuart to Billson, April 3, 1952, Uganda 1908–54, Women's Library, 3AMS/D/49; Aidan Southall and Peter Gutkind, *Townsmen in the Making: Kampala and Its Suburbs* (Kampala: East African Institute of Social Research, 1957), 193–94.

24. Gerald McElligott, "Venereal Diseases in the Tropics," *British Journal of Venereal Diseases* 27 (1951): 125; Uganda Protectorate, *1951 Annual Medical Report* (Entebbe: Government Printer, 1952); Uganda Protectorate, *1952 Annual Medical Report* (Entebbe: Government Printer, 1953); Lyons, "Sexually-Transmitted Diseases"; Tuck, "Syphilis," 164–69. Similar shifts in STI prevention policy toward self-conscious modernity and responsibility developed in interwar England. See Francesca Moore, "'A Mistaken Policy of Secretiveness': Venereal Disease and Changing Heterosexual Morality in Lancashire, UK, 1920–1935," *Historical Geography* 43 (2015): 37–56. See also Roger Davidson, *Dangerous Liaisons: A Social History of Venereal Disease in Twentieth-Century Scotland* (Amsterdam: Brill, 2000).

25. Davidson, *Dangerous Liaisons*; O. P. Arya and John Bennett, "Venereal Disease in an Elite Group (University Students) in East Africa," *British Journal of Venereal Disease* 43 (1967): 275–79; Arya and Bennett, "Attitudes of College Students in East Africa to Sexual Activity and Venereal Disease," *British Journal of Venereal Diseases* 44 (1968): 160–66; Arya and Bennett, "What Do the Educated Want to Know about

VD? An Analysis of the Questions Asked by University and College Students in Uganda," *Uganda Medical Journal* 2 (1973): 91–103.

26. Denis Burkitt to Sir Harold Himsworth, MRC, January 21, 1963; External scientific staff, Mr. Denis Burkitt, Makerere College Medical School, NA, FD12/882; John Bennett, "The Social Determinants of Gonorrhoea in an East African Town," *East African Medical Journal* 39 (1962): 332–42; V. Ongom, "Prevalence and Incidence of Venereal Diseases in Military Communities in Uganda," *East African Medical Journal* 47, no. 9 (1970): 479–83; Aaron Masawe, "Syphilis in Uganda: The History, Clinical Features and Cellular Immunity" (MMed diss., Makerere University Kampala, 1971), 34; Arya and Bennett, "Venereal Disease"; Uganda Protectorate, *1952 Annual Medical Report*. See Lyons, "Sexually-Transmitted Diseases," 141.

27. Jack Davies, "Pathology of Central African Natives: Mulago Hospital Post Mortem Studies," *East African Medical Journal* 24, no. 8 (1947): 289–303; Davies, "Causes of Death in African Children," *East African Medical Journal* 25 (1948): 228; Dr. Evans, diary of 1953 visit to Uganda, Wellcome Archive, A.3/1 PP/PRE; Tuck, "Syphilis," 227. Adrian Mindel and Claudia Estcourt, "Syphilis," in *Sexually Transmitted Diseases: Vaccines, Prevention and Control*, ed. Lawrence Stanberry and David Bernstein (Cambridge: Academic Press, 2000), 388, noted that between 1917 and 1941 Yale Medical School autopsies found 9.7 percent of patients displayed evidence of syphilis.

28. Mengo maternity registers, 1907–39, Albert Cook Library, Kampala. The extent to which Mulago's doctors shed assumptions of African hypersexuality before the 1940s should not be exaggerated. Michael Tuck found that European patients with the same clinical signs and serology as Africans were less likely to be diagnosed as syphilitic in the interwar period. "Syphilis," 227.

29. Uganda Annual Medical Report, 1953, Nsambya Hospital Registers, Kampala; Int. HW, Bristol, July 31, 2008.

30. See, for example, Bukoba District Annual Report, 1926, Tanzania National Archives (TNA), Dar es Salaam, 215/77/A; Bengt Sundkler, *Bara Bukoba: Church and Community in Tanzania* (London: Hurst, 1980). See Derek Peterson, *Ethnic Patriotism and the East African Revival: A History of Dissent* (Cambridge: Cambridge University Press, 2012).

31. Birgitta Larsson, *Conversion to Greater Freedom? Women, Church and Social Change in North-Western Tanzania under Colonial Rule* (Uppsala: University of Uppsala, 1991), 96.

32. Bukoba District Annual Report, 1925, TNA, 1733/3:46 (AB40); Bukoba District Annual Report, 1919, TNA, 1733/5 (AB48), p. 8.

33. Larsson, *Conversion to Greater Freedom*, 107–8.

34. Arthur Culwick, "The Population Problem in the Bukoba District," 1938, Bukoba, University of Dar es Salaam, EAF CORY 239, pp. 7–9.

35. Bukoba District Annual Report, 1948, TNA, 215/2237.

36. East African Medical Survey, *Annual Report, 1952* (Nairobi: East African High Commission, 1953), 23–32. In the early 1950s birth rates for the indigenous

inhabitants of both Buganda and Buhaya were similarly low, but the subfertility of the Ganda was masked by the high fertility of immigrant groups, who made up almost half of Buganda's population by this time.

37. Bukoba District Annual Report, 1925 (Bukoba subdistrict), TNA, 1733/3:46 (AB40); Bukoba District Annual Report, 1928, TNA, 215/77/B; Tanganyika Territory, Annual Medical Report 1928, TNA Library; Tanganyika Territory, *Annual Report of the Medical Department 1941* (Dar es Salaam: Government Printer, 1942); Tanganyika Territory, *Annual Report of the Medical Department 1943* (Dar es Salaam: Government Printer, 1944).

38. Bukoba District Annual Report, 1928, TNA, 215/77/B; Arthur Culwick and Geraldine Culwick, *The Culwick Papers, 1934–1944: Population, Food and Health in Colonial Tanganika*, ed. Veronica Berry (London: Academic Books, 1994), 173; "Official Correspondence Relating to Constitutional Matters, Politics and Land, Including Notes and Memoranda by Hans Cory, 1950–58," District Commissioner to Provincial Commissioner, April 10, 1951, Bukoba, UDSM, EAF CORY 21; William Laurie, "A Pilot Scheme of Venereal Disease Control in East Africa," *British Journal of Venereal Diseases* 34 (1958): 21.

39. Bukoba District Annual Report, 1923, TNA, 1733/8 (AB10), pp. 18–19.

40. John Iliffe, *East African Doctors* (Cambridge: Cambridge University Press), 40; Bukoba District Annual Report, 1948, TNA, 215/2237; Annual Report for the Bukoba District for the Year 1946, TNA, 215/2070.

41. A. Donne, editor of *Mambo Leo*, to Secretary of Native Affairs, September 21, 1930, TNA, 19153, vol. 1, *Venereal Disease: Anti-venereal Measures*; Larsson, *Conversion to Greater Freedom*, 107–9; Hans Cory and Morwenna Hartnoll, *Customary Law of the Haya Tribe, Tanganyika Territory* (London: Cass, 1971), 104–5; Bengt Sundkler, "Marriage Problems in the Church in Tanganyika," *International Review of Missions* 34 (1945): 253–55; Hans Cory, "The Haya Tribe and the Incidence of Venereal Disease, Bukoba 1938–48," typescript, UDSM, EAF CORY 104, p. 10; Culwick, and Culwick, *Culwick Papers*, 44–50; A. Culwick, "Population Problem," 9.

42. Peterson, *Ethnic Patriotism*.

43. Tim Harris, *Donkey's Gratitude: Twenty-Two Years in the Growth of a New African Nation; Tanzania* (Durham: Pentland, 1992), 261–65; "Official Correspondence," UDSM.

44. Hope Trant, "Not Merrion Square: Anecdotes from a Woman's Medical Career in Africa," Weston Library, Oxford, MSS.Af.s.1872(143), p. 128; Laurie, "Pilot Scheme," 18; William Laurie and Hope Trant, *East African Medical Survey, Monograph No. 2: A Health Survey in Bukoba District, Tanganyika* (Nairobi: East African High Commission, 1954), 4–5.

45. Laurie and Trant, *East African Medical Survey*, 135–41; "Official Correspondence," UDSM; Int. HL, Maruku, June 17, 2000; Int. JBK, Ijumbi, August 11, 2000; Annual Report for the Bukoba District for the year 1953, TNA, 215/2700; District Medical Officer to Provincial Medical Officer, monthly report,

West Lake, May 1957, June 6, 1957, TNA, Acc. 71 M. 1/1, Medical General, vol. 2; West Lake Provincial Annual Report 1960, TNA, 967.822.1; Annual Report for the Bukoba District for the year 1957, TNA, 215/3449; Int. VK, Bukoba, June 27, 2000.

46. Roy Billington, "Neurosyphilis in Uganda: A Comparison of Two Five-Year Periods," *East African Medical Journal* 43, no. 11 (1966): 469–73; Masawe, "Syphilis in Uganda," 14. For Buhaya, see "Annual Report, Bukoba District Council Medical Services, 1966," January 30, 1967, Mwanza Provincial Archives, MISS/DN/53.

47. Priscilla Reining and Audrey Richards, "Report on Fertility Surveys in Buganda and Buhaya, 1952," in *Culture and Human Fertility*, ed. Frank Lorimer et al. (Paris: UNESCO, 1954), 351–404; E. Kibukamusoke to Audrey Richards, May 31, 1967, 16/48, Richards Papers; Uganda Protectorate, *Uganda Census 1959: African Population* (Entebbe: Ministry of Economic Affairs, 1960); Uganda, *Report on the 1969 Population Census* (Entebbe: Ministry of Planning and Economic Development, 1971); Emmanuel Kaijuka et al., *Uganda Demographic and Health Survey, 1988/1989* (Columbia, MD: Ministry of Health–Uganda/Institute for Resource Development/Macro Systems, 1989), 19; Uganda Protectorate, *African Population of Uganda Protectorate: Geographical and Tribal Studies* (1948; repr., Nairobi: East African High Commission, 1953); Januario Nabaitu, Cissy Bachengana, and Janet Seeley, "Marital Instability in a Rural Population in South-West Uganda: Implications for the Spread of HIV-1 Infection," *Africa* 64, no. 2 (1994): 243–51.

48. Roushdi Henin and Bertil Egero, "1967 Population Census of Tanzania: A Demographic Analysis," Bureau of Resource Assessment and Land Use Planning Research Notes 19, UDSM, 1972; Roushdi Henin, *National Demographic Survey of Tanzania, 1973*, 6 vols., Dar es Salaam: Tanzania Bureau of Statistics, 1973), 2:32; National Bureau of Statistics and ORC Macro, *Tanzania Demographic and Health Survey, 1991–02* (Calverton, MD: National Bureau of Statistics/ORC Macro, 1993), 53–58; L. Mtimavalye et al., "Infertility among Women in Five Rural and Two Urban Districts of Tanzania," *Journal of Obstetric and Gynecology in East and Central Africa* 3 (1984): 125–29; Ulla Larsen, "Primary and Secondary Infertility in Tanzania," *Journal of Health and Population in Developing Countries* 3 (2003): 1–15; Larsen, "Childlessness, Subfertility, and Infertility in Tanzania," *Studies in Family Planning* 27, no. 1 (1996): 18–28.

49. East African Medical Survey, *Annual Report, 1951* (Nairobi: East African High Commission, 1952), 66; William Brass, "The Estimation of Fertility Rates from Ratios of Total to First Births," *Population Studies* 8, no. 1 (1954): 74–87; Henin, *National Demographic Survey*, 1:215–38, 3:1–134, 6:75; Larsen, "Childlessness," 20–27. The EAMS had used eight rather than five years as the measure of subsequent sterility, but the change is unlikely to have affected the results significantly.

50. East African Medical Survey, *Annual Report, 1953* (Nairobi: East African High Commission, 1954), 12–13.

51. Other examples of societies where crises of subfertility provoked social reactions that were likely to accelerate STI transmission include the Dobe !Kung (when fear of sterility becomes acute, "the woman often tries conception with another partner, thereby ensuring the transmission of the disease [gonorrhea] to others") and the Nzakara ("Ainsi les populations inféondes se trouvent prisonnières un cycle: stérilité → mobilité des femmes → maladies vénérienne [Infertile populations become trapped in a cycle: sterility leads to female mobility, which leads to STIs]). Nancy Howell, *Demography of the Dobe !Kung* (London: Academic Press, 1979), 180; Jean Hurault, "Un ouvrage méconnu: Infécondité en Afrique Noire d'Anne Retel-Laurentin," *Cahiers d'études africaines* 27, nos. 105–6 (1987): 177–85. See also Anne Retel-Laurentin, *Un pays à la dérive: Une société en régression démographique; Les Nzakara de l'est centrafricain* (Paris: Delarge, 1979).

52. Laurie and Trant, *East African Medical Survey*, 37–38.

53. Int. M, Bukoba, 1998.

54. Int. VKB, Busindi, 2000; Int. VM, Kanyangereko, June 16, 2000; Int. GK, Nkindo, August 2000; Int. HL, Maruku, June 17, 2000; Int. YK, Kikukwe, August 2000. See Larsson, *Conversion to Greater Freedom*, 103–21.

55. Cook, *Medical Vocabulary*; Cecil Hackett, "On the Origin of the Human Treponematoses (Pinta, Yaws, Endemic and Venereal Syphilis)," *Bulletin of the World Health Organization* 29, no. 1 (1963): 7–41; Zeller, "Establishment," 400–401; Jack Davies, "'The History of Syphilis in Uganda," *Bulletin of the World Health Organization* 15 (1956): 1052–53; Tuck, "Syphilis," 52–68; Ferdinand Walser, *Luganda Proverbs* (Berlin: Reimer, 1982), proverb 1663; Int. HW, Bristol, July 31, 2008.

56. Haya students of Saint Andrew's Teacher Training College, Korogwe, to the Secretary of the Council of Buhaya, July 6, 1961, Mwanza Provincial Archives, L5/II/B.

57. Int. MM, Ruhija, August 2000, b. 1932.

58. Int. TM, Busindi, August 2000, b. 1935.

59. Priscilla Reining, "The Haya: The Agrarian System of a Sedentary People" (PhD diss., University of Chicago, 1967), 86–87. It is indicative of the limited value of the Kahn test before its refinement that the East African Medical Survey, *1952 Annual Report* (Nairobi: Government Printer, 1952): 32, noted that, having tested six hundred women, surveyors found that a positive Kahn result "had no apparent association with the fertility of the women."

60. G. A. Macgregor, "The Incidence of Syphilis among Antenatal Women Attending Kagondo and Bukoba Hospitals' Maternity and Child Welfare Clinics," Medical Officer Bukoba, March 1942, Bukoba District Book, Weston, Library Oxford.

61. See, for example, Int. AC, Rubaa-Rubya, August 2000; Int. AM, Busindi, August 2000; Int. MM, Ijumbi, August 2000; Int. SKN, Maruku-Butailuka-Kasha, August 2000, b. 1938. Women also inserted herbs to aid conception and act as a perfume.

62. Int. WR, Rubya, June 21, 2000. See also Int. VPB, Busindi, 2000; and Int. KK, Bibanja, June 15, 2000.

63. Reining, "Haya of North-Western Tanzania," 218–19; Int. YK, Kikukwe, August 2000; Int. PB, Maruku, August 2000; Int. JBK, Ijumbi, August 11, 2000; Int. SK, Rubya, June 21, 2000; Int. N, Katongo, 1998; Int. GK, Nkindo, August 2000.

64. A. Richards and P. Reining, "Report on Fertility Surveys in Buganda and Buhaya, 1952," UDSM CORY 373; Laurie and Trant, *East African Medical Survey*, 37; Henin, *National Demographic Survey*, 2:78, 32.

65. East African Medical Survey, *1951 Annual Report* (Nairobi: Government Printer, 1951); East African Medical Survey, *Annual Report*, 67. A full 9 percent of all cases were coinfected with both gonorrhea and syphilis—these were shared equally between the two conditions in the calculation used in the discussion. In Buganda by the 1970s STI clinics were again regarded as male spaces to such an extent that a female VD clinic was opened at Mulago. Masawe, "Syphilis in Uganda," 29–31.

66. Ian Phillips, "A Guide to Antibiotic Treatment of Gonorrhoea in Uganda," *Makerere Medical Journal* 1, no. 3 (1968): 105; Phillips et al., "Antibiotic Sensitivity of Gonococci in Kampala," *East African Medical Journal* 46 (1969): 38–45.

67. Government of Uganda, *Annual Reports of the Ministry of Health, 1963–9* (Entebbe: Government Printer, 1964–70); Arya and Bennett, "Venereal Disease." Alternatively, the higher incidence of other STIs may simply have reflected superior diagnostic capacity around Kampala.

68. Uganda, *1952 Medical Report* (Entebbe: Government Printer, 1953).

69. Southall and Gutkind, *Townsmen in the Making*, 88–89; Lucy Mair, *Native Marriage in Buganda, International Institute of African Languages and Cultures Memorandum XIX* (Oxford: Oxford University Press, 1940), 32; Int. FN, Butanga, August 29, 2004; Peter Gutkind, "African Urban Family Life: Comment On and Analysis of Some Rural-Urban Difference," *Cahiers d'études africaines* 10 (1962): 202; Cyril Crocker et al., "A Study of Knowledge, Attitudes, and Practices of Family Planning in Uganda, East Africa," *Journal of Reproductive Medicine* 7, no. 5 (1971): 235–38. Marital stabilization should not be confused with moral purity. The frequent partner exchange that was symptomatic of the smuggling culture associated with the outbreak of HIV in the early 1980s was already well established in Buhaya's border settlements by 1967. Divisional Executive Officer to all Assistant Divisional Officers and all Village Executive Officers, March 2, 1967, Missenyi, Mwanza Provincial Archives, F37/54.

70. Int. FGD, Kisubi Kiwulwe, September 4, 2004; Int. KJK, Kitala, August 31, 2004; Int. IST, Kagezi village, Masaka, August 21, 2004; Int. FGD, Takajunge, August 26, 2004.

71. Arya and Bennett, "Venereal Disease"; Arya and Bennett, "Attitudes of College Students."

72. E. Barongo, Deputy General Secretary TANU to Shell Muhanna MP, January 18, 1962, MPA, L5/II/B; Sospeter Matola Matovu to Secretary, Tanganyika African Club Nairobi Branch, January 10, 1963, MPA, L5/II/B.

73. See, for example, Int. MM, Ruhija, August 2000; Int. TM, Busindi, August 2000; Int. SKN, Maruku-Butailuka-Kasha, August 2000; Int. PMJ, Rubya, August 9, 2000; Int. MM, Kanoni-Kamachumu, August 2000; Int. CN, Kanoni, August 2000; Int. GK, Nkindo, August 2000; Int. FK, Kikukwe, August 2000; Int. KM, Kikuku-Kanyigo, August 2000; District Medical Officer to Secretary of the Council of Buhaya, August 18, 1959, MPA, M20/8 Maternity, 1959–72.

74. There are notable similarities with the experience of the United Kingdom, where the interwar STI program laid the foundations for the National Health Service. See John Eyler, *Sir Arthur Newsholme and State Medicine, 1885–1935* (Cambridge: Cambridge University Press, 1997), 277–94.

75. See, for example, Int. RK, Takajjunge, August 26, 2002; Int. CNSM, Butanga, August 26, 2004; and William Schneider, *The History of Blood Transfusion in Africa* (Athens: Ohio University Press, 2013).

Chapter Nine

"A Wise Provision of Nature for the Prevention of Too Many Children"

Evidence from the Australian Colonies

Janet McCalman and Rebecca Kippen

Doctors, scholars, politicians, and moralists have always had much to say about venereal disease, as have feminist historians and historians of eugenics and medical discourse. But rarely do we hear the voices of the afflicted, nor engage with the lived reality of the penalties of sex. Yet the relevant evidence can be found in medical records or reconstructed from population data to enable us to focus on the experiences endured by the afflicted and those rendered infertile. While the history of elite discourses matter, we need to know more about who, where, and why men and women became sick from sex and what it did to their lives. In this chapter we explore the lives from four marginalized populations in early colonial Australia: the family Furlong over four generations, convict women transported to Tasmania, Aboriginal women in Victoria, and women admitted to the charity Melbourne Women's Hospital.

A Family History

On November 7, 1883, the resident medical officer in the infirmary of the Melbourne Women's Hospital made his clinical observations of Maria Furlong (née Robinson). She was thirty-four years old and had married fifteen years before, at the age of nineteen.[1] The resident medical officer was delicate about Maria's condition, heading the page with the diagnosis of pregnancy and umbilical hernia, lest the prying eyes of the ladies of the hospital Committee of Management raise awkward questions. Hence, her face bore "stigmata," but he did not specify of what nature. She now was "very flabby," even though she was "fairly healthy" and had a "good sanguine complexion." She was experiencing a difficult pregnancy with pains in her back between the shoulders. She had been vomiting for seven days and on admission was "very weak, with a feeble pulse, breathing fast and oppressed." Four days later she miscarried a six-month-old fetus that had been "some time dead." By November 24, thirteen days after the miscarriage, she was discharged with the hernia "very much less tense—lying loosely outside." She was advised "to avoid hard food and strong *drink*."[2]

The hernia was not a red herring. It killed her six months later, after she suffered an intussusception of the bowel for a month at home.[3] It would have been an agonizing death. She was a heavy drinker, but then she had reason to be. She had reported to the resident medical officer the year before that she had borne nine children and suffered eight abortions, and she was about to have her ninth miscarriage. Birth registrations can be found for only six of those children, so perhaps she had three stillbirths in addition to nine miscarriages.[4] By the time of her death in 1884, she had just two surviving children from those eighteen conceptions: Caroline, ten years old; and Maria Louisa, five years old. Her firstborn, William, died in infancy in 1867; Charles died next in 1872, at eleven months, of diarrhea; Frederick, her second-born, died in 1875, six years old, of croup; and the second William died in 1876, at seven days, from exhaustion and diarrhea. Maria Louisa was to die at age ten, from typhoid, in 1889. Only Caroline lived into adulthood; she never married and died in poverty at the age of seventy-four, as a "cake maker," having been apprenticed as a bookbinder (figure 9.1).[5]

Their father, William Lawrence Furlong, was a printer, son of a surgeon from Mauritius. He had a cultivated signature and was well read. After the death in 1884 of his first wife, Maria, he moved into government employment as a "battery man" on the railways, where he had security and could style himself a "civil servant." He married Mary Ellen Carrigg in 1887 and started a second family, fathering six daughters over the next ten years: Mary,

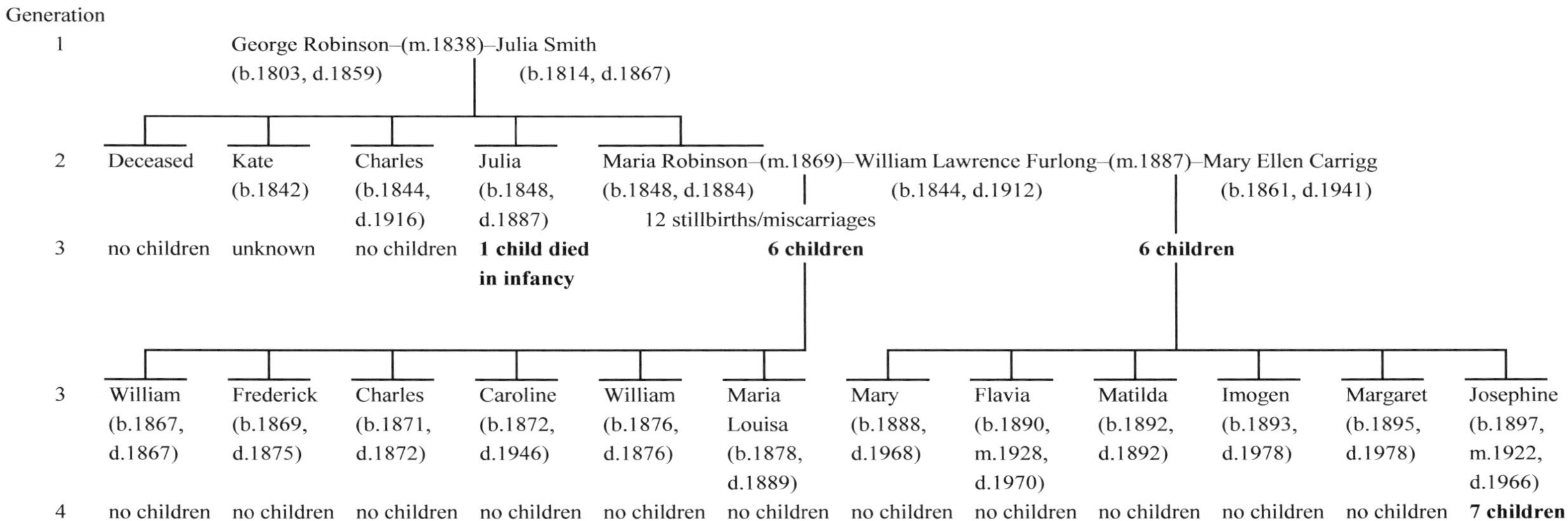

Figure 9.1. George Robinson and Julia Smith family tree.

Flavia, Matilda, Imogen, Margaret, and Josephine.[6] Only Matilda perished in infancy. Like their older half sister Caroline, the five survivors were apprenticed as bookbinders. Flavia married in her late thirties and had no children. Mary, Imogen, and Margaret remained single, living into their ninth decade all together in a cottage in the inner city.[7] Just one daughter of William and Mary Ellen—the last-born, Josephine—could be found to have had children.[8] The seed of William Lawrence Furlong—twenty-four conceptions over two relationships and thirty years—produced just one family in the third generation (figure 9.1). Was there also a "taint" feared in this second family?

William Lawrence Furlong must have met his first wife, young Maria Robinson, soon after his arrival as a free immigrant in 1865. She was then a habitué of the Eastern Market in the rough end of Melbourne, with theaters, louche hotels, and brothels. Her mother had died in early 1867, and in July of that year Maria gave birth to William's first child, a son, named for his father; the child died five hours after birth.[9]

By February 1868 Maria was lodging with a "well-known disorderly character Elizabeth Trembath," probably as a base for continued prostitution. Trembath accused her of stealing three pounds, ten shillings, and Maria was sentenced to two months in jail.[10] In March 1869 Maria was again convicted, this time with vagrancy, along with four other women and a young man, for being "constantly around the Eastern Market." The women received three months in jail and the young man, six.[11] Maria was pregnant with her second child and must have been released early to give birth. The delivery took place in May 1869 at 25 Little Napier Street, Fitzroy, the home of William Furlong. Three months later Maria and William married at Saint Patrick's Cathedral, Melbourne.[12]

So why was young Maria already a vagrant and a prostitute and lodging with a notorious and dissolute woman who was rarely out of the courts? Maria was the daughter—according to the story she had given William Furlong—of a Tasmanian whaler, George Robinson, and his wife, Julia, whose maiden name she did not know. George Robinson, a mat maker, died of gangrene of the lungs in 1859 in Hobart, Tasmania, abandoned by his wife and children.[13] Julia Smith had been born in Athlone, County Meath, and at the age of twenty-one, and already a widow, she was convicted for the second time for theft in London at the Old Bailey and transported to Van Diemen's Land for seven years.[14] She had been "on the town," or a public prostitute, in London for twelve months, according to the police. She arrived on the *Westmoreland* in 1836 and received permission to marry George Robinson two years later.[15] She had five children with him, four of whom were still alive at the time of her death: Kate born in 1842, Charles in 1844, and twin girls, Maria and Julia, in 1848.[16] Kate disappears from sight, but Charles appeared in Melbourne in 1868—a bad year for the family—charged with burglary and sentenced to five years hard labor on the roads. He rehabilitated himself in later life, married late at the age of fifty-seven, and became a stepfather in the process. His marriage lasted until his death at the age of seventy-two—one family success story, if not a reproductive one.[17]

Maria's twin, Julia, fared not so well. Likewise racking up convictions for larceny and a two-year sentence in 1867 for stealing, in 1870 she lost her only baby at twelve months from extended diarrhea.[18] A year later, as a "woman of the town," she was sentenced to three years' prison for manslaughter when she stabbed her de facto in the neck during a drunken fight. She was in prison again in 1887, when she was transferred to the Yarra Bend Lunatic Asylum, where at age thirty-nine, she died of "cerebral softening" (a likely indicator of tertiary syphilis).[19] As for their mother, Julia Senior, she had been convicted for drunkenness soon after marriage in Hobart.[20] Like many former convict women who had been on the town before transportation, she could not resist the rich pickings in gold rush Victoria and by 1857 was running a disorderly house in Romeo Lane, the haunt of Vandemonian prostitutes in Melbourne.[21] In her final years her crimes were drunk and disorderly conduct, and she died, also of "softening of the brain," in Melbourne Hospital in January 1867. She was fifty-four.[22]

This tragic family history is one of syphilis and its legacy over two generations of transmission and possibly even longer psychic effects. This was a family that faded away. Just one of the third generation had children, out of twenty-five conceptions and thirteen recorded live births (see figure 9.1). It had all begun with Julia Smith, who had been just one of the hundreds of thousands of Irish-born women who found themselves unsupported and on the streets of English and Scottish cities in the nineteenth century, and who had nothing to sell in that marketplace other than their bodies. Like many of the toughest convict women, she regarded her daughters as capital and prostituted them also, perhaps as had happened to herself.

Convict Women and the Penalty of Gender

Convict women like Julia Smith, transported to Van Diemen's Land between 1803 and 1853, provide a window into the impact of sexually transmitted disease on life courses and on fertility. The detailed gaze of the "paper panopticon" that managed the penal colony has left us with a remarkable record of captive lives. Through the Founders and Survivors Ships Project, online genealogical and historical records have enabled the reconstitution of twenty-five thousand convict lives—before, during, and after sentencing—out of the sixty-eight thousand transported to Van Diemen's Land.[23] Servitude imposed a penalty on all convict lives, but far more so for women. In particular, women who had been "on the town" before transportation, according to their convict and police records, suffered an extreme mortality penalty, which isolated them as a subpopulation at high risk of venereal disease.[24]

The sex imbalance in the colony, with men outnumbering women six to one at the peak, ensured that most convict women married.[25] Indeed, the penal authorities encouraged convict marriages as a reward for good behavior and in the interests of orderly, permanent settlement.[26] However, even though largely married, convict women transported before the age of twenty-five years, and thereby young enough to build families in the colony, had a high incidence of acquired or secondary lifetime infertility. Figure 9.2 shows the fertility distribution of English- and Irish-born convict women, transported between the age of twenty and twenty-five years over the period 1820 to 1853, with the sample further restricted to those known to have married after transportation and known to have died after the age of fifty years. The population groups are classified by country of birth (England or Ireland) and whether they were noted as having been "on the town" at the time of conviction. Around one-third of young women convicts had "on the town" noted on their records.[27]

There are significant variations between the four population groups. English-born women who had been on the town have the highest levels of infertility, at 31 percent, followed by Irish on-the-town women at 25 percent. English women not noted to have been on the town still had high levels of childlessness, at 17 percent, suggesting that perhaps they also were subject to infertility from sexually transmitted infections. Only the Irish-born women, not on the town, had relatively low infertility of 8 percent.

The fertility data point to the extreme vulnerability of the most deprived girls and women in nineteenth-century society. In addition, young convicts, particularly young women convicts, were far more likely than their social peers to have lost both parents. This suggests dislocation of the household and a life on the streets or on tramp, particularly at a time from the late eighteenth century, where internal migration to cities was taking people away from their native parishes, where the Old Poor Law provided supported for children without fathers.[28]

Girls without protective fathers and "respectable connections" were more vulnerable to sexual abuse. *My Secret Life* testifies to the harassment suffered by unprotected and destitute children in the streets, lanes, and fields of

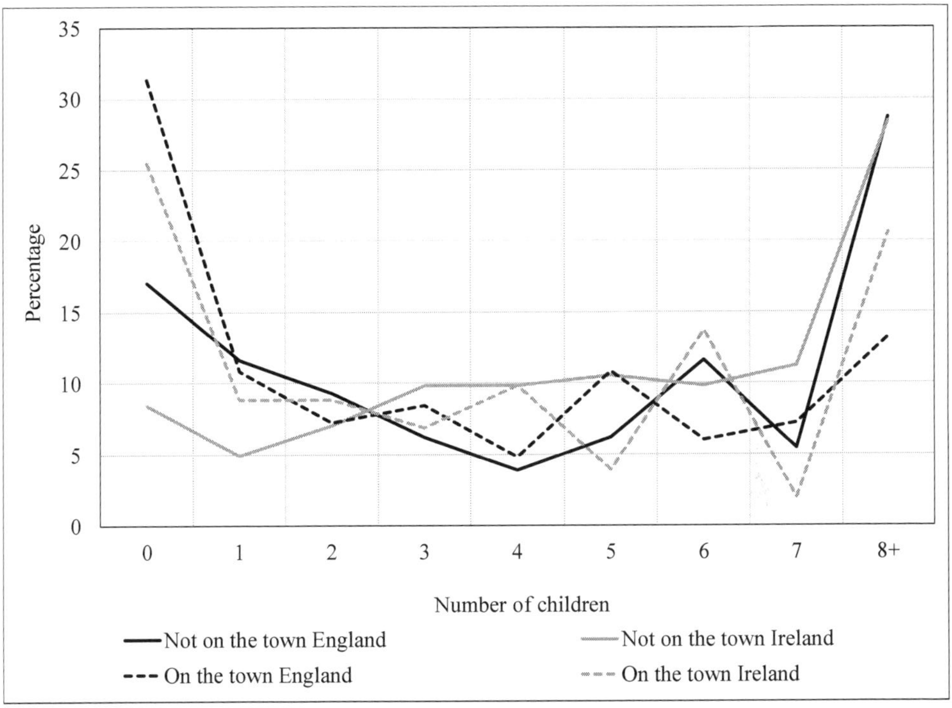

Figure 9.2. Distribution of the number of children (completed fertility), from a sample of convict women, ages twenty to twenty-four, transported to Tasmania from 1820 to 1853, who married after transportation and survived to age fifty; sorted by country of birth and "on the town" status (n = 599). Author calculations using data from McCalman and Kippen, Founders and Survivors data set.

Britain: a pattern of child sexual abuse that would be replicated by some former convicts in the Australian colonies.[29] Mary Ann Pryke was transported in 1846 aboard the *Sea Queen* at the age of sixteen to "remove her from bad connections." In the 1841 census her father was absent from the household in Bury Saint Edmunds. By the 1851 census her mother was described as a widow; cohabiting with her, her two adult sons, and one remaining daughter were two prostitutes. Two doors down prostitutes were also listed in the census. This was the red-light district of Bury Saint Edmunds. Mary Ann committed petty larcenies, but in 1844, when she was fourteen, she furiously resisted being raped one night by a George Edwards until he ran off. Edwards was sentenced to two years in jail with hard labor.[30] As a convict, Mary Ann was pugnacious, and on release, married to Humphrey Short, she continued to have a criminal career in Melbourne, running a brothel, drinking, and fighting. Only two boys of their five children survived childhood; neither was literate and both continued their parents' criminal careers.[31] Mary Ann, however, died at the age of thirty-five from syphilitic caries in the skull.

Mary Holehouse, per the *Tory* in 1845, ran a brothel with her husband, John Clay, behind an oyster shop in Ballarat East. Just six of her sixteen children survived infancy and childhood.[32] One daughter was raped at the age of six in the Charlie Napier Hotel by a "decently dressed lad of seventeen or eighteen years." Medical evidence was tendered that although there were indications that an assault had taken place, the child either was not a virgin or had a congenital absence of a hymen. The decent-looking lad received a sentence of eighteen months, although the judge declared he deserved a whipping.[33]

Mary Kinnear, born in Dublin, was convicted in Perth, Scotland, while her siblings were in Dundee and transported on the *Margaret* in 1843. At the age of thirty-three, she had been five years on the town, and the ship surgeon noted that she was "inclined to be insolent." Under sentence she was unruly, angry, and drunken, and she was found to be taking men to her bed. In consequence she spent thirty days in solitary confinement with pitch-dark total sensory deprivation and only two buckets for company.[34] On release she survived in Hobart by prostitution, but syphilis was eating at her body. At the coronial inquiry into her death in May 1852 from exposure, want, and disease, Thomas Harper testified,

> I have known her for six or seven years. She got her living by prostitution. The last time I saw her alive was on Friday evening last between nine and ten o'clock—she was in John Burns house lying in front of the fire—she was quite pale and her face was quite cold but she was sensible—I touched her face and she said "Oh Tommy do not hurt me"—I left her and did not see her again till the following morning when she was dead. She did not complain of anything when I saw her on the Friday evening—She appeared to be dying. She was covered with vermin and had an old coarse rug over her. It was Burns' wife fetched me in to her—She was destitute—She used to sit on a stone at top of the court and creep into a hole under Burns house at night. Burns and his wife treated her as kindly as their circumstances permitted.[35]

Early infection with venereal disease was common among the very poor, especially as young virgins were prized as a cure for syphilis.[36] Margaret Cosgrave (*Waverley*, 1847) was convicted of attempting to lure a child into her brothel in Melbourne for an eager customer.[37] Others, like Mary Lochrie (*Margaret*, 1843) and Bet Morgan (*America*, 1831), prostituted their daughters.[38] Many women who had been "on the town" bore no children or just one, and few of these babies survived. Anywhere children were out of sight of their caregivers, if they were poor, they were vulnerable to rape, and rarely was the criminal responsibility borne by the rapist, especially if the child came from a "rough" family. As Louise Jackson argues, the ravished child had suffered a loss of innocence, consigning them, even as victims, to the morally dangerous class.[39] The trade—or white slave market—in child sex was widespread in Victorian society, both at home and in the colonies.

The Old Poor Law had provided a safety net for those without families to support them, but by the end of the eighteenth century its provisions were breaking down in the face of internal migration, urbanization, and population growth.[40] The radically revised Poor Law of 1834 criminalized poverty and replaced an entitlement with confinement and isolation. Safety derived from being part of a stable household, either as a family member, an apprentice, or a servant; being "on the town" meant not just being a prostitute but being a public woman without protectors, available to all takers. Henry Mayhew reported that the police counted about eight thousand such "public women" in London in 1857.[41] The sex trade was complex, especially in major cities, from high-class courtesans or "exclusives" to "dressed women" resourced by brothel keepers to those who kept their own apartments to "clandestine" prostitutes or "sly women" to, at the bottom, "park women," who were too diseased to solicit in daylight. Many of these escaped police observation. Women "on the town" were sleeping and eating where they could, taking customers to "night houses" or "introducing houses."[42] The sexual exchange nearly always involved alcohol and food, and the outcome could often be larceny from the intoxicated person. This was a perilous existence, and vulnerability to violence, alcohol addiction, and sexual exploitation was embodied in destitute and convict women's reduced survival and low fertility.

Aboriginal Women in Colonial Australia

However, there was another group in colonial Australia who was even more defenseless against sexual predation and violence: Aboriginal women and girls.[43] Aboriginal Victorians suffered a catastrophic population collapse between 1788 and 1900, from an estimated sixty thousand people in the southeast corner of the continent to just six hundred by the time of federation in 1901. Murder, abduction of females, and infectious diseases from smallpox and tuberculosis to syphilis and gonorrhea effected a near genocide on what had been a collection of culturally rich Aboriginal societies that had survived for at least fifty thousand years.[44]

Today, while the population who identify as having an Aboriginal heritage in Victoria is approaching forty thousand people, there are no "full blood" Victorian Aboriginal people still alive.[45] Australia is a rich, developed nation that enjoys eighth place out of 188 on the Human Development Index ranking of life expectancy, but the average life expectancy of indigenous Australians is a full ten years less, matching those countries that rank at the fiftieth percentile. Indigenous Australians do worse than do the average inhabitants of Sri Lanka or Vietnam and still suffer the lowest life expectancy of any indigenous people living within a developed country.[46]

The Koori Health Research Database is a reconstitution of the Aboriginal population of Victoria from the 1840s to the mid-1980s, built from vital registrations and the records of the Victorian Aboriginal Protection Board in its various manifestations.[47] It documents the embodied impact of colonization and government policy on Aboriginal Victorians through their mortality and fertility and demonstrates the widening of the notorious gap between indigenous health and well-being and that of the rest of the population.[48] The total database comprises 7,900 individuals, of whom 495 were non-Aboriginal people married to Aboriginal spouses. Fertility analyses of the records of Aboriginal Victorian (Koori) women born 1900–1929 and who survived to fifty years, reveal a marked heaping at zero births and at eight or more births. In contrast, the completed fertility of the general Australian female population born over the same period shows a peak percentage at two births (figure 9.3). This suggests a high level of secondary or acquired infertility in socially vulnerable Aboriginal girls and young women, while the population recovery has come from a relatively small number of very large families; one woman had more than two hundred great-grandchildren.[49]

Aboriginal fertility was not a concern of the colonial medical profession in Victoria, however. Indeed, any reference at all to Aboriginal people and their health had ceased in the colonial medical literature by 1870. The Aborigines were a "dying race," and the role of colonial authorities was to "smooth their pillow." Early explorers had remarked on the visible presence of what they assumed was syphilis spread by whalers and sealers making landfall, and skin eruptions that looked like smallpox seemed to move down the river systems.[50] European diseases therefore penetrated Aboriginal communities even before white settlement in 1835, and the sexual exploitation of Aboriginal women grew with the expansion of Melbourne and the coastal settlements. While some frontier relationships were consensual and perhaps enabled individual women to survive, most left a legacy of psychic and physical damage that shattered morale and stymied any chance of Aboriginal people rebuilding their communities.[51] The early Aboriginal protectors in the colony

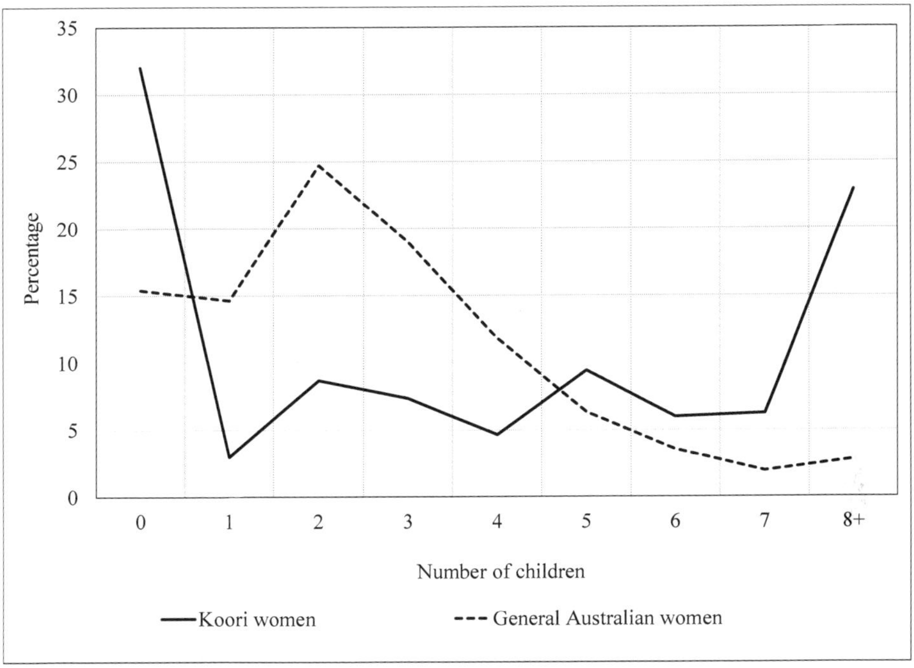

Figure 9.3. Distribution of the number of children (completed fertility), from a sample of Koori women born from 1900 to 1929 and who survived to age fifty (n = 171) and general Australian women born from 1900 to 1929. Author calculations using data from McCalman et al., Koori Health Research Database; and "Women by Age by Children Ever Born," 1999, special tabulation of the 1981 Australian Census of Population and Housing, Australian Bureau of Statistics, Canberra.

observed the signs of syphilis in the 1860s, and Rev. John Green, manager of Coranderrk Aboriginal Station, was open about its prevalence and its impact on infant mortality.[52] Thus, the loss of women to white abductors and venereal infection had a catastrophic effect on Aboriginal fertility, except for the fortunate few who were able to bear children and from whom the core population of Aboriginal Victoria is now descended.[53]

Case Histories of Impoverished Women at the Melbourne Women's Hospital

Aboriginal women and "morally compromised" convict women were victims of structural violence, where they had no entitlement to protection from institutions, family, husbands, employers, and the wider community.[54] In a patriarchal society women without adequate male breadwinners or personal wealth were even more vulnerable than lone males who were similarly without resources or entitlements of any kind. To understand the biology of this embodied gender penalty, we return to the Melbourne Women's Hospital in the second half of the nineteenth century.

The Melbourne Women's Hospital (today the Royal Women's) was established in 1856 as the Melbourne Lying-In Hospital and Infirmary for the Diseases Peculiar to Women and Children. Modeled on the Edinburgh Lying-In Hospital and the Dublin Rotunda, it was committed to detailed medical record keeping from the beginning, and, more by chance than design, much of that archive has survived. The midwifery records from 1857 to 1900 provide information on a population of impoverished colonial people, predominantly overseas-born until the late 1870s, around half of whom were single at the time of their recorded confinement. The most significant factor in determining birth weight and infant survival was whether the mother was supported or unsupported, either by a husband or an extended family. Similarly, for those babies who survived infancy, it was girls who suffered more than boys from growing up in extreme poverty, the lowest socioeconomic group suffering a gender penalty in survival that disappeared once households had left the casual, irregular economy.[55] But it is in the gynecological records that we can glimpse the toll that poverty and vulnerability took on fertility.

The infirmary case records from 1883 to 1909 are intact, transcribed into leather-bound volumes. They contain case notes, a surgical record, and, sometimes, detailed nursing notes. They cover a critical period in the history of medicine of the impact of germ theory and laboratory analysis, antisepsis, and asepsis; improved pathological understanding from the laparotomy; and the new surgical techniques afforded by instruments like the curette. The hospital initiated its own nurse training in 1862 and became a university teaching hospital in 1865. Its consultants were leaders in the colonial medical profession, editing medical journals and participating in the collegial medical life of clinical meetings and conferences. Melbourne's Women's Hospital was the outstanding hospital of its type in the Australasian colonies, benefiting, as did both colonial Victoria and South Australia, from the forced immigration of talented medical men who had contracted tuberculosis. Melbourne and its institutions had become a laboratory for modern scientific ideas and modern social reform. It was no colonial outpost.

The hospital was a charity hospital from the beginning, run on voluntary principles with subscribers providing recommendations for admission. It was intended to provide safe obstetric care for the many women left abandoned in gold rush Melbourne or who were too poor to have a safe place for childbirth. From its inception the founding doctors had insisted that unmarried women be freely admitted, even though this was not the practice in England. The case histories open a remarkable window into the intimate lives of the poor, into the realities of childbearing and female maladies, and into the human, private face of venereal diseases. They cannot collectively tell us about the incidence of sexually transmitted infections and their effects on fertility, but they can tell us about the experience and hint at prevalence and etiology. They enable us to see behind the statistics and to understand causation. Even death certificates are generally unhelpful in identifying lives damaged by venereal disease.[56]

Detailed hospital records of gynecological cases are relatively rare in the historical archive. Even worse, patients with infectious diseases, in particular venereal diseases, were often not meant to be admitted: hence the assertion of "umbilical hernia" as Maria Furlong's most serious problem. References to venereal disease in case histories were often oblique. In 1887, however, the resident medical officer was frank about Mrs. Davis, born in London, who had advanced syphilitic disease of the rectum, vagina, and uterus and who was treated with rest and irrigation with corrosive sublimate lotion (one in one thousand) for three weeks. She was discharged relieved. She had married at twenty-one, more than sixteen years before, and had just one pregnancy twenty years ago when unmarried and one abortion five or six years ago.[57]

The case notes enable us to be privy to the private lives of the poor. They tell of women who brought on miscarriages by heavy lifting; of the fifty-two-year-old mother of seven (all borne by the age of twenty-six) who strained herself lifting buckets of quartz at the gold diggings; and of the sixty-two-year-old Yorkshire-born mother of eleven, who was in acute pain after using an eighteen-pound hammer working red hot iron as a blacksmith (it was likely that she had cancer).[58] Some patients were foulmouthed. Lena Scott "created a disturbance and used revolting language" in October 1884 and departed after thirty days' recuperation after an Emmet operation for a lacerated cervix. A decade later she was a suburban brothel owner with a young pimp and was ordered to leave town.[59] A young mother, from the remote mountain-locked gold town of Walhalla, was suffering from a "lacerated and eroded cervix" and had "some abortions"; she claimed her name was Mrs. Thunderbolt. She too left after a couple of days because she "couldn't bear being separated from her husband."[60] The greatest burden of disease in the hospital wards was the "sickness of women," what is now known as pelvic inflammatory disease. Its causes were various: complications of miscarriage, in particular missed abortions that had remained untreated; induced abortion; childbirth injuries and malpractice; puerperal infection; tuberculosis; and, of course, venereal disease.

In the modern world, where half a million women die each year in childbirth, disability and continuing gynecological morbidity constitute a huge burden of suffering on women in countries with poor health services.[61] In these circumstances venereal disease remains an unknown quantity, underreported particularly where it is most prevalent and women's status is worst. In the past most women delivered at home, under the care of relatives, friends, wise women, and, if they were lucky, skilled midwives. Doctors and their instruments were sometimes called at the last minute to women exhausted and distressed by obstructed labors and when injuries were inevitable. But only those fortunate enough to have a doctor or to be in hospital could hope to have their tears sutured and their wombs repositioned.

Mrs. Sullivan, age sixty, after eleven pregnancies and ten carried to term, had been living for nine years with her womb protruding outside the vagina. Its surface was ulcerated, but, after rest and topical treatment, the introduction of a wooden pessary gave her "great comfort."[62] What the casebooks suggest is the immense burden among the poor and neglected of maternal chronic morbidity and acquired infertility.

Mildred Evans, age nineteen, was one of hundreds of pregnant Tasmanian girls who fled to Melbourne in the second half of the nineteenth century. She was just fourteen when she had her baby and had been quite well until the birth. It was a very long labor, and she made a "tedious recovery"; "always since [she] has had pains in the left side and back" and had intermenstrual discharge. Now there were suppurating glands at the base of her neck, and she looked "tired and worn, and had lost weight lately." She had tuberculosis, but she also had a chronic pelvic infection. She had an Emmet operation for a "lacerated cervix" at the Melbourne hospital, and Dr. Walter Balls-Headley this time performed another. After a month in the hospital, she was discharged "cured" to a convalescent home.

Mildred is untraceable in the historical record—she must have given, as did many of the patients, a false name to the hospital. But her condition, what they diagnosed as a "lacerated cervix," was in fact a gross infection of the uterus and appendages that was breaking through in ulcers. There may have been a laceration at her confinement, but the infection raging now inside her was perhaps a sequela of that long labor, perhaps a venereal infection and certainly complicated by tuberculosis of the glands (scrofula).[63] The Emmet operation was developed by the innovative US gynecologist Thomas Emmet for repair of the cervix by stripping and suture, but while it could repair clean tears, if there was chronic infection behind the lesion, then, as happened with Mildred, it soon broke down. It was the procedure du jour in the 1880s.[64]

Mrs. Barnes, age twenty-nine, of Collingwood, had never been well since her first and only confinement, after which she remained weak, with pains in the loins, and then suffered an early miscarriage ten months later. Then, in August 1880 (she remembered the time well), she got a yellow discharge, followed by copper-colored spots, and her womb became ulcerated. She was sick for three months, and in 1881 came into the hospital for an Emmet. She had been attending the outpatient clinic for months and now was to have her second Emmet for a "big laceration of the uterus" in August 1884. Mrs. Kingham, age twenty-eight, of Windsor, had four children and two abortions since she married at twenty-two. She had always been well until the second abortion on March 17, four and a half months earlier, which left her "very weak." She had severe pain in the left side, which was worse on walking or exertion, plus, in her own words, "headaches and tremblings." The "laceration" of the cervix was described as having a ragged and thickened anterior lip.[65]

Maggie Riley, age twenty-one, lived in the red-light district of Little Lonsdale Street. She was very sick. She had borne two children, the last just two weeks before, and now she had cellulitis. She was "thin and anaemic," but after treatment with hot foments, the cellulitis subsided. Next she seemed to come down with bronchitis, and the hospital staff realized that she had tuberculosis. She weighed seven stone four pounds (101 lbs) and had a curvature of the spine. After careful nursing for ten weeks, the raised patches of infection all over her body had faded, her chest expansion had improved, and she had put on four pounds. She was sent to the convalescent home.[66]

In Dr. Stephen Burke's casebook for 1884, the largest proportion of patients were between the ages of twenty and twenty-four years, and, overall, 63 percent were under the age of thirty. With those under twenty-five years, tuberculosis and venereal disease, often from abuse, were the most significant, but dysmenorrhea (severe menstrual pain) and infertility also brought many to the hospital. They were treated with painful, lacerating surgery to enlarge the cervical os in the mistaken belief that their pain was due to a blockage; endometriosis was not recognized.

Rose Shepherd, a fourteen-year-old domestic servant, had hurt her back nine months before while lifting a ten-gallon boiler, and she had pains ever since. She was diagnosed with a contracted os, and a metrotomy to enlarge it was performed. At fourteen she was no longer a virgin.[67] The metrotomy, another surgical favorite since the 1840s, was carried out with an instrument that had multiple blades that expanded with a spring to incise the cervix.[68] It was often performed without anesthetic, and the packing of the os to expand it would have caused many to faint. It also contributed to later cervical incompetence if the unfortunate ever fell pregnant.[69]

Changing Practice at the Melbourne Women's Hospital

The largest single group at the Melbourne Women's Hospital comprised those over twenty, suffering the effects of mismanaged childbirth and abortion, and this became more prevalent with age. The most insidious was the missed abortion, where a woman experienced flooding but did not seek medical care to remove the products, often out of ignorance or lack of access to care. The retained products then became the seat of infection. Induced abortion was being noticed more and commented on, as new technologies—curettes and especially the Higginson's syringe, which the hospital sold for half price at its dispensary—expanded techniques beyond contrived falls down stairs and the vast trade in herbal remedies for "irregularity."[70] As the birthrate fell with the fertility transition, so calls on the hospital to treat postabortal sepsis rose as women sought to limit their pregnancies. Venereal diseases and postpartum and postabortal sepsis combined to present the most significant caseload to the hospital, all of it impacting on fertility. And as women aged, so did the morbidity associated with childbearing increase, often aggravated by the privations of poverty.

The Melbourne gynecologists followed the British practice in the removal of ovaries and remained conservative about complete removal except in cases of severe disease.[71] When Maggie Barry, age twenty-three, presented in 1888 with a free yellow discharge since the time of her marriage, and with possibly one missed abortion six months after marriage and no pregnancies since, the surgery of choice for Dr. Balls-Headley remained the Emmet's repair, with corrosive douches and the passing of a sound through the outer os to measure success.[72]

Dr. Balls-Headley, like many, as Michael Worboys has shown, was slow to accept germ theory and had resisted the adoption of antiseptic midwifery at the hospital in the mid-1880s on the grounds that a better class of patient would immediately improve the maternal death rate.[73] However, he was the first among the consultants to use the term *salpingitis* in a case in late 1887 for a patient with a severe postpartum infection.[74] The young resident surgeon, Dr. John Dunbar Hooper, who had challenged the senior consultants by publishing a devastating case analysis of a hundred consecutive deliveries under his watch in the winter of 1887 to win the argument for antiseptic midwifery, was himself a leading consultant a decade later. In

1898 he performed a double oophorectomy on a Mrs. J. of Collingwood. She had had one child seven years before, just after her marriage, and two abortions since. She had always been well until the birth of her child; now she had bearing-down pain, headaches, and heavy bleeding. By 1898 the procedure was to dilate and curette first, before making a medial incision. The right tube and ovary were full of pus, with adhesions that made removal difficult. The left-side appendages were much enlarged and adhered to the anterior surface of the uterus and the bowel. The adhesions were eventually broken down. She survived and lived to be eighty-four.[75] The surgeons were reluctant to remove both ovaries and by 1900 often tried to leave something behind, particularly in the cases of young women.[76] Dr. Rothwell Adam was particularly careful to obtain patients' consent for the removal of ovaries.[77]

The turning point in the understanding of the sickness of women emerged at the 1889 Intercolonial Medical Congress in Melbourne. The chair of the Gynaecology Section, Dr. Ferdinand Batchelor from Dunedin, New Zealand, in his presidential address condemned the attachment to the speculum as the means of understanding pelvic disease, when a bimanual pelvic exploration could reveal the interrelatedness of diseased pelvic organs. Lawson Tait in England had used laparotomy to reveal the significance of tubal disease that spread through the peritoneum, building masses of adhesions that pushed the uterus out of position. Dr. Felix Meyer, newly elected an honorary at the Melbourne Women's Hospital, then spoke of the role of "unscientific" and hasty obstetrics in cervical laceration pelvic infection. Dr. Balls-Headley responded that the lacerated cervix was not under discussion, and in any case lacerations of the cervix were "a wise provision of Nature for the prevention of too many children."[78]

In 1894 Balls-Headley expanded on his neo-Darwinian interpretation of maternal morbidity in his book *The Evolution of the Diseases of Women*, the first major gynecological work published by an Australian practitioner. It was also a philosophical treatise, and he paid tribute to Charles Darwin, Herbert Spencer, Arthur Schopenhauer, Charles Letourneau, and August Bebel, among others. Humanity advanced through evolution and the survival of the fittest, he argued, and disease was a mechanism for eliminating the unfit. However, fitness could be promoted by the better regulation of society and improving the position of women. He was among the first medical writers to link social and psychological factors to gynecological disease, but his social diagnosis of the dangers to women's health was an interesting mix: a falling marriage rate, leaving too many spinsters to wither; unwarranted mental cultivation through the education of women and girls; tight lacing; excessive tea drinking; and venereal disease (a product of less than universal marriage).

For his suffering charity patients at the Women's Hospital, he felt sympathy for their excessive physical labors and errant husbands who joined trade unions and went on strike. Finally, state socialism, as exemplified in the colony of Victoria and indeed Australasia: "has induced the expectation that the State is to be looked to for relief. . . . The result is the burdening of the taxpayers, the repression of the old British energy, the pauperisation of the country, and the deficiency of marriage."[79] Balls-Headley was writing at the peak of the worst depression in Victorian history, generated by unrestrained land speculation and fraud.

The laboratory was also bringing change. Albert Neisser had identified the gonococcus in 1879, but it was not until the appointment of a pathologist, C. H. Mollison, in 1892 that the University of Melbourne laboratory began to make a difference and that medical students were trained in bacteriology. Medical leaders, particularly in Victoria, were becoming increasingly obsessed with venereal disease and race suicide in a new white nation marooned in an Asian world. Within a decade the number of laboratory tests increased sixfold. The subsequent arrival of the Wassermann test also emboldened the key campaigners—Dr. James Barrett and Professor Harry Allen—to seek a government trial of syphilis as a notifiable disease in 1910. After twelve months the reported incidence for the whole of Melbourne was 0.5 percent, nothing like their expectations. In 1913 a test of one hundred consecutive admissions to the obstetric ward of the Women's Hospital in 1913 revealed ten positives and six partials. To make matters worse, an autopsy revealed that a patient who had died of eclampsia showed signs of congenital syphilis. The doctors concluded that every obstetric patient should be given a Wassermann test, but the authorities baulked at the expense.[80] The Women's Hospital doctors, including progressives like Felix Meyer, were to become "soft" (i.e., nonhereditarian) eugenicists, convinced by their exposures to the miseries of the poor that social ills were best avoided by improving the fitness of the race through antenatal care, better sexual knowledge, and birth control. The child and maternal health service and antenatal hospital clinics succeeded where more aggressive eugenicists like Professor Richard Berry, obsessed with the social evil of the "high-grade moron," failed to convince the state Parliament to pass eugenic legislation.[81]

What mattered for the public patients in the Women's Hospital was that once their pus-filled tubes were perceived to have probably come from a sexually transmitted infection, their treatment over time became harder and less sympathetic. The surgeons hesitated less in removing diseased fallopian tubes, although most preferred to preserve some ovarian tissue to avoid adverse psychological effects. A culture of surgical intervention, without consent, in a woman's "best interests" became entrenched. Still in the 1960s incomplete abortions that presented on Monday mornings—known as "scrape day"—were curetted without anesthetic, often in the corridors because of the long lines. The hospital became notorious for its caseload of postabortal sepsis and between 1933 and 1945 pioneered emergency bedside pathology to diagnose gas gangrene of the uterus. It was routine to assume that every woman who presented with an incomplete abortion had attempted to induce it. And it was equally routine to assume that every woman who presented with infertility at the infertility clinic had suffered a sexually transmitted infection. One specialist confessed later that once he had a laparoscope, he discovered to his surprise that only a third of the Women's Hospital infertility patients showed signs of a venereal infection.[82] Like too many consultants of his era, he never bothered to publish the results.

Infertility, Poverty, and Structural Violence

At the clinical level it was very difficult to determine whether acquired infertility was due only to venereal disease or to complications of delivery or abortion, and so it remains for us at a demographic level. What we can say is that pelvic inflammatory disease and birth injuries inflicted great suffering on women and must have had a significant impact on fertility over the life course. Morbidity, and in particular the risk of venereal disease, was directly related to women's level of control over their lives and the supports and entitlements they could call on. Those cast out of respectable society by extreme poverty, delinquency, or ethnicity were at greatest risk, but poverty itself condemned child-bearing women to botched deliveries, birth injuries, and chronic infection, which also compromised their fertility. These findings are similar to those of Phillips Cutright and Edward Shorter, who showed that the lower completed fertility of US nonwhite women born between 1867 and 1935 could be explained by both higher rates of venereal disease and higher maternal morbidity.[83] What these data from the Australian colonies reveal is something of the experience of impaired fertility of their poorest and most marginalized and abused women: the very poor, the homeless, and, above all, the colonized indigenous people, for whom acquired infertility for a long time imperiled their very survival as a people, just as it did in Melanesia and the wider Pacific.[84]

Notes

1. Victorian Marriage Certificate (VMC), 1869/2916.

2. Stephen Burke, casebook no. 1, November 7, 1883, Honorary Physician Labour Ward Casebook of the Women's Hospital and Infirmary for Diseases of Women hereafter cited as HPLWC), VPRS 17390, Public Records Office, Victoria, 9.

3. Victorian Death Certificate (VDC), 1884/4187.

4. Victorian Birth Certificates (VBC), 1867/13926, 1869/14653, 1871/1530, 1872/22555, 1876/15327, 1878/22848.

5. VDC, 1867/7930, 1872/6501, 1875/6804, 1877/853, 1889/988, 1946/12178.

6. VMC, 1887/2617; VBC, 1888/20295, 1890/21147, 1892/21657, 1893/21100, 1895/16227, 1897/13709.

7. VDC, 1892/13339, 1970/15446, 1968/23299, 1978/21951, 1978/5912.

8. VDC, 1966/9308.

9. VDC, 1867/7930.

10. *Age* (Melbourne), January 7, 1867; *Age*, February 21, 1867.

11. *Argus* (Melbourne), March 15, 1869.

12. VBC, 1869/14653; VMC, 1869/2916.

13. Peter Gunn and Rebecca Kippen. *Household and Family Formation in Nineteenth-Century Tasmania, 1838–1899: Deaths*. Computer file. Canberra: Australian Data Archive, The Australian National University, 2016. http://doi.org/10.4225/87/57f495e147d70.

14. Van Diemen's Land became Tasmania in 1853.

15. Founders and Survivors: Australian Life Courses in Historical Context, 1803–1920 (hereafter cited as FAS), accessed February 17, 2019, www.foundersand-survivors.org/, Julia Smith, *Westmoreland*, 1836, ai65749.

16. VDC, 1867/2399.

17. VMC, 1901/1374; VDC, 1916/7017.

18. VDC, 1870/886.

19. *Age*, December 17, 1867; Marion Button, Victorian Prisoners Index (Females), VPRS 12798, Public Record Office, Victoria.

20. *Colonial Times* (Hobart), November 26, 1844.

21. *Argus*, May 13, 1857.

22. VDC, 1867/2399.

23. Janet McCalman and Rebecca Kippen, Founders and Survivors: Life Course Ships Project, data set of 25,000 convicts transported to Van Diemen's Land (Tasmania) on 126 convict ships, 1812–53 (2017), https://doi.org/10.4225/03/59ed402437518; Janet McCalman et al., "Building a Life Course Dataset from Australian Convict Records: Founders and Survivors; Australian Life Courses in Historical Context, 1803–1920," in *Population Reconstruction*, ed. Gerrit Bloothooft et al. (Heidelberg: Springer, 2015): 285–98.

24. Rebecca Kippen and Janet McCalman, "Wages of Sin and Penalties of Gender: Mortality and Causes of Death of Convict Men and Women Transported to Van Diemen's Land, 1812–1853" (paper presented at the Australian and New Zealand Society for the History of Medicine Biennial Conference, Sydney, June 30–July 4, 2015).

25. Rebecca Kippen and Peter Gunn, "Convict Bastards, Common-Law Unions and Shotgun Weddings: Premarital Conceptions and Ex-nuptial Births in Nineteenth-Century Tasmania," *Journal of Family History* 36, no. 4 (2011): 387–403.

26. Kirsty Reid, *Gender, Crime and Empire: Convicts, Settlers and the State in Early Colonial Australia* (Manchester: Manchester University Press, 2007).

27. Christine Leppard-Quinn, "Labelling the Transported Prostitute: An Exercise in Textual Archaeology," *Tasmanian Historical Studies* 18 (2013): 35–59.

28. Rebecca Kippen and Janet McCalman, "Convicts and Families: Parental Loss and Family Formation of Young Convicts Transported to Van Diemen's Land (Tasmania), 1841–1853," 2018, *The History of the Family*, https://doi.org/10.1080/1081602X.2018.1513855.

29. "Walter," *My Secret Life*, ed. Gershon Legman (1890; repr., New York, Grove, 1966); *Geelong Advertiser*, September 16, 1853, 2; *Star* (Ballarat), February 19, 1854, 4.

30. *Suffolk Chronicle, or Weekly General Advertiser and Country Express*, March 23, 1844, 5.

31. FAS, Mary Ann Pryke, *Sea Queen*, 1846, ai57717.

32. FAS, Mary Holehouse, *Tory*, 1845, ai33537.

33. *Ballarat Star*, February 15, 1866, 2; *Argus*, February 26, 1866, 6.

34. FAS, Mary Kinnear, *Margaret*, 1843, ai40482.

35. SC195/1/30 Inquest 2728, Tasmanian Archives and Heritage Office.

36. Victorian Parliamentary Papers, *Select Committee upon a Bill for the Prevention of Contagious Diseases* (Victoria, 1878), vol. 8; see also, for discussion of legal cases involving infection of children with venereal disease, Victoria Bates, *Sexual Forensics in Victorian and Edwardian England Age, Crime and Consent in the Courts* (Basingstoke: Palgrave, 2016), chap. 2.

37. Names and dates in parentheses after convicts' names are the ships individuals arrived on and the year of arrival. *Age*, February 2, 1864, 6. By that time Margaret Cosgrave of 1847 had become Margaret Blackford.

38. *Argus*, October 13, 1856, 5; *Colonial Times*, March 4, 1845, 3. Mary Lochrie became Mary Ann Harrrold, and Bet Morgan became Bet Naylor.

39. Louise A. Jackson, *Child Sexual Abuse in Victorian England* (London: Routledge, 2000).

40. Sara Horrell, Jane Humphries, and Hans-Joachim Voth, "Destined for Deprivation: Human Capital Formation and Intergenerational Poverty in Nineteenth-Century England," *Explorations in Economic History* 38 (2001): 339–65.

41. Michael Mason, *The Making of Victorian Sexuality* (Oxford: Oxford University Press, 1994), 76–80.

42. Henry Mayhew, *London Labour and the London Poor* (London: Dover, 1861), 1:213, 477–79.

43. Marilyn Lake, "Frontier Feminism and the Marauding White Man," *Journal of Australian Studies* 20, no. 49 (1996): 12–20; Penelope Edmonds, *Urbanizing Frontiers: Indigenous Peoples and Setters in Nineteenth Century Pacific Rim Countries* (Vancouver: University of British Colombia Press, 2010), 145–49.

44. Len Smith et al., "Fractional Identities: The Political Arithmetic of Aboriginal Victorians," in *Indigenous Peoples and Demography: The Complex Relationship between Identity and Statistics*, ed. Per Axelsson and Peter Sköld (New York: Berghahn Books, 2011): 15–31; Len Smith, "How Many People Had Lived in Australia before It Was Annexed by the English in 1788?," in *The Aboriginal Population Revisited*, ed. Gordon Briscoe and Len Smith (Canberra: Aboriginal History Monograph, 2002): 9–15.

45. Smith et al., "Fractional Identities."

46. United Nations, *Human Development Report, 2015* (New York: United Nations Development Program, 2015); Australian Institute of Health and Welfare, *The Health and Welfare of Australia's Aboriginal and Torres Strait Islander Peoples: 2015* (Canberra: AIHW, 2015).

47. McCalman et al., Koori Health Research Database, 2018, https://doi.org/10.4225/03/5a9779c80f529.

48. Janet McCalman et al., "Colonial Health Transitions: Aboriginal and 'Poor White' Infant Mortality Compared, Victoria, 1850–1910," *History of the Family* 16, no. 1 (2011): 62–77.

49. Janet McCalman et al., "The Colonization of Victoria and the Koori Health Research Database" (paper presented at the European Social Science History Conference, Valencia, Spain, March 30–April 2, 2016).

50. Peter Dowling, "What Charles Sturt Saw in 1830: Syphilis beyond the Colonial Boundaries," *Health and History* 19, no. 1 (2017): 44–59.

51. Penelope Edmonds, "The Intimate Urbanising Frontier: Native Camps and Settler Colonialism's Violent Array of Spaces around Early Melbourne," in *Making Settler Colonial Space: Perspectives on Race, Place and Identity*, ed. Tracey Banivanua Mar and Penelope Edmonds (Basingstoke: Palgrave Macmillan, 2010), 129–54.

52. Victorian Parliamentary Papers, 1877–78, *Royal Commission on the Aborigines*, Parliament of Victoria.

53. Janet McCalman et al., "Origins of 'The Gap': The History of the Demographic Transition in Aboriginal Victoria" (unpublished manuscript, 2019).

54. Paul Farmer, "On Suffering and Structural Violence: A View from Below," *Race/Ethnicity: Multidisciplinary Global Contexts* 3, no. 1 (2009): 11–28.

55. Janet McCalman, Ruth Morley, and Gita Mishra, "A Health Transition: Birth Weights, Households and Survival in an Australian Working-Class Population Sample Born 1857–1900," *Social Science and Medicine* 66, no. 5 (2008): 1070–83.

56. Janet McCalman, *Sex and Suffering: Women's Health and a Women's Hospital; The Royal Women's Hospital, Melbourne, 1856–1996* (Baltimore: Johns Hopkins University Press, 1999). The remainder of this chapter draws on this monograph.

57. Walter Balls-Headley, casebook no. 2, December 17, 1887, HPLWC, 98.

58. Burke, casebook no. 1, December 14, 1885, HPLWC, 13; Thomas Rowan, casebook no. 2, February 1, 1887, HPLWC, 29.

59. Balls-Headley, casebook no. 1, October 15, 1884, HPLWC; *Mercury and Weekly Courier* (Melbourne), December 7, 1893.

60. Balls-Headley, casebook no. 2, October 6, 1887, HPLWC, 88.

61. Tabassum Firoz et al., "Measuring Maternal Health: Focus on Maternal Morbidity," *Bulletin of the World Health Organization* 91, no. 10 (2013): 794–96.

62. Burke, casebook no. 1, December 5, 1884, HPLWC, 87.

63. Balls-Headley, casebook no. 2, January 16, 1889, HPLWC, 161.

64. *British Medical Journal* 15 (January 1887): 109–10.

65. Balls-Headley, casebook no. 1, August 6, 1884, HPLWC, 73, 63.

66. Gerald Henry Fetherston, casebook no. 2, February 9, 1888, HPLWC, 57.

67. Burke, casebook no. 1, June 20, 1884, HPLWC, 101.

68. James Young Simpson, "Dilation and Incision of the Cervix Uteri in Cases of Obstructive Dysmenorrhea," in *The Obstetric Memoirs and Contributions of James Y. Simpson* (Edinburgh: Royal College of Physicians of Edinburgh, 1856), 288–91.

69. McCalman, *Sex and Suffering*, 40–42.

70. Ann Larson, *Growing Up in Melbourne: Family Life in the Late Nineteenth Century* (Canberra: Demography Program, Australian National University, 1994), 56–59; letter to the editor, *Australian Medical Gazette*, February 1883, 108.

71. "Normal Ovariotomy: Battey's Operation; Tait's Operation," *British Medical Journal* 1367 (March 1887): 576–77.

72. Balls-Headley, casebook no. 2, November 28, 1888, HPLWC, 150.

73. Michael Worboys, *Spreading Germs: Disease Theories and Medical Practice in Britain, 1965–1900* (Cambridge: Cambridge University Press, 2000).

74. Balls-Headley, casebook no. 2, October 1, 1887, HPLWC, 84.

75. Hooper, casebook, July 13, 1898, HPLWC; VDC: 1949/12954.

76. Rothwell Adam, casebook, March 31, 1900, HPLWC; Hooper, casebook, March 31, 1900, HPLWC.

77. Adam, casebook, June 24, 1899, HPLWC; Adam, casebook, February 16, 1898, HPLWC.

78. McCalman, *Sex and Suffering*, 120.

79. Walter Balls-Headley, *The Evolution of the Diseases of Women* (London: Elder, 1894), 32.

80. McCalman, *Sex and Suffering*, 132–37.

81. Similarly, in Britain the "hard," hereditarian eugenicist position was tested and found wanting in scientific support by the famous 1904 Interdepartmental Enquiry into Physical Deterioration, which instead recommended a range of environmental measures to improve child health among the poor: Simon Szreter, *Fertility, Class*

and Gender in Britain, 1860–1940 (Cambridge: Cambridge University Press, 1996), 207–37.

82. Szreter, *Fertility, Class and Gender*, 223–31, 357–58.

83. Phillips Cutright and Edward Shorter, "The Effects of Health on the Completed Fertility of Nonwhite and White U.S. Women Born between 1867 and 1935," *Journal of Social History* 13, no. 2 (1979): 191.

84. These data mirror the impact of sexually transmitted diseases on other colonized people in the Pacific, as discussed by Tim Bayliss-Smith, chap. 6; see also chapter 7 by Roy F. Scragg, chap. 7, both in this volume.

Part Four

Infertility and the Specter of Venereal Diseases in Modern Europe

Chapter Ten

"The Archenemy of Fertility"

Gonorrhea and Infertility, Germany 1870–1935

Christina Benninghaus

In March 1929 Maria Meyer was discharged from the university hospital in Tübingen, where she had been treated for infertility. At thirty-four years of age, Meyer had been married for seven years to a shopkeeper and had never conceived. Years before she had undergone surgery at a hospital in Konstanz; now she had been treated with conventional therapies, including the application of light, heat, and water. For diagnostic and therapeutic purposes, an abrasion of her uterus had been performed. An insufflation of her tubes had shown that these were patent. Everything seemed to be okay. But, upon leaving the hospital, Meyer told the doctors that her parents tormented her. They believed that she would not conceive because her husband had infected her with gonorrhea. To counter such accusations, the doctors provided Maria Meyer with a certificate stating that repeated tests and examinations had not shown any signs of an infection.[1]

That gonorrhea could lead to infertility in both men and women was common knowledge by the end of the 1920s. For decades the German public had been told that in many, even the majority of, cases of a sterile marriage the husband was to blame, either for infecting his wife with gonorrhea or for being sterile himself. In this chapter I ask how the notion that gonorrhea could lead to infertility was developed, debated, modified, and popularized.

How did people like Maria Meyer's parents come to associate childlessness with gonorrhea?

As is well known, the debate started when German-born Emil Noeggerath published a short book on "latent gonorrhea" in 1872, arguing that infections with gonorrhea were far more dangerous than hitherto believed.[2] His views were not easily accepted, but they also proved difficult to dismiss. Research by Michael Worboys and more recently by Elliott Bowen and Anne Hanley has stressed that the identification of the gonococcus by Albert Neisser in 1879 did little to close the debate in Britain; instead, competing views on the existence of latent gonorrhea coexisted until at least the turn of the century.[3] Skepticism seems to have been especially marked among British gynecologists, and it took decades of research and debate and the intervention of feminists before the Royal Commission on Venereal Disease in 1916 acknowledged the dangers posed by gonorrhea, especially to women's health and fertility (see chapter 12, in this volume).

Worboys and Bowen each refer to the example of latent gonorrhea to criticize the notion of a laboratory revolution. Bacteriological tests proved very difficult and of little practical relevance when it came to diagnosing and treating latent gonorrhea in women. Victoria Bates shows that bacteriological tests were also hardly used in Britain in turn-of-the-century criminal court cases.[4] In this chapter I approach the topic of latent gonorrhea from a different perspective. Not only is my research focused on Germany, where bacteriology was far more readily embraced than in Britain; I am also predominantly interested in medical debates on the connection between gonorrhea and infertility and in the ways in which their results were communicated to the public.[5] Medical knowledge about the dangerous nature of gonorrhea, this chapter will argue, was firmly established by the turn of the century. Among German experts, it was generally accepted that gonorrhea could lead to infertility in both men and women, and this knowledge influenced infertility diagnosis and treatment. It also shaped perceptions of infertility. Already in the 1890s and especially after the turn of the century, public health campaigners warned their audiences about the dangers associated with gonorrhea. However, campaigns to fight venereal disease continued to devote more attention to syphilis, a disease causing more spectacular and gruesome symptoms and therefore far better suited for frightening audiences into abstinence, prophylaxis, or treatment.

Somewhat surprisingly, unintended childlessness caused by gonorrhea was not even turned into a public health concern when the German public started to obsess with the declining birthrate shortly before World War I. Health propaganda from the 1920s presented venereal disease as a widespread health issue, but not as a demographic threat. Only later, when health politics were redefined to serve the biopolitical aims of National Socialism, was infertility cast as a public health concern. By this time, however, sexually transmitted diseases were in rapid decline, and new methods of infertility diagnosis and treatment were affecting the experiences of patients.

Latent Gonorrhea and Infertility

Emil Noeggerath's claims were bold. In 1872, in a book apparently put together somewhat hastily over the summer, he set out to revolutionize medical approaches to gonorrhea.[6] At this time catching "the clap" (*Tripper* was the equivalent colloquial German term) was perceived as unpleasant but not particularly dangerous. It was apparently an extremely common experience, especially among younger urban middle-class men, including medical students. Noeggerath now presented it as a severe health issue. He argued that it was particularly dangerous for women, among whom it could cause severe pelvic inflammation, which in turn could result in infertility. In his subsequent 1876 paper presented to the first meeting of the American Gynecological Society, Noeggerath stressed that gonorrhea could also lead to male sterility by causing obliterations of the spermatic ducts and inflammation of the testes.[7]

At the time of publication, Noeggerath was a well-established gynecologist.[8] Born in 1827, Noeggerath had studied medicine in his hometown of Bonn before undergoing additional clinical training at Berlin, Vienna, Prague, and Paris. He had briefly worked as an assistant doctor at the university hospital in Bonn and had set up private practice. In 1857 Noeggerath emigrated to the United States, where he joined a closely knit community of German doctors practicing in New York's Lower East Side and mainly catering for immigrants from Europe. A member of the Collegium of the Physicians of the German Dispensary of the City of New York, Noeggerath had access to the latest medical literature. But, apart from this, his resources were limited, especially when compared to the research possibilities of professors and graduate students at medical faculties in Germany—probably the main intended audience for his book. Why, we might wonder, was Noeggerath in a position to see connections hidden to others? Why was he confident that he could and should establish a new disease entity?

Noeggerath's interest in gonorrhea seems to have developed out of his thriving gynecological practice. Time and again he was consulted by women suffering from pelvic inflammations. These conditions, while rarely life threatening, could be extremely painful and could cause long-term suffering, especially when turning into a chronic condition. Menstruation would often be irregular and very painful, and sexual intercourse could become unbearable. Abdominal pain could be constant or could peak during attacks accompanied by high fever and general weakness, and quite a number of these patients would experience reproductive difficulties.

To explain these cases Noeggerath developed the idea of "latent gonorrhea" resulting in acute, chronic, and recurrent pelvic inflammations. He was convinced that gonorrhea was caused by a microorganism, which in men would lead to symptoms typically associated with gonorrhea—discharge and itching—and which during sexual intercourse would be passed on to women, where it might or might not lead to an acute inflammation and accompanying symptoms. Apart from this, however, the microorganism could also hide in the male or female genital tract and could proliferate later when conditions for its spread were more favorable. In women this could be during pregnancy or after the birth of a child. While causing relatively little harm when restricted to the urethra, the infection could also spread to the uterus, the fallopian tubes, the ovaries, and the peritoneum in women and to the testes in men, causing painful inflammation and sterility.

Noeggerath's theory of latent gonorrhea, while resting on bacteriological thinking, was first and foremost based on clinical observations and meticulous record keeping. From the case histories he published it can be seen that Noeggerath was a particularly attentive—indeed, one could say obsessive—examiner.[9] His published case histories show that he had kept extensive records that documented the patient's history, including detailed notes on the results of (repeated) examinations. Noeggerath routinely used a speculum to visually examine the vagina and the cervix. He determined the position and size of the uterus and the size of the ovaries by bimanual pelvic examination and carefully noted details on discharge, swellings, and adhesions that pointed to past inflammation. Some of his patients had already seen a number of experts and had been in treatment for years. From the case histories, some of which fill three narrowly printed pages, it appears that Noeggerath listened carefully to patients' accounts and complaints. Some of the case histories document years of suffering with recurrent bouts of pelvic inflammation and rather futile attempts to avoid a renewed attack. Only in one case did Noeggerath record that a patient—not surprisingly, a young English woman—was reluctant to consent to being examined and refused the repeated use of the speculum.[10]

Noeggerath also took samples of discharge and studied them under the microscope. And he grew cultures using an incubator. Convinced that gonorrhea was caused by a specific microorganism, he had hoped to be able to find proof that the cases he saw were connected to the disease. But his results were not conclusive. In his 1872 publication, he mentioned a fungus, which he had been able to cultivate, but in 1876 he dropped the claim that this might be the pathogen causing gonorrhea.[11] Presenting fifty case histories and a statistic on infertility, he hoped to convince his readers that latent gonorrhea not only existed but posed a severe health threat.

Noeggerath's clinical skills were a precondition for seeing the pattern he would come to call "latent gonorrhea," but these observations were possible only because he saw a rather peculiar group of patients. Three aspects are worth stressing. First, compared to other physicians, Noeggerath was likely to witness more cases of gonorrhea transmitted from husband to wife. Not only was gonorrhea especially common in urban areas such as New York, but Noeggerath also based his account on patient records from his private practice. These patients almost invariably belonged to the middle class. They subscribed to a sexual culture marked by a much-criticized double standard. While women were expected to enter marriage without prior sexual experiences, men were allowed to solicit prostitutes.[12] In some cases Noeggerath had witnessed how young women whom he had seen as a family doctor quickly developed signs of gonorrhea after marrying a man known to have been infected but declared healthy.

Second, as the case histories suggest, Noeggerath often managed to talk to the husbands of his patients, and in a number of cases he could even do a sperm test. Such personal encounters were possible because many of his patients lived in New York and because Noeggerath did home visits, if necessary. Interaction with husbands of private patients was probably part of normal business, for example, when settling bills or discussing treatment options. Judging by the published case histories, these middle-class men were not particularly tight-lipped when asked about their sexual experiences. Hence, when suspecting an infection with gonorrhea, Noeggerath actually could and often did talk to the husband while other experts, such as gynecologists based in spa towns in Germany, would usually have had to rely on the woman's testimony alone.

Third, Noeggerath saw a comparatively high proportion of especially desperate cases of pelvic inflammatory disease. Considered an expert, he treated women who were chronically ill and had already exhausted other options. Some had seen famous gynecologists such as Friedrich Wilhelm Scanzoni, James Marion Sims, or Thomas Addis Emmet. They had undergone surgery, spent time at European spas, and been treated with pessaries or massages. For some, painful pregnancies resulting in miscarriages or extremely difficult deliveries had been followed by life-threatening infections, recovery from which took months. Others suffered from recurrent inflammations, often extremely painful, which seemed to come out of the blue and which Noeggerath could only treat with opium and chloroform. Such cases were extremely frustrating. These were women from Noeggerath's own social stratum who did not have to do heavy work—who could rest, eat well, take the waters—but who still could not be cured (see chapter 9 for an account of such suffering also at this time among women in Australia entirely lacking these social advantages). Latent gonorrhea—even if hard or impossible to cure—provided an explanation.

But Noeggerath not only was a perceptive examiner, trusted practitioner, daring surgeon, and attentive clinical observer; he also regarded medicine as a scientific endeavor. He drew up statistics and participated in postmortems; he published and presented cases to the New York Obstetrical Society and employed laboratory methods. Perhaps most important, Noeggerath kept up with current developments in medicine and was probably even eager to leave his mark. His father, Johann Jacob Noeggerath, had held the chair in mineralogy at Bonn. Emil Noeggerath came to the United States to take a position at a newly founded medical school—a job that, however, did not materialize. Once in New York he joined forces with another young German doctor, Abraham Jacobi, who would later be regarded as one of the founding fathers of pediatrics. Together they published *Contributions to Midwifery, and Diseases of Women and Children*, a volume in which they tried to capture the state of the art in their disciplines. Between them they had scrutinized English, German, French, Italian, and some other European medical journals so that they could offer their US readers "the essence of all that is dispersed in hundreds of publications."[13]

For Noeggerath medicine was a collective scientific undertaking. And it seems likely that he kept up with the latest developments in the emerging field of bacteriology. To think that the symptoms he observed in his patients could be caused by a specific microorganism—Noeggerath spoke of a fungus—was not far-fetched. At the time research on the connection between infections and microorganisms flourished.[14] Research by Edwin Klebs on soldiers killed during the Franco-Prussian War had shown that septicemia following gunshot wounds developed only when certain microorganisms were present.[15] Other infections like typhus, puerperal fever, and diphtheria were also regarded as linked to bacteria. But to identify the pathogen responsible for a specific disease was another matter.

Noeggerath could see the effects of gonorrhea because he relied on a broad spectrum of evidence and combined methods that might be characterized as representing the laboratory, the clinic, and traditional bedside medicine.[16] He did not attempt to separate these ways of knowing, each of which had its limitations. Instead, he explained his sophisticated methodology in the following way in the introduction to his book:

> I have tried to make the fabric that is here offered for examination dense and durable by way of intertwining the different strands in an appropriately complementary way and not too sparsely so that each of them helps to solidify the whole. I would have hoped to add to this research by adding twice as many case histories because, as will become apparent, it is only through seeing a large number of similar case histories that we can prove our interpretation.[17]

Debating Latent Gonorrhea

Noeggerath's ideas did not meet with great enthusiasm. This was not surprising. Because his theories were based on clinical observations, other doctors needed time to reconsider the cases they saw in their own practice in the light of Noeggerath's theory. For some the existence of latent gonorrhea made perfect sense. Others were skeptical.[18] Even Noeggerath's supporters, however, thought that he had overstated his claim.[19] Many doctors knew from personal as well as professional experience that gonorrhea could be cured. When Noeggerath presented his finding to the American Gynecological Society in 1876, a Dr. Johnson from Washington, DC, related the results of an ad hoc study he had conducted: "I may state that in conversation with twenty different physicians, who acknowledged having had gonorrhea in early life, in no single case had any such symptoms, as have been referred to, been developed in their wives, and all have had quite large families of children."[20]

In his attempt to raise awareness, Noeggerath had clearly exaggerated the dangers posed by gonorrhea. He had included cases that could easily be explained by other causes and that were now held against him.[21] But Noeggerath was criticized not only because his evidence did not seem entirely sound. There were larger issues at stake. If Noeggerath was right, the medical approaches to gonorrhea and to pelvic inflammation had to be changed. Warning male patients who had caught the clap, and possibly also would-be brides, would have appeared as crucial.[22] Conventional forms of treating women experiencing discharge and pelvic pains or complaining about infertility had to be reconsidered. Noeggerath was especially critical of surgical treatments that were dangerous because they could spread germs to noninfected parts of the female reproductive organs. To agree to Noeggerath's ideas about gonorrhea meant to accept that many cases of gonorrhea in women could have been avoided had doctors and their male patients acted more responsibly. This was explosive stuff. If Noeggerath was right, women had to be warned. They had to be made aware that they had misplaced their trust, both in doctors and husbands.[23] Given that Noeggerath's claims were unfamiliar and far-reaching and that they threatened to challenge existing hierarchies and well-ingrained practices of medical treatment, it is not exactly surprising that they were resisted. This would change only slowly, as pathological research on gonorrhea gained ground. As noted, several historians have stressed that the identification of the gonococcus by Neisser in 1879 did not make much of a difference to the diagnosis of gonorrhea, especially in Britain. In fact, it took years before the pathogenicity of gonococci had been proven. They were difficult objects to study, because they were not easily stained, because they looked just like other cocci, because they would not grow on the media normally used to cultivate microorganisms, and because they did not cause inflammation in animals. Hence, a number of ethically problematic experiments on humans were designed to prove that gonococci were indeed the pathogen that caused gonorrhea.[24] And very often such experiments were not even successful.[25]

Diagnostic problems persisted, especially when it came to women.[26] To estimate the effects of gonorrhea on the fertility of both men and women proved even more difficult. Doctors interested in this question used different approaches. Traugott Kroner, to give an example, studied the postpartum period of women whose newborn babies had shown signs of blennorrhea. According to his results, these mothers rarely experienced any signs usually associated with postpartum gonorrhea.[27] Enoch Heinrich Kisch, spa doctor in Marienbad and professor at the University of Prague, started a survey among his patients, correlating infertility and gonorrhea of husbands. Apparently, there was no positive link.[28]

One of the major problems in proving Noeggerath's claim that gonorrhea could lead to pelvic inflammation was to show that gonococci could actually invade deeper layers of tissue. One of the best-known experts on gonorrhea—Ernst Bumm, who in 1885 developed a method to cultivate gonococci using human blood serum—was convinced that gonococci could infect only the mucous membrane and could not lead to inflammation of the peritoneum. Bumm had studied the histology of membranes infected by gonorrhea by using tiny slices of the conjunctivas of newborns whose infection with gonorrhea had lasted for a certain number of days.[29] Reading Bumm's study, it becomes obvious how very difficult research on gonorrhea was and how contradictory the results.

With regard to infertility, a study by Ernst Wertheim, published in 1891, made a real difference.[30] Wertheim analyzed pus and tissue taken from the fallopian tubes of women who were undergoing surgery at the university hospital in Prague. He could demonstrate that gonococci were indeed present in the infected tubes. By the 1890s a consensus started to emerge. In medical handbooks gonorrhea was now increasingly reported as one of the major causes of infertility. While Noeggerath was criticized for having exaggerated the importance of gonorrhea, the existence of latent gonorrhea and the dangers due to infections were now generally accepted.

Gonorrhea and Male Sterility

While debates on the causal relation between gonorrhea and female infertility continued, another of Noeggerath's suggestions quickly gained purchase among German doctors. In 1871 he had started not only to inquire into the medical history of his sterility patients' husbands but to propose sperm testing. In 1872 he could draw on five, and in 1876 on fourteen, cases in which men known to have suffered from gonorrhea in the past were now living in a sterile marriage and had consented to a test. In half of these cases, the semen, collected in a condom during intercourse and brought to Noeggerath's practice shortly afterward, did not contain any spermatozoa. "The gentlemen from whom these last-mentioned specimens were obtained were to all appearance healthy men, some of them unusually large and vigorous, their sexual functions unimpaired," Noeggerath noted.[31] Only in three out of fourteen cases did the spermatozoa look normal, although most men reported that their infections with gonorrhea had not been complicated by an epididymitis. It appeared that, just as in women, gonorrhea was more dangerous in men than hitherto believed.

That gonorrhea could lead to infertility if the infection spread to both testes had already been shown, in fact several decades earlier, by other authors.[32] And Noeggerath was not the only one to advocate sperm testing. Already in 1868 his US colleague James Marion Sims had proposed to consider male sterility in cases of involuntary childlessness.[33] In Germany the method became more widely accepted after a professor from the University of Gießen, Ferdinand Adolf Kehrer, published results of a systematic investigation into the causes of sterility that he had conducted between 1876 and 1879. In an earlier publication Kehrer had already suggested that in about a quarter of all sterile marriages, azoospermia in the husband was the major cause of unintended childlessness.[34] To prove his point he started to collect forty cases in which both partners could be examined. The forty men who had their sperm analyzed were merchants, shopkeepers and artisans. A handful of them—mostly owners of an estate or a factory—probably belonged to the upper classes. Kehrer carefully noted the exact dates on which the tests were conducted and provided short case histories, adding medical details and a short sexual biography for each of his patients. In fourteen cases the semen was found to contain no spermatozoa; in two cases the men turned out to be impotent. Kehrer concluded that in more than a third of all sterile marriages the problem probably resided with the husband and encouraged his fellow doctors to consider sperm testing whenever they were asked for help in cases of childlessness.[35]

Over the following years Kehrer's study was often cited. As I have argued elsewhere, the growing medical interest in male sterility can be partly explained by the frustration felt by many doctors when diagnosing and treating female infertility.[36] What was difficult in women—to assess the fertility of an individual and to offer a meaningful prognosis—was comparatively easy in men, if fertility was equated with the existence of an abundance of moving spermatozoa in the semen, if a microscope was at hand, and if men were willing to provide a sperm sample.

Perhaps the enormous popularity of German medicine and, more specifically, of modern scientific approaches to medicine—certainly at its height during the 1880s—helped to persuade patients. In any case resistance to sperm testing seems to have been limited, especially among urban, middle-class men. Between 1883 and 1887, to give an example, a well-known gynecologist in Hamburg was seen by 2,500 women, of whom 76 were private patients specifically seeking infertility treatment. In 46 of these 76 cases, a sperm test was conducted, 15 husbands rejected a test, and 15 were not available for test or treatment because they lived abroad or were absent on business. The semen of 21 men did not contain any spermatozoa, usually because of a past infection with gonorrhea; 6 men were impotent; and 15 women had been infected by their husbands. Only in 12 cases was the sperm considered normal.[37] Clearly, men were often responsible for the childlessness of a marriage, with gonorrhea being the most important cause.

It is impossible to know how many gynecologists or even ordinary family doctors offered or insisted on sperm testing. But a shift in attitudes can easily be gleaned from contemporary publications. Alexander Peyer's popular *Die Microscopie am Krankenbette* (*Atlas of Clinical Microscopy*), first published in 1884, started to include a chapter on sperm testing in its fourth edition, published in 1897, because the issue was now seen as "of great practical importance."[38] Likewise, two medical handbooks exclusively devoted to infertility and published in 1885 and 1886, respectively, had been reluctant to accept that gonorrhea was a major cause of infertility, arguing that it was so widespread that it could not have much of an impact, as so many men and women reproduced successfully in spite of being infected.[39] However, when publishing a second edition of his handbook in 1895, one of the authors introduced a new chapter on gonorrhea. Thus, by the last decade of the nineteenth century, the importance of gonorrhea as a major cause of infertility in men and women was increasingly regarded as an established fact.[40]

But just how dangerous gonorrhea really was continued to be a mystery. The issue was seen as calling for more clinical attention and more research. Alongside medical research based on autopsies and clinical material, a large follow-up study was conducted, which was later often cited. It was based on an attempt to reconstruct the reproductive lives of men who during their military service had been treated for gonorrhea at the army hospital in Hannover. Using medical records, the author, chief staff surgeon Benzler, traced 3,000 men and followed their military careers. He excluded those who returned to be treated for a second infection. Other men had died, emigrated, or remained single. Although the army and police bureaucracy cooperated, only 474 complete reproductive histories could be compiled, with records reaching back to the 1870s. They included cases like those of "musketeer G," who fathered an illegitimate son before joining the army in 1873. He was treated for gonorrhea when joining the army but did not show any sign of a new infection during his three years of service. He got married in 1879 and again in 1892 but had no children in either of these marriages.

Benzler differentiated between patients with "simple gonorrhea," those with a one-sided inflammation of the testes, and those with double-sided inflammation. In the first and largest group, which comprised 363 marriages, 38, or 10.5 percent, had remained childless, while 63, or 17.3 percent, had only one child. In the second group 26 out of 111, or 23.4 percent, were childless, and 15, or 13.5 percent, had only one child. In the third group 10 out of 24 marriages, or 41.7 percent, were childless and 5, or 20.8 percent, had only one child. Epididymitis, the author concluded, was clearly detrimental to the fertility of a marriage.[41]

Studies on Britain have suggested that male sterility was regarded as a rare condition and that doctors were reluctant to even consider its possibility.[42] For Germany nothing could be further from the truth. By the turn of the century, if not earlier, ordinary gynecologists were encouraged to undertake a semen analysis, which was presented as easy to do even for those with "little experience in microscopy."[43] While the treatment of male sterility was regarded as the prerogative of the urologist, repeated sperm testing was seen as part of a comprehensive sterility diagnosis to be administered by the gynecologist.[44] It was even debated whether a doctor who operated on a woman to combat infertility would not be liable for negligence if he had not insisted on a sperm test before.[45] Although the subdiscipline of andrology had not yet developed, male reproductive bodies did not fly under the radar of medical attention in Germany. Quite to the contrary.

Warning the Public

From the late 1880s onward, the emerging consensus that gonorrhea was an infectious disease caused by gonococci, which could cause severe pelvic inflammations in women and infertility in both sexes, was taken up in popular health-advice literature. Such literature was in high demand and reached all but the poorest segments of a now fully literate society. A medical handbook for ordinary women, *Das Weib als Gattin und Mutter*, the second edition of which was published in 1889, stated that men were more likely to be responsible for the childlessness of a marriage because they often had been infected with a venereal disease that caused their semen to become "watery" and that reduced the number of spermatozoa.[46] In her *Frauenbuch*, a medical self-help book for women first published in 1896 and quickly selling some forty thousand copies, Hope Bridget Adams, one of the very first female doctors practicing in Germany, devoted special attention to gonorrhea. Lengthy chapters with seemingly endless illustrations detailed the symptoms and consequences of the infection as it affected different organs. With regard to its effects on fertility, Adams cited the usual figures: she estimated that in seven out of ten infertile marriages the problem was caused by the husband either because he was sterile himself or because he had infected his wife with gonorrhea.[47] While the heavily illustrated *Frauenbuch* was rather expensive, a short brochure titled *Eheglück!*, published in 1889, contained those parts of the book dealing with contraception, venereal disease, and infertility. A two-page table listed curable and incurable causes of infertility in women and men. Adams encouraged her readers to think of infertility as an avoidable and curable condition. Unintended childlessness was "not a punishment by god, nor a mysterious physical condition or fate, unfathomable and beyond relief, but the result of identifiable and avoidable causes." Three-quarters of the causes of infertility could be erased if only gonorrhea was dealt with.[48]

Even readers not particularly looking for health advice on sexual matters could encounter the new theories concerning male sterility and its relationship to gonorrhea in contemporary encyclopedias. While the article on infertility in the fourth edition of *Meyers Konversationslexikon*, published in 1889, had referred only to women, the supplement published in 1890 included an entry on "Unfruchtbarkeit (Sterilität), männliche" (Infertility [Sterility], male). It stated that male infertility had recently received growing attention and that it could be caused by syphilis, tuberculosis, or cancer but was mainly due to inflammation following an infection with gonorrhea. Readers were informed that sterility was different from impotence and that it could be caused by aspermatism (the lack of semen) or by azoospermia (the lack of spermatozoa in the semen). The latter condition was said to be much more common and something that could be assessed only if the "seemingly completely normal semen" was examined under a microscope.[49]

With the formation of the Deutsche Gesellschaft zur Bekämpfung der Geschlechtskrankheiten (German Society for Combating Venereal Disease) in 1902, the dangers of gonorrhea were even more widely discussed. Talks, leaflets, and exhibitions, later also films, were used to point out the dangers associated with venereal diseases, to deter from pre- and extramarital sex, especially with prostitutes, and to stress the trustworthiness of doctors and their ability to provide adequate treatments.[50] Whether the public should also be advised on prophylactics was controversial. Medical experts were certain that condoms and chemical disinfectants were effective.[51] But to distribute such information to possible consumers could be and indeed was seen as promoting pre- and extramarital sex and prostitution. As Lutz Sauerteig has shown, the rift between advocates of moral reform who wanted to solve the problem of venereal diseases by fighting prostitution and other forms of nonmarital sex and hygienists interested in pragmatic solutions went right through the German Society for Combating Venereal Disease.[52] However, compared to Britain and France (see chapter 11, in this volume), the German public appears to have been much more likely to receive practical advice on how to avoid an infection with the help of condoms and chemical disinfectants, which were sold in pharmacies.[53] Doctors were keen to gain a monopoly of treating venereal diseases. Hence, both sexes were encouraged to see a doctor (and not to rely on quack medicine) as soon as they discovered signs of an infection. Apparently, such advice was not without its effects, as the number of clients seeking help in local clinics for venereal disease went up during and after exhibitions.[54]

After World War I, during which many soldiers had been offered prophylactics and had received treatment for venereal diseases, health advice became ever more sophisticated. In the aftermath of the war, the Hygiene Museum in Dresden put together several versions of a traveling exhibition on venereal disease, which proved very successful and was apparently seen by some 1.7

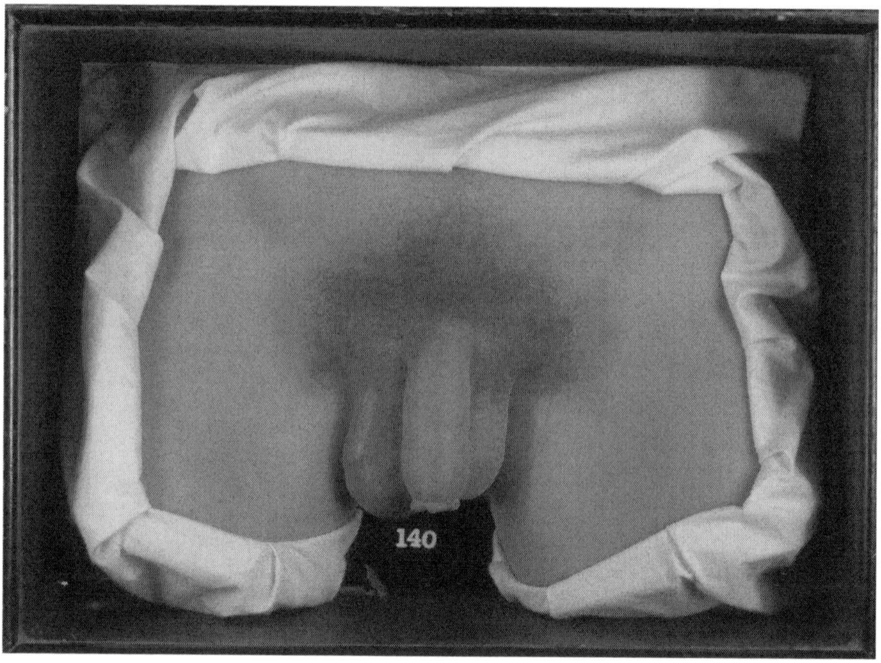

Figure 10.1. Anatomical wax model in display case, used in a commercial exhibition on venereal diseases, end of nineteenth century. Deutsches Hygiene-Museum Dresden (DHMD), 2011/13.

million Germans in cities and towns all over the country. Suited to be shown in small and large spaces, these exhibitions comprised a variety of different media, including wall charts, wax models, and preparations. A particularly striking medium utilized to show possible effects of syphilis were life-size models in wax depicting human genitalia or other body parts exhibiting the sores and ulcers produced by syphilis. The symptoms and consequences of gonorrhea paled in comparison.[55] Figure 10.1 shows a wax model produced for a commercial exhibition that toured German fairgrounds around 1900. It represents male genitalia and shows the symptoms of a gonorrheal infection that has spread to the right testicle.

The following images (figs. 10.2 to 10.6) were produced by the German Hygiene Museum, one of the most important players in early twentieth-century German health education. Apart from traveling exhibitions on venereal disease, the museum also produced wall charts, models, pamphlets and slide shows, and other materials, which could be bought or borrowed by health educators.[56] The museum cooperated closely with the Deutsche Gesellschaft zur Bekämpfung der Geschlechtskrankheiten (German Society for Combating

Venereal Diseases) and followed a pragmatic approach that presented venereal diseases as diagnosable, preventable, and curable. To increase trust in medicine, audiences were informed about methods of diagnosis. Relevant images showed gonococci as seen through a microscope (fig. 10.2) and the inside of healthy and infected urethrae as seen by the doctor during examination.[57]

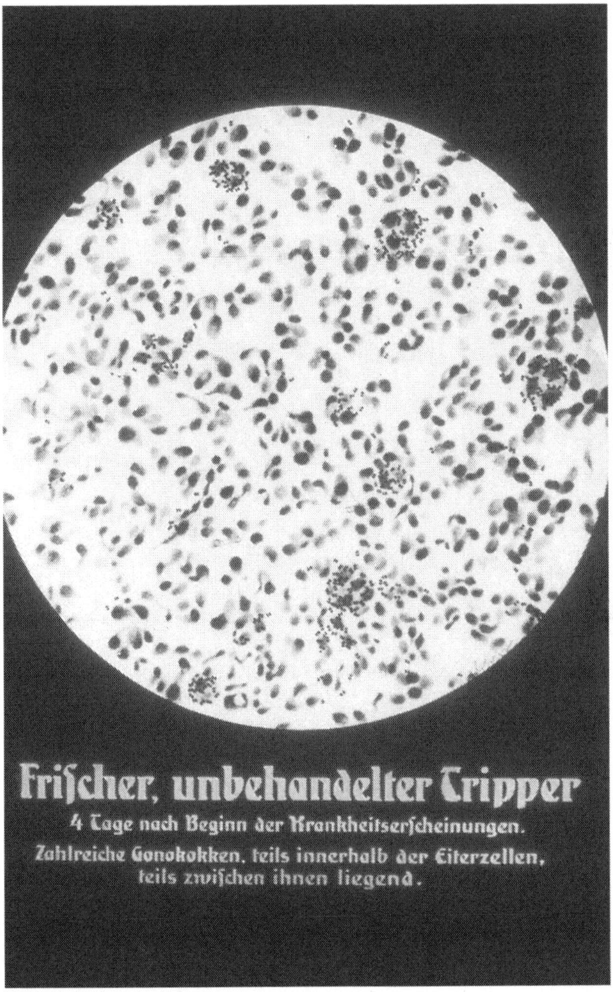

Figure 10.2. "Fresh, untreated gonorrhea. Four days after the start of disease symptoms showing many gonococci." Microscopic image used as part of a slide show, ca. 1919, to accompany talks on venereal disease. The image points to the worrisome proliferation of gonococci but also to the medical possibility of detecting them. DHMD, 1999/994.

Audiences were offered detailed information about sexual physiology and the devastating effects gonorrhea could have on male and female bodies (figs. 10.3 and 10.4).

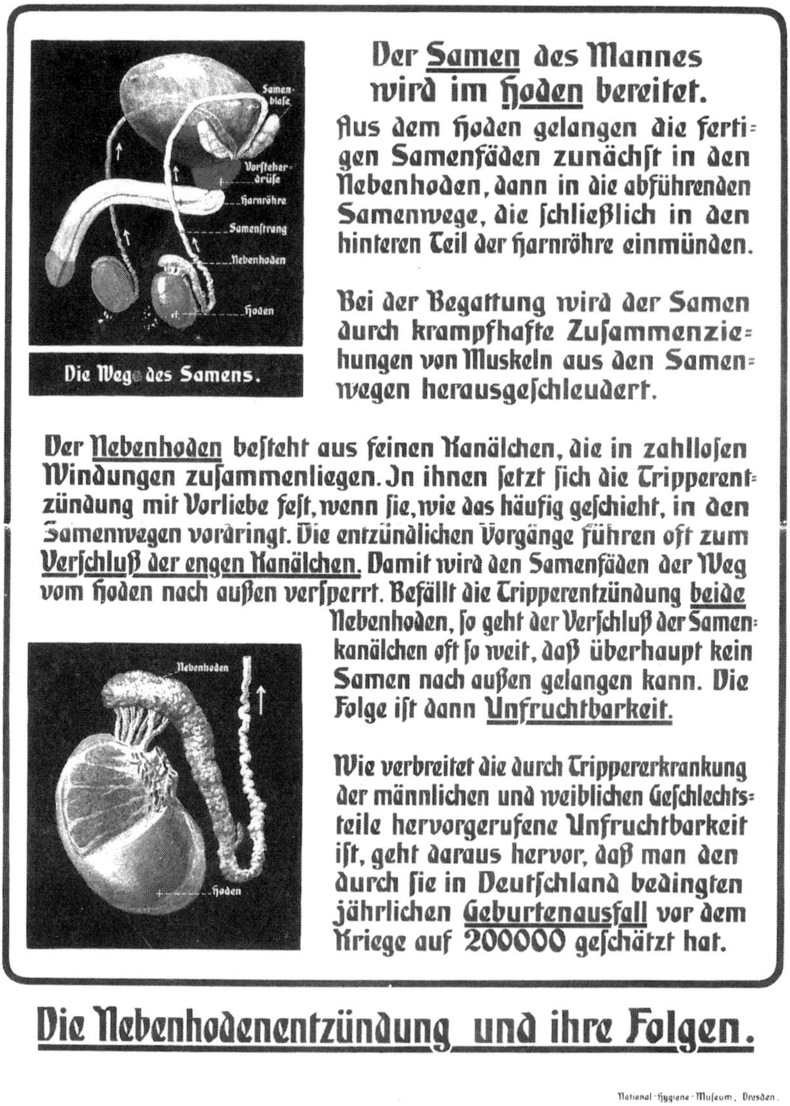

Figure 10.3. "Epididymitis and its consequences," ca. 1919. Photograph of a poster publicized during the 1920s, explaining and visualizing possible effects of gonorrhea on the testes. Infertility is mentioned and the figure of two hundred thousand children not born because of gonorrhea each year is quoted as a pre–World War I estimate. DHMD, 2015/462.

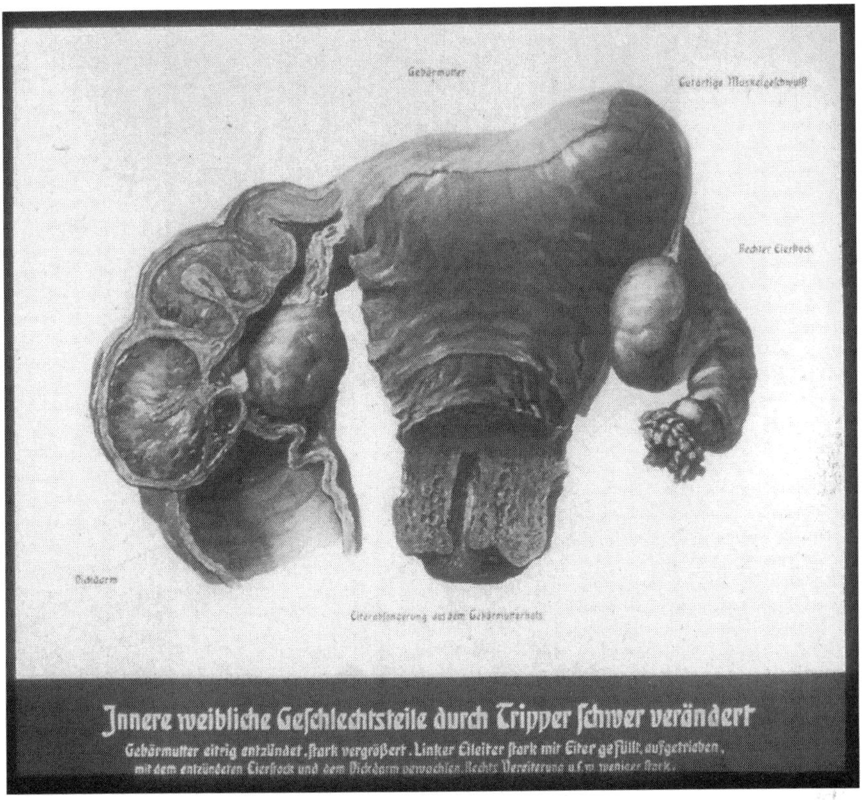

Figure 10.4. "Inner female genitals severely altered by gonorrhea." Image used as part of a 1920s slide show on venereal disease and also in publications. Uterus and fallopian tubes appear filled with pus. The lay public is invited to share the medical view of venereal disease. DHMD, 1999/945.

Chart diagrams were used to illustrate the spread of venereal diseases. In figure 10.5, for example, absolute numbers reported for one month were used to calculate hypothetical rates of infection for different age groups. These rates of infection were added to arrive at a figure representing the probability of having been infected with gonorrhea at least once in one's life-time. For men between forty and fifty, this method resulted in a probability of 160 percent. Not surprisingly, critics believed these estimates to be exaggerated.[58]

Statistical evidence (based on the study by Benzler mentioned earlier) on the connection between gonorrhea and both absolute sterility ("keine Kinder") and one-child sterility ("nur ein Kind") is shown in figure 10.6. Occasionally demographic effects of gonorrhea were mentioned. A poster on "Epididymitis and its consequences" (fig. 10.3) claimed 200,000 births lost

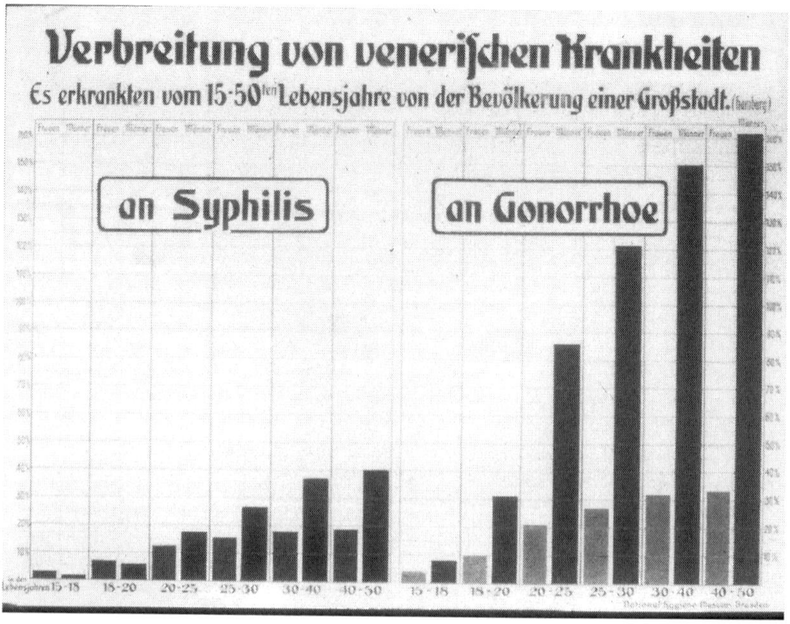

Figure 10.5. Spread of venereal diseases for inhabitants of Hamburg, according to age. A bar chart used in a 1920s slide shows indicative frequencies of infection with syphilis and with gonorrhea for women (left column) and men (right column). No source or date are given, but the figures appear to have been based on a controversial survey conducted in 1913. As explained in this chapter's text, this was a propaganda chart and its method of construction did not produce statistically valid indicators. DHMD, 1999/982.

annually. Unlike later Nazi health propaganda, this statistical information was not visualized as a nationalist message.

The exhibitions assured their audiences that venereal diseases could be cured, but only with the help of doctors. A rise in the number of patients seeking help from local health-advice centers was seen as the best indicator of success. The exhibitions also included information on possible forms of prophylaxis—a feature that was not always easily accepted by local partners, with whom the museum needed to cooperate.[59]

It was only in the mid-1920s that a wall chart was designed that visualized unintended childlessness.[60] Along with the image of a blind man, a woman is shown who apparently has been crippled and rendered infertile by gonorrhea. The text explicitly states that gonorrhea frequently causes sterility in men and women (fig. 10.7). Weimar health advice included vivid depictions of sexually transmitted diseases, with

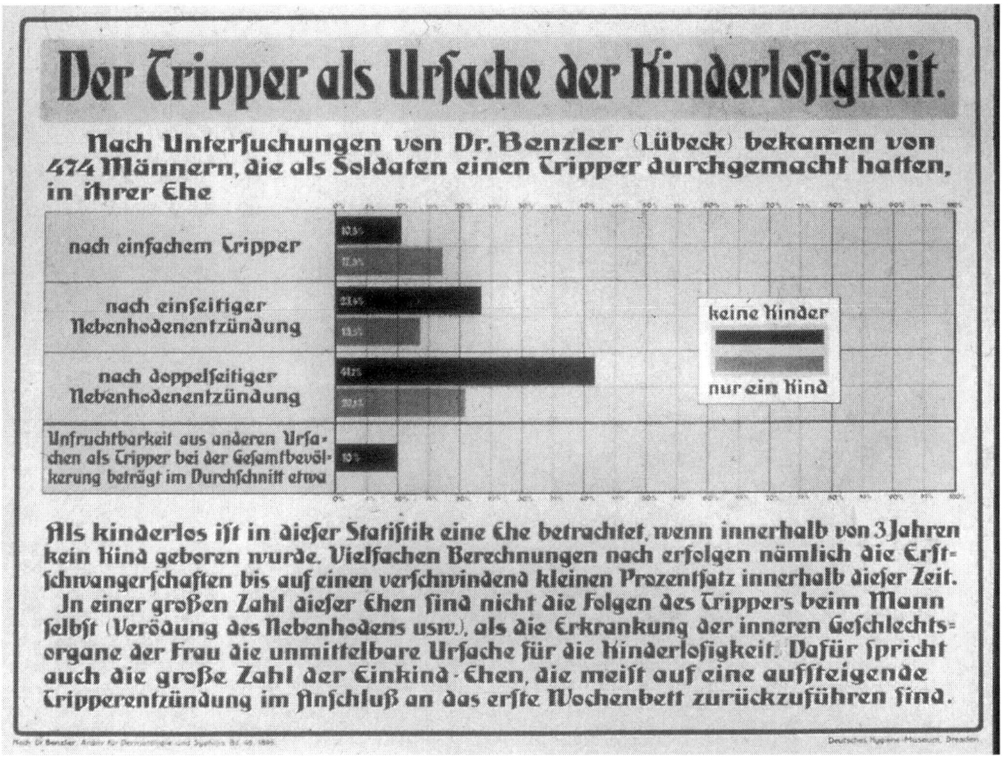

Figure 10.6. "Gonorrhea as cause of childlessness." A bar chart presenting the data collected by Dr. Benzler. The chart differentiates in the upper three rows between men who had had, first, "simple clap," second, one-sided epididymitis, and, third, double-sided epididymitis. At the bottom in the fourth row, a bar representing "infertility not caused by gonorrhea" is added, which shows that "simple gonorrhea" did not carry a high risk of infertility. DHMD, 1999/1623.DHMD, 1999/982.

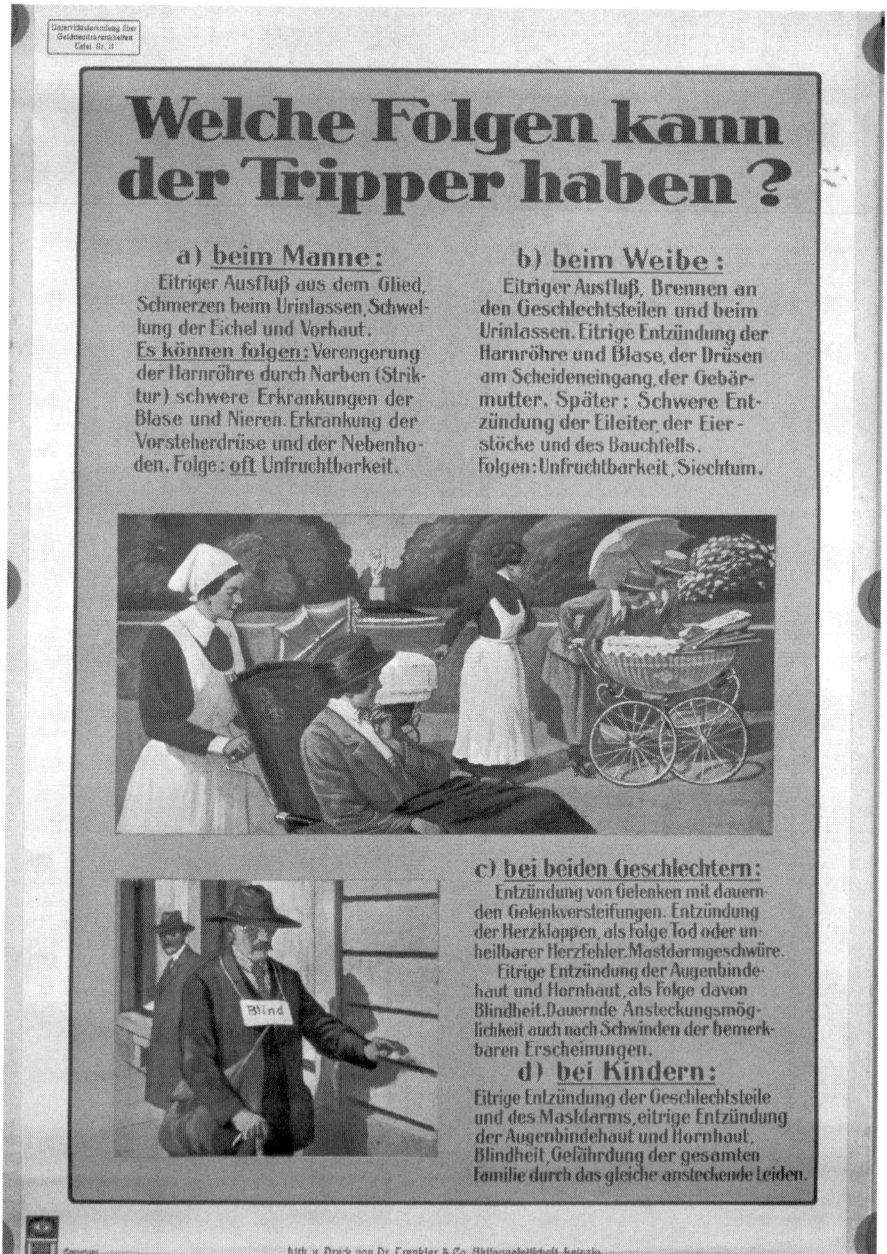
Welche Folgen kann der Tripper haben?
a) beim Manne:
Eitriger Ausfluß aus dem Glied, Schmerzen beim Urinlassen, Schwellung der Eichel und Vorhaut.
Es können folgen: Verengerung der Harnröhre durch Narben (Striktur) schwere Erkrankungen der Blase und Nieren. Erkrankung der Vorsteherdrüse und der Nebenhoden. Folge: oft Unfruchtbarkeit.
b) beim Weibe:
Eitriger Ausfluß, Brennen an den Geschlechtsteilen und beim Urinlassen. Eitrige Entzündung der Harnröhre und Blase, der Drüsen am Scheideneingang, der Gebärmutter. Später: Schwere Entzündung der Eileiter, der Eierstöcke und des Bauchfells.
Folgen: Unfruchtbarkeit, Siechtum.
c) bei beiden Geschlechtern:
Entzündung von Gelenken mit dauernden Gelenkversteifungen. Entzündung der Herzklappen, als Folge Tod oder unheilbarer Herzfehler. Mastdarmgeschwüre.
Eitrige Entzündung der Augenbindehaut und Hornhaut, als Folge davon Blindheit. Dauernde Ansteckungsmöglichkeit auch nach Schwinden der bemerkbaren Erscheinungen.
d) bei Kindern:
Eitrige Entzündung der Geschlechtsteile und des Mastdarms, eitrige Entzündung der Augenbindehaut und Hornhaut, Blindheit, Gefährdung der gesamten Familie durch das gleiche ansteckende Leiden.
Blind

Figure 10.7. "Which are the possible consequences of gonorrhea? A: for men, B: for women, C: for both sexes, D: for children." Wall chart from 1925. The column on men mentions infertility as a frequent consequence of gonorrhea. DHMD, 1995/25.

syphilis taking center stage. Those images and texts dealing with gonorrhea presented eye infections of newborns and sterility in both men and women as possible, even frequent, consequences. That the parents of Maria, from whose case record I quote at the beginning of this chapter, were concerned was not surprising: they had had ample opportunities to pick up information on the relationship between venereal disease and sterility.

Demographic Concerns, Birth Control, and Venereal Disease

Around 1912 public attention in Germany was captured by a hitherto rarely discussed phenomenon: the drop in the birthrate.[61] The "Geburtenrückgang"—the decline in the number of children annually born per every thousand in a population—was an international phenomenon. In Germany it had started during the late 1870s. Slow at first, the development had not caused much concern. After all, Germany's population was growing extremely fast, much faster than those of France or Britain, and the birthrate was merely returning to what would have been normal in earlier decades. It was only after 1910 that the now clearly accelerating decrease of the birthrate began to be perceived as a problem: Was Germany to follow into the footsteps of France, where two children per family were becoming the norm? And could and should such a development possibly be averted by progressive population politics?

The ensuing debate was heated and multifaceted. It formed part of what Edward Ross Dickinson has recently called a "brawl" about everything connected to sexuality, which engaged a great many German intellectuals in the decades before World War I.[62] They tried to understand and to evaluate what appeared to be a revolution in sexual norms and behaviors. Still influenced by traditional religious ideas and practices but increasingly also by socialism, sex reform, feminism, and consumer culture, millions of German couples had to negotiate reproduction under rapidly changing economic conditions and found themselves living family lives very different from those of their parents. Not surprisingly, contemporaries sought for explanations and disagreed violently when it came to assessing the current situation and to contemplating future developments.

One of the questions raised as soon as debates about the decline in the birthrate started was whether the development could be attributed to degeneration and venereal disease. But these issues remained marginal and were quickly put aside. Influential studies like those by Julius Wolf and Jean Borntraeger mentioned venereal diseases but devoted their attention almost exclusively to socioeconomic factors.[63] When, in 1912, the Prussian government launched a survey to investigate the possible causes of the drop in the birthrate, it explicitly asked whether part of the decline was due to health issues or degeneration. The survey was based on a preliminary report of which three thousand copies were distributed to provincial and regional governments, regional medical advisory boards, and medical associations, who were asked to respond to the report by providing detailed information on demographic developments and changes in reproductive behavior. And so they did.[64] When the final report, or *Denkschrift*, was published in 1915, questions remained, but a general consensus had been reached. While two regional medical advisory boards had pointed to venereal diseases as a contributing factor, all reports agreed that the drop in the birthrate had to be attributed mainly to an extremely widespread, popular drive toward a deliberate reduction in the number of children.[65] The reports mentioned many factors, from urbanization, secularization, women's emancipation, the spread of consumer culture, socialism, a lack of adequate housing, and continuous economic hardship to the ready availability of contraceptives, but at the heart of the phenomenon they saw a sea change in attitudes toward sexuality and reproduction. Though to varying degrees, couples from all social classes and milieus had apparently started to drastically reduce the number of their children by relying on (combinations of) contraceptives, coitus interruptus, abortions, and abstinence. If something was to be done about this development, population policies had to target attitudes and social conditions, not germs.

With regard to the possible importance of gonorrhea, the *Denkschrift* echoed a position put forward by Alfred Blaschko, one of Germany's most eminent venereologists. In a paper on *Geburtenrückgang* and venereal disease published in 1913, Blaschko elaborated on the sterilizing effects of gonorrhea and syphilis.[66] Using available studies, he estimated that 350,000 German couples were childless because of prior infections with venereal disease. However, while he certainly advocated further campaigns, he was also convinced that the drop of the birthrate needed to be understood as a cultural revolution that, as he pointed out, was affecting not only Germany but Western Europe. Blaschko believed that, contrary to his earlier assessments, rates of venereal disease were coming down and that VD-induced infertility therefore could not explain the drop in the birthrate. His text shows that he perceived the situation as rather dangerous: not because infertility was spreading but because conservative antivice campaigners and officials used the drop in the birthrate to demand a ban on contraceptives.

For all their disagreements with regard to the significance of the drop in the birthrate, most politicians and experts seem to have tacitly agreed that venereal disease was not a major factor. When they debated possible remedies, increased medical services or advice centers for those experiencing reproductive difficulties or intensified research on causes and treatment of infertility were normally not mentioned. Although it was acknowledged that infertility was widespread, affecting hundreds of thousands of couples, it was not cast as a major public health issue, not even at a time when the drop in the birthrate captured the popular imagination.

Venereal Disease and Infertility in Nazi Health Propaganda

Biology and medicine were central to National Socialism.[67] With the nation imagined as a body under threat from internal and external enemies, health education was increasingly brought under direct state control.[68] Not the health of the individual but the current and future well-being of the race was presented as the central objective that—if necessary—would trump the interests of individuals. Attention to the body politic and the expectation that eugenics could be used to improve nation and race were not new, nor were they exclusively used by National Socialists. Historians have pointed to international connections and to continuities and changes in biopolitics between Weimar and Nazi Germany.[69] It is beyond the scope of this chapter to map the changes in sexual and social policies brought about by National Socialism after 1933. However, a glimpse at materials from anti-VD campaigns designed and distributed by the German Hygiene Museum illustrates the comparatively liberal stance taken by important Weimar health educators.

After the Nazis had come to power in 1933, the German Hygiene Museum rapidly aligned itself with the political aims and aesthetic preferences of the new regime.[70] About half of its former scientific staff, many of them Jewish, was sacked. Instead of concentrating on individual health, the museum now propagated forms of racial thinking. How did this play out when it came to anti-VD propaganda? When we compare pre- and post-1933 health education materials, it becomes obvious that some motives used in earlier exhibitions were reused and adapted. For instance, the bar chart shown in figure 10.6, which was originally produced in the 1920s (and in fact used data collected in 1898), was reissued during the Nazi period, but the bottom bar was removed in a purposeful attempt to dramatize the threat of gonorrhea. Other motives were newly introduced.

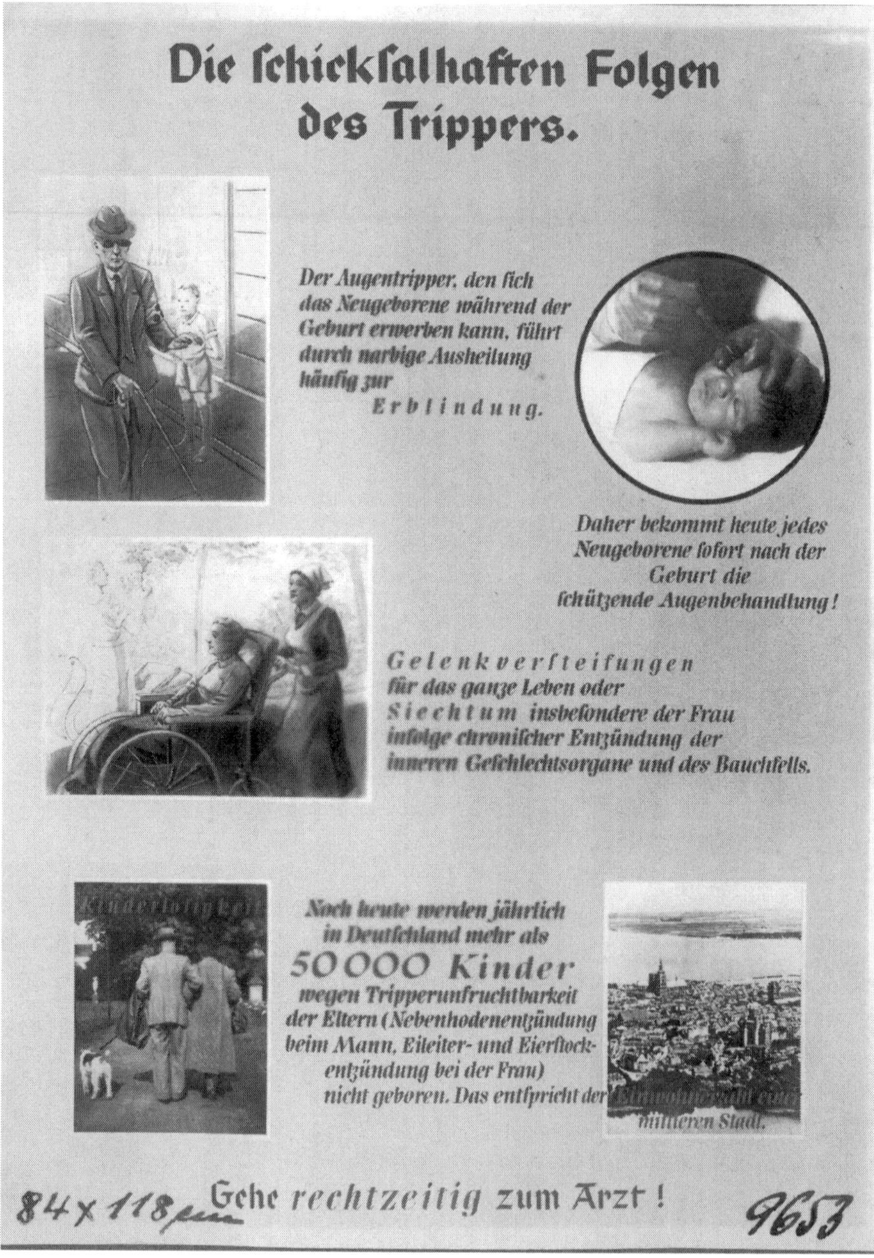

Figure 10.8. "The fateful consequences of gonorrhea." Redesigned wall chart from 1938. The bottom part now shows a childless couple and the image of a middle-sized town and argues that fifty thousand children a year were not being born owing to a gonorrhea infection in men or women. DHMD, 1994/587.

The wall-chart warning against the dangers of gonorrhea was redesigned in 1938 (see fig. 10.8). The heading was changed from a question about possible consequences of gonorrhea to a statement about *fateful* outcomes. Potentially useful information about symptoms was excluded. The wall chart not only informed about the dangers of ophthalmia neonatarum but showed how Credé's prophylaxis was performed, euphemistically presenting it as "protective eye treatment." The image in the middle continued to underline that gonorrhea could lead to infirmity. Infertility is invoked by the contrasting image of a mother with child bathed in golden light. At the bottom of the wall chart we find a new component: the information that gonorrhea can lead to infertility due to epididymitis and inflammations of tubes and ovaries is framed by two images. The one on the left shows a childless couple while the one on the right is meant to visualize the number of children not born due to gonorrhea—fifty thousand per year—by depicting a town with a comparable number of citizens.

The new motif of the childless old couple was also introduced in other materials. Figure 10.9 depicts such a couple. Seated by a window with only a potted plant to care for, the old couple watch their peers, who get to play with their grandchildren in an idyllic garden.

While this image appealed to the interest of the individual who would enjoy the benefits of having children and grandchildren, other wall panels underlined the racial consequences of venereal diseases. Figure 10.10 shows a flock of empty cradles surrounding a lonely woman, while other parts of the image show children crippled by syphilis or point to the economic loss of manpower.

Such images clearly marked a shift in the message presented by health campaigns. While viewers were invited to contemplate the individual hardship that could be brought about by an infection, the images also conveyed that venereal diseases endangered the nation and that individuals had a responsibility toward their *Volk*.

Conclusion: Not Invisible, but Marginal

Around 1900 gonorrhea was generally believed to be the "archenemy of fertility," a view frequently presented to medical students, medical practitioners, and the general public.[71] In this chapter I have explored how the idea that gonorrhea was a major cause of infertility developed and circulated and how it was supported, spread, questioned, and redefined. I have followed developments in medicine, in political debates concerning the drop in the birthrate, and in popular health advice. While these discourses were connected, they

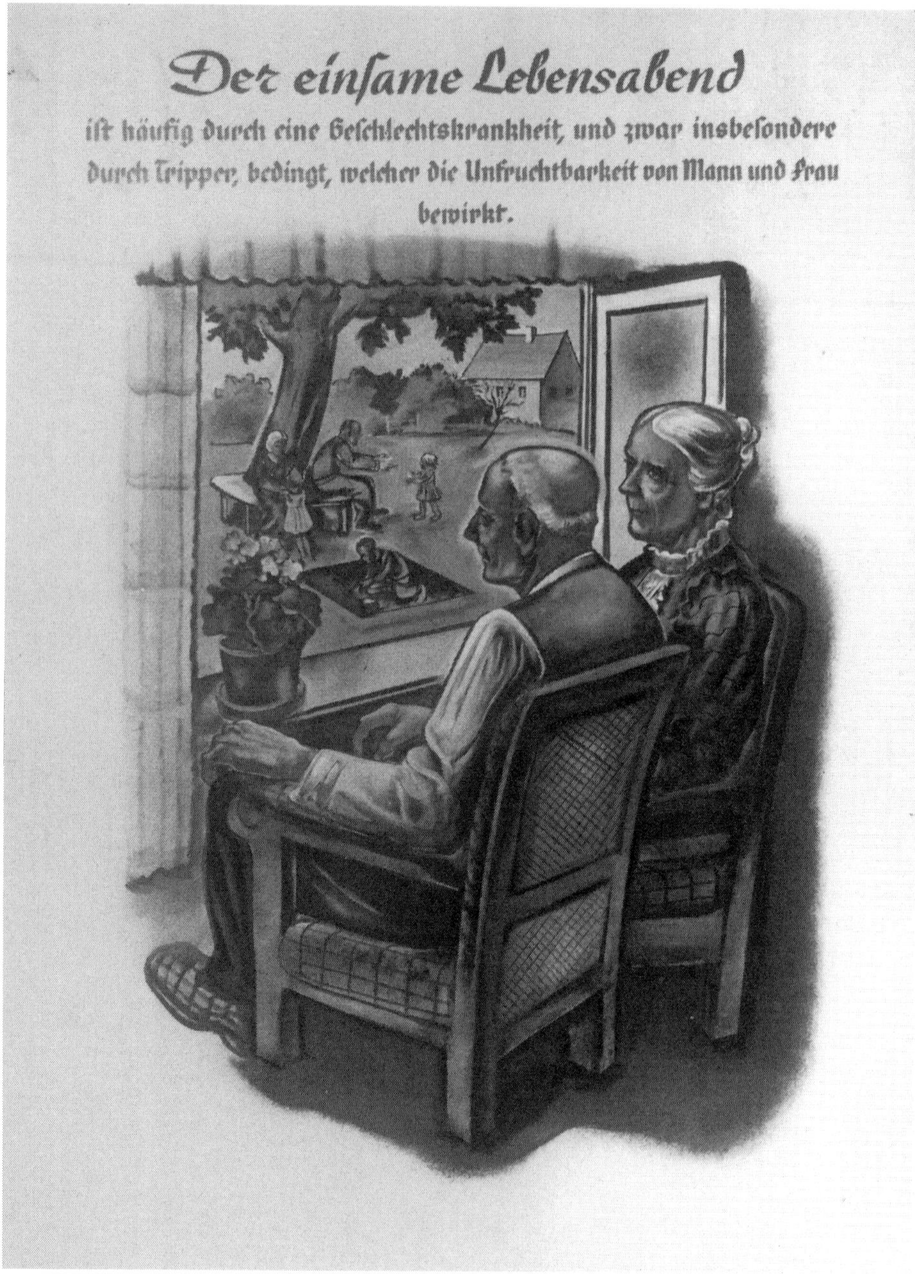
Der einſame Lebensabend
iſt häufig durch eine Geſchlechtskrankheit, und zwar insbeſondere
durch Tripper, bedingt, welcher die Unfruchtbarkeit von Mann und Frau
bewirkt.

Figure 10.9. “Lonely old age is often the result of a venereal disease, especially gonorrhea, which causes infertility in both men and women.” Wall chart from an exhibition on “The War on Cancer,” which toured Germany between 1939 and 1944 and which included a section on infectious diseases. DHMD, 2001/248.7.

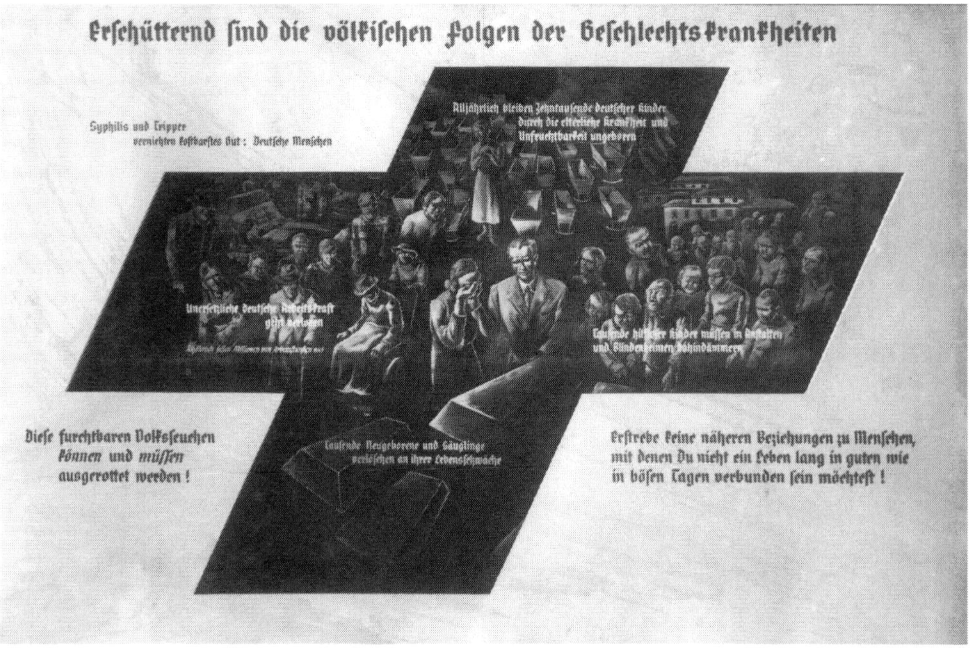
Erschütternd sind die völkischen Folgen der Geschlechtskrankheiten
Syphilis und Tripper
vernichten kostbarstes Gut: Deutsche Menschen
Alljährlich bleiben Zehntausende deutscher Kinder
durch die elterliche Krankheit und
Unfruchtbarkeit ungeboren
Tausende Neugeborene und Säuglinge
verlöschen an ihrer Lebensschwäche
Diese furchtbaren Volksseuchen
können und müssen
ausgerottet werden!
Erstrebe keine näheren Beziehungen zu Menschen,
mit denen Du nicht ein Leben lang in guten wie
in bösen Tagen verbunden sein möchtest!

Figure 10.10. Photograph of a wall panel from a 1938 exhibition on "Health in Everyday Life," which clearly reflects Nazi biopolitics. "Harrowing are the racial consequences of venereal diseases. Syphilis and gonorrhea destroy precious goods: German people. Every year tens of thousands of German children remain unborn due to parental illnesses and infertility." DHMD, 2006/477.8.

followed different agendas and trajectories. They did not mirror an actual increase in the spread of disease, nor can they be seen as a continuous unfolding of biopolitical concerns. Instead, they were driven by developments and actors within their respective fields.

When Noeggerath developed his theory of latent gonorrhea, he was not driven by public health or demographic concerns. His interest in gonorrhea grew out of his encounters with difficult cases impossible to cure, which he interpreted in the light of budding bacteriological disease theories. His fellow doctors in Germany—while critical with regard to the figures Noeggerath had proposed—generally accepted that gonorrhea could lead to infertility, once bacteriological research had established that gonococci could spread beyond the mucus membrane. German doctors were particularly intrigued by the possibility of diagnosing sterility and latent gonorrhea in men. Given that infections with gonorrhea were common among adolescent and adult men, the idea that gonorrhea might often be latent and that it could seriously endanger an innocent bride significantly expanded doctors' sphere of influence. Armed with microscopes, they performed repeated examinations on seemingly healthy patients, aimed at assessing men's health and fertility. They found male infertility (the absence of spermatozoa) in a significant proportion of infertile marriages.

Around 1900 public health campaigns to combat venereal disease were launched. They invariably included information on gonorrhea and its detrimental effects on fertility in both sexes. But syphilis was clearly presented as more important. This was partly connected to the characteristics of health campaigns as media products. Because of its terrifying and easily visualized nature, syphilis was much better suited for frightening audiences into changing their sexual behaviors. While less widespread than gonorrhea, syphilis produced enormous costs for health insurers, who had to pay for treatment and sick leave. And the apparent phenomenon of "congenital syphilis" raised the fear that it could affect the future generation, a problem that was not believed to pertain to gonorrhea. Furthermore, with the introduction of salvarsan and neosalvarsan, syphilis could actually be cured, if patients were willing to comply. Hence, health campaigners had good reasons to concentrate on syphilis.

Shortly before World War I, debates about the drop in the birthrate gripped the attention of the German public. The question of whether or not gonorrhea played a part in what to many seemed like a threat to the nation's health and future was, however, quickly put aside: while gonorrhea was regarded as a major cause of infertility, it could not explain the recent drop in the birthrate. According to medical expertise, the continued campaigns to combat venereal disease had actually been successful, leading to a decline in new infections. The drop in the birthrate was attributed to another factor: a truly revolutionary change in attitudes to reproduction.

Throughout the first third of the twentieth century, health advice mentioned that gonorrhea could lead to infertility, but it was only during the Nazi period that health propaganda constructed gonorrhea as a racial threat and public health concern. At this time, however, medical approaches to infertility had long shifted, with emphasis instead on the multiplicity of factors of infertility, especially in women, including hormonal, psychological, and constitutional factors.[72]

For those like Maria Meyer and her husband, who experienced reproductive difficulties, and even for her parents, who had probably ignored the frequent call to ask future sons-in-law for a health certificate, the heightened awareness of gonorrhea as a possible or even frequent cause of sterility added a further layer of shame to the experience of infertility. While Maria Meyer and her peers often had access to medical services, the plight of involuntarily childless couples did not receive much public attention. Even marital advice centers, which proliferated during the 1920s and which provided many couples with contraceptives, do not appear to have been keen on helping those who could not have children. Infertility remained a primarily private affair until Nazi biopolitics politicized reproduction in all its facets.

Notes

Research for this article was supported by a M4Human Fellowship of the Gerda Henkel Foundation.

1. Universitätsarchiv Tübingen, Bestand 317/853, case 97.

2. Emil Noeggerath, *Die latente Gonorrhoe im weiblichen Geschlecht* (Bonn: Cohen & Sohn, 1872).

3. Michael Worboys, "Unsexing Gonorrhea: Bacteriologists, Gynecologists and Suffragists in Britain, 1860–1920," *Social History of Medicine* 17, no. 1 (2004): 31–59; Elliott Bowen, "Limits of the Lab: Diagnosing 'Latent Gonorrhea,' 1872–1910," *Bulletin of the History of Medicine* 87, no. 1 (2013): 63–85; Anne Hanley, "'The Great Foe to the Reproduction of the Race': Diagnosing and Treating Infertility Caused by Venereal Diseases," in *The Palgrave Handbook of Infertility in History*, ed. Gayle Davis and Tracey Loughran (London: Palgrave Macmillan, 2017), 335–58.

4. Victoria Bates, "'So Far as I Can Define without a Microscopical Examination': Venereal Disease Diagnosis in English Courts, 1850–1914," *Social History of Medicine* 26, no. 1 (2012): 38–55.

5. Debates on venereal disease have been reconstructed and analyzed in a number of historical studies. For Germany, see Lutz Sauerteig, *Krankheit, Sexualität, Gesellschaft: Geschlechtskrankheiten und Gesundheitspolitik in Deutschland im 19. und frühen 20. Jahrhundert* (Stuttgart: Steiner, 1999); Sauerteig, "'The Fatherland Is in Danger, Save the Fatherland!' Venereal Disease, Sexuality and Gender in Imperial and Weimar Germany," in *Sex, Sin and Suffering: Venereal Disease and European Society since 1870*, ed. Roger Davidson and Lesley A. Hall (London: Routledge, 2004), 76–92; and Petra Ellenbrand, *Die Volksbewegung und Volksaufklärung gegen Geschlechtskrankheiten in Kaiserreich und Weimarer Republik* (Marburg: Görich & Weiershäuser, 1999). New research by Anita Gertiser and by Anja Laukötter has stressed the necessity of interpreting health education with regard to genre, conventions, audiences, and (commercial) purposes. See Gertiser, *Falsche Scham: Strategien der Überzeugung in Aufklärungsfilmen zur Bekämpfung der Geschlechtskrankheiten (1918–1935)* (Göttingen: Vandenhoeck & Ruprecht, 2015); and Laukötter, "Medien der Sexualaufklärung: Forschungsstand und Forschungsperspektiven," *NTM Zeitschrift für Geschichte der Wissenschaften, Technik und Medizin* 20, no. 3 (2012): 225–32. See also Christian Bonah and Anja Laukötter, "Introduction:

Screening Diseases; Films on Sex Hygiene in Germany and France in the First Half of the 20th Century," *Gesnerus* 72, no 1 (2015): 5–14. Studies by Britta McEwan and Annette Timm on Vienna and Berlin alert us to local traditions and infrastructures in health education. See McEwan, *Sexual Knowledge: Feeling, Fact and Social Reform in Vienna, 1900–1934* (New York: Berghahn Books, 2012); and Timm, *The Politics of Fertility in Twentieth-Century Berlin* (Cambridge: Cambridge University Press 2010).

6. Noeggerath, *Latente Gonorrhoe.*

7. Emil Noeggerath, "Latent Gonorrhea, Especially with Regard to Its Influence on Fertility in Women," *Transactions of the American Gynecological Society* 1 (1876): 268–300.

8. The most detailed account of Noeggerath's life and work is Paul Diepgen,"Emil Noeggerath und die Gynäkologie in der zweiten Hälfte des 19. Jahrhunderts," *Archiv für Geschichte der Medizin* 20, no. 3 (1928): 198–232. Unfortunately, it is not clear how Diepgen gathered the information he used for this article. He seems to have spoken to Noeggerath's family, but he certainly did not have access to US materials. Information on Noeggerath's life is taken from Diepgen's account if not otherwise stated.

9. Noeggerath experimented with different diagnostic methods, such as using probes of different shapes to examine the urethra of men. He also developed a method of gynecological examination for which a finger was introduced into the bladder.

10. Noeggerath, *Latente Gonorrhoe*, case 9, pp. 26–28. On debates regarding the use of the speculum, see Kathryn Yeniyurt, "When It Hurts to Look: Interpreting the Interior of the Victorian Woman," *Social History of Medicine 27, no. 1 (*2014): 22–40.

11. Noeggerath, *Latente Gonorrhoe*, 4.

12. The "double standard" in sexual matters was much criticized by late nineteenth- and early twentieth-century moral reform movements. For an early study, see Keith Thomas, "The Double Standard," *Journal of the History of Ideas* 20, no. 2 (1959): 195–216.

13. Emil Noeggerath and Abraham Jacobi, *Contributions to Midwifery, and Diseases of Women and Children, with a Report on the Progress of Obstetrics, and Uterine and Infantile Pathology in 1858* (New York: Baillière Brothers, 1859).

14. Felix Victor Birch-Hirschfeld, "Die neuern pathologisch-anatomischen Untersuchungen über krankmachende Schmarotzerpilze," *Schmidt's Jahrbücher der in- und ausländischen Medicin* 155 (1872): 97–109.

15. Edwin Klebs, *Beiträge zur pathologischen Anatomie der Schusswunden nach Beobachtungen in den Kriegslazarethen in Carlsruhe 1870 und 1871* (Leipzig: Vogel, 1872).

16. Bedside, hospital, and laboratory medicine have been characterized as three distinct forms of medical thinking or even three medical cosmologies. However, as John V. Pickstone has suggested, these different ways of knowledge production are

better understood not as successive but as nested: older concepts are partly integrated into newer ones. Noeggerath embodies what in Pickstone's terminology would be an analytical approach: he gathered cases and data that he would analyze to gain new insights. Laboratory techniques were part of this endeavor of analysis but were not (much) used for experimentation. On the difference between natural history, analysis, and experimentation, see Pickstone, *Ways of Knowing: A New History of Science, Technology and Medicine* (Chicago: University of Chicago Press, 2000). On the difference between biographical medicine, medical analysis, and experimentation, see Pickstone, "Commentary: From the History of Medicine to a General History of 'Working Knowledges,'" *International Journal of Epidemiology* 28 (2009): 646–49.

17. Noeggerath, *Latente Gonorrhoe*, vii. The original German reads as follows: "Das Gewebe, welches hier zur Prüfung vorliegt, habe ich versucht derb und haltbar zu machen, dadurch, dass ich die einzelnen Fäden nicht zu sparsam, in passender Weise so ineinander gewunden, dass jeder einzelne zur Solidificierung des Ganzen beiträgt. Ich hätte gewünscht, der Arbeit durch fortgesetzte Beobachtung, wo möglich die doppelte Anzahl von Fällen beifügen zu können, da zur Beweisführung, bis jetzt, wie aus dem Folgenden sich ergeben wird, nur eine grosse Masse von gleichlautenden Krankheitsgeschichten, das nötige Material liefern kann."

18. When Carl Hennig presented comparable cases to the Gesellschaft für Geburtshülfe (Society of obstetrics) in Leipzig in November 1873, a "very lively debate" ensued, in which almost everybody opposed Hennig's conclusion that gonorrhea could cause severe infections, especially in women recovering from childbirth. "Mittheilungen aus der Gesellschaft für Geburtshülfe in Leipzig," *Archiv für Gynäkologie* 6 (1874), 518.

19. Angus MacDonald, "Latent Gonorrhea in the Female Sex, with Special Relation to the Puerperal State," *Edinburgh Medical Journal* 18, pt. 2 (January–June 1873): 1086–104.

20. Noeggerath, "Latent Gonorrhea, 298.

21. Heinrich Fritsch presented several case histories that suggested that gonorrhea could, indeed, have devastating consequences, but that these were far less common than Noeggerath had suggested. See "Zur Lehre von der Tripperinfektion beim Weibe," *Archiv für Gynäkologie* 10 (1876): 470–78.

22. As the president of the American Gynecological Society suggested regarding Noeggerath's paper, "If these views are true, a modification of this paper should be found in every Sabbath school library throughout the land." *Transactions of the American Gynecological Society* 1 (1876): 293.

23. As one of the discussants in New York, a Dr. Trenholme from Montreal, put it, "We, upon our side of the line, look upon it as rather a reproach not to have a large family; and if our Canadian ladies found out that their sterility was dependent upon the former condition of their husbands, I do not know what would take place." *Transactions of the American Gynecological Society*, 1 (1876): 293–94.

24. Especially with regard to US debates, see Thomas G. Benedek, "Gonorrhea and the Beginnings of Clinical Research Ethics," *Perspectives in Biology and Medicine* 48, no. 1 (2005): 54–73.

25. On human experiments using gonococci in Germany, see Marion Maria Ruisinger, "'Erlaubt ist, was neu, was anregend, was interessant ist . . .' Gynäkologische Forschung im Zeichen der Mikrobiologie," in *Herausforderungen: 100 Jahre Bayerische Gesellschaft für Geburtshilfe und Frauenheilkunde*, ed. Christoph Anthuber et al. (Stuttgart: Thieme, 2012), 36–46.

26. See, for example, Albert Döderlein,"Die gonorrhoischen Erkrankungen der weiblichen Geschlechtsorgane," in *Kurzes Lehrbuch der Gynäkologie*, ed. Otto Küstner, 4th ed. (Jena: Fischer, 1910), 429–43, esp. 437.

27. Traugott Kroner, "Über die Beziehungen der Gonorrhoe zu den Generationsvorgängen," *Archiv für Gynäkologie* 31 (1887–88): 252–64.

28. Enoch Heinrich Kisch, *Die Sterilität des Weibes*, 2nd ed. (Vienna: Urban und Schwarzenberg, 1895), 268–69.

29. Ernst Bumm, *Der Mikro-Organismus der Gonorrhoischen Schleimhauterkrankung "Gonococcus-Neisser,"* 2nd ed. (Wiesbaden: Bergmann, 1887).

30. Ernst Wertheim, "Die ascendirende Gonorrhoe beim Weibe: Bakteriologische und klinische Studien zur Biologie des Gonococcus Neisser," *Archiv für Gynäkologie* 42 (1891): 1–86.

31. Noeggerath, "Latent Gonorrhea," 287–88.

32. M. Gosselin, "Novelle études sur l'oblitération des voies spermatique et sur stérilité consecutive à l'épididymite bilatérale," *Archives Générales de Médicine* 5 (1847): 257–70; Thomas Blizard Curling, "Observations on Sterility in Man; with Cases," *British and Foreign Medico-chirurgical Review* 33 (1864): 494–508.

33. James Marion Sims, "Illustrations of the Value of the Microscope in the Treatment of the Sterile Condition," *British Medical Journal* 2, nos. 409–10 (1868): 465–66, 492–94.

34. Ferdinand Adolf Kehrer, "Operationen an der Portio vaginalis," *Archiv für Gynäkologie* 10 (1876): 431–58.

35. Ferdinand Adolf Kehrer, "Zur Sterilitätslehre," in *Beiträge zur klinischen und experimentellen Geburtskunde und Gynäkologie*, ed. Ferdinand Adolf Kehrer (Giessen: Roth, 1879–80), 76–139.

36. Christina Benninghaus, "Beyond Constructivism? Gender, Medicine and the Early History of Sperm Analysis, Germany 1870–1900," *Gender and History* 34, no. 3 (2012): 647–76.

37. The study from which these statistics are taken was based on Ludwig Prochownik's files but was conducted independently. Throughout the following decades it was often quoted. The authors stated that they had set out to refute Kehrer's and Paul Fürbringer's claims regarding the spread of gonorrhea and its consequences but reached the conclusion that the disease was in fact very common and that it posed a real threat to the reproductive capacities of both men and women. See

H. Lier and S. Ascher, "Beiträge zur Sterilitätsfrage," *Zeitschrift für Geburtshilfe und Gynäkologie* 18 (1890): 262–323.

38. Alexander Peyer, *Die Microscopie am Krankenbette* (Basel: Benno Schwabe, 1884). The fourth edition was published in 1897, under the title *Atlas der Mikroskopie am Krankenbette (Harnsedimente, Harnröhrenausflüsse, Spermatorrhoe, Abnormitäten der Samenflüssigkeit)* (Basel: Schwabe, 1897), plate 88.

39. P. Müller, *Die Sterilität der Ehe: Entwicklungsfehler des Uterus* (Stuttgart: Enke, 1885); Enoch Heinrich Kisch, *Sterilität des Weibes, ihre Ursachen und ihre Behandlung* (Vienna: Urban und Schwarzenberg, 1886).

40. Kisch, *Sterilität des Weibes* (1895).

41. Dr. Benzler, "Sterilität und Tripper," *Archiv für Dermatologie und Syphilis* 45 (1895): 33–56.

42. Hanley, "Great Foe," in Davis and Loughran, *Palgrave Handbook of Infertility*, 335–58.

43. Richard Schaeffer, "Über weibliche Sterilität," *Die ärztliche Praxis* 20, no. 10 (1907): 109–12. In his paper, which was originally presented to the Schöneberger Ärzteverein (Schöneberg doctors' association) in Berlin in April 1907, the author tactfully warned his male audience that while they could always practice using their own sperm, two fellow doctors had become quite depressed when realizing that their own sperm lacked spermatozoa (110).

44. Ernest Fraenkel in Breslau, to give an example, kept track of two hundred cases of infertility, diagnosed and treated from 1903 onward. Fraenkel, himself a well-known gynecologist, collaborated with urologists who, on his behalf, did sperm tests on fifty-nine men. "Klinische Beiträge zur Pathologie und Therapie der weiblichen Sterilität," *Sammlung Klinischer Vorträge, Neue Folge* 460–61 (1907): 63–104.

45. Ludwig Pincus, "Wichtige Fragen zur Sterilitätslehre," *Archiv für Gynäkologie* 82 (1907): 188–210, esp. 205. Between 1885 and 1907 Pincus had seen 491 couples complaining about infertility. Sperm tests had shown that in 119 cases the cause of sterility seemed to rest with the husband (see statistics on page 195).

46. Richard Weber (that is, Jakob Ruhemann), *Das Weib als Gattin und Mutter, seine naturgemäße Bestimmung und seine Pflichten* (Berlin: Steinitz, 1889), 108.

47. Hope Bridget Adams, *Das Frauenbuch: Ein ärztlicher Ratgeber für die Frau in der Familie und bei Frauenkrankheiten* (Berlin: Schwarz, 1896).

48. Hope Bridget Adams, *Eheglück! Die Hygiene des Geschlechtslebens von einer praktischen Ärztin* (Berlin: Schwarz, 1899), 25.

49. "Unfruchtbarkeit (Sterilität), männliche," in *Jahres-Supplement, 1890–1891*, vol. 18 of *Meyers Konversationslexikon*, 4th ed. (Leipzig: Bibliographischen Instituts, 1890–91, p. 952.

50. On the Deutsche Gesellschaft zur Bekämpfung der Geschlechtskrankheiten, see Sauerteig, *Krankheit, Sexualität, Gesellschaft*; and Ellenbrand, *Volksbewegung*.

51. Döderlein, "Gonorrhoischen Erkrankungen," in Küstner, *Kurzes Lehrbuch der Gynäkologie*," 429–43, esp. 438.

52. Lutz Sauerteig, "Moralismus versus Pragmatismus: Die Kontroverse um Schutzmittel gegen Geschlechtskrankheiten zu Beginn des 20. Jahrhunderts im deutsch-englischen Vergleich," in *Neue Wege in der Seuchengeschichte*, ed. Martin Dinges and Thomas Schlich (Stuttgart: Steiner, 1995), 207–48.

53. See, for example, the pamphlet *Die Geschlechtskrankheiten* (Venereal disease), published by the Central Commission of Health Insurers in 1900 and written by the dermatologist and activist Alfred Blaschko. It could be bought for only fifteen pfennigs, and, according to Sauerteig, it went through eighteen editions and sold seven hundred thousand copies. See also Felix Block, *Wie schützen wir uns vor den Geschlechtskrankheiten und ihren üblen Folgen?*, 3rd ed., Flugschriften der Deutschen Gesellschaft zur Bekämpfung der Geschlechtskrankheiten, (Leipzig: Barth, 1908), which gave detailed instructions on the use of the bactericide Protargol and was sold for thirty pfennigs.

54. Thomas Steller, "Volksbildungsinstitut und Museumskonzern: Das Deutsche Hygiene-Museum, 1912–1930" (PhD diss., University of Bielefeld, 2014), 194.

55. On visual strategies employed to scare audiences, see Gertiser, *Falsche Scham.*

56. Thomas Steller, "Seuchenwissen als Exponat und Argument: Ausstellungen zur Bekämpfung der Geschlechtskrankheiten des Deutschen Hygiene-Museums in den 1920er Jahren," in *Infiziertes Europa: Seuchen im langen 20. Jahrhundert*, ed. Malte Thiessen, Beihefte zur Historischen Zeitschrift, NF 64 (Munich: Oldenbourg Wissenschaftsverlag, 2013), 94–114.

57. Dr. Eugen Emanuel Galewsky, *Ausstellung: Die Geschechtskrankheiten und ihre Bekämpfung; Führer durch das Gebiet der Geschlechtskrankheiten* (Dresden, National-Hygiene-Museum 1919), 7. The section dealing with syphilis informed about the Wassermann test.

58. For a critical discussion of these figures, see Hans Haustein, "Statistik der Geschlechtskrankheiten," in *Soziale Bedeutung, Statistik und Bekämpfung der Geschlechtskrankheiten*, ed. Hugo Hecht and Hans Haustein (Berlin: Springer, 1927): 980–81.

59. On the exhibitions and the conflicts regarding information on condoms and disinfectants, see Steller, "Volksbildungsinstitut und Museumskonzern," 181–99.

60. Stories of individuals and families wrecked by syphilis were a prominent presence in plays, novels, and films used to warn against the dangers of venereal disease (see Gertiser, *Falsche Scham*). Gonorrhea and infertility were comparatively unspectacular. But see Hans von Hoffensthal, *Lori Graf* (Berlin: Fleischl, 1909), for a novel in which a middle-class man infects his wife with gonorrhea, which renders her infertile.

61. Population discourses have received much scholarly attention. See, for example, Patrick Krassnitzer and Petra Overath, eds., *Bevölkerungsfragen: Prozesse des Wissenstransfers in Deutschand und Frankreich* (Cologne: Böhlau, 2007); and Rainer Mackensen and Jürgen Reulecke, eds., *Das Konstrukt "Bevölkerung" vor, im und nach dem "Dritten Reich"* (Wiesbaden: Sozialwissenschaften, 2005). For an excellent comparison of debates in France and Germany, see Christiane Dienel, *Kinderzahl*

und Staatsräson: Empfängnisverhütung und Bevölkerungspolitik in Deutschland und Frankreich bis 1918 (Münster: Westfälisches Dampfboot, 1995). See also Cornelie Usborne, *The Politics of the Body in Weimar Germany: Women's Reproductive Rights and Duties* (Basingstoke: Macmillan, 1992). Timm, *Politics of Fertility*, offers a rather teleological narrative on German debates on demography and venereal disease.

62. Edward Ross Dickinson, *Sex, Freedom, and Power in Imperial Germany, 1880–1914* (Cambridge: Cambridge University Press, 2014).

63. Julius Wolf, *Der Geburtenrückgang: Die Rationalisierung des Sexuallebens in unserer Zeit* (Jena: Fischer, 1912); Jean Borntraeger, *Der Geburtenrückgang in Deutschland, seine Bewertung und Bekämpfung* (Berlin: Schoetz, 1912).

64. Geheimes Staatsarchiv Preußischer Kulturbesitz (GstA), I. HA Rep. 76 Kultusministerium VIII B Nr. 2006. The reports fill three voluminous files. While they contain interesting details such as locally distributed advertisements by chemists selling contraceptives or letters from individual doctors, many answers were clearly influenced by the original 1912 report, which had accompanied the questionnaire. Paul Weindling provides a statistical overview of the responses. See *Health, Race and German Politics between National Unification and Nazism, 1870–1945* (Cambridge: Cambridge University Press, 1989). Some of the advertisements and photographs that accompanied the reports are reprinted in Anna Bergmann, *Die verhütete Sexualität: Die medizinische Bemächtigung des Lebens* (Hamburg: Rasch und Röhring, 1992), 174, 177, 180, 181.

65. Ministerium des Innern, *Denkschrift über die Ursachen des Geburtenrückganges und die dagegen vorgeschlagenen Maßnahmen* (Berlin, 1915). A copy can be found in GStA Berlin, I. HA Rep. 76 Kultusministerium VIII B Nr. 2022.

66. Alfred Blaschko, "Geburtenrückgang und Geschlechtskrankheiten," *Zeitschrift für Bekämpfung der Geschlechtskrankheiten* 14, no. 11 (1913): 393–455. For another attempt to estimate the importance of gonorrhea as a cause of infertility, see Sigismund Peller, "Die soziale Bedeutung der Gonorrhöe," *Das österreichische Sanitätswesen* 38 (1913): 84–97. Trying to summarize the available studies, Peller concluded that gonorrhea was believed to be responsible for between one-seventh and five-sixths of all sterile marriages (96). He was appalled by these discrepancies and called for more comprehensive research. According to his estimate, about one-third of all cases of involuntary childlessness were due to gonorrhea. See also Richard Schaeffer, "Statistische Beiträge zum Geburtenrückgang in Deutschland," *Zeitschrift für Geburtshilfe und Gynäkologie* 74 (1913): 636–77. Schaeffer concentrated on the question of abortions and argued that these had not increased. He also denied that a rise in venereal disease could explain the drop in the birthrate.

67. Cornelie Usborne, "Social Body, Racial Body, Woman's Body: Discourses, Policies, Practices from Wilhelmine to Nazi Germany, 1912–1945," *Historical Social Research* 36, no. 2 (2011): 140–61; Weindling, *Health, Race and German Politics*; Robert Jütte et al, *Medizin und Nationalsozialismus: Bilanz und Perspektiven der Forschung* (Göttingen: Wallstein, 2011).

68. On health education in Weimar and Nazi Germany, see Sebastian Weinert, *Der Körper im Blick: Gesundheitsausstellungen vom späten Kaiserreich bis zum Nationalsozialismus* (Berlin: De Gruyter, 2017).

69. Edward Ross Dickinson, "Biopolitics, Fascism, Democracy: Some Reflections on Our Discourse about 'Modernity,'" *Central European History* 37, no. 1 (2004): 1–48.

70. Peter E. Fässler, "Eine symbiotische Beziehung? Zur Kooperation zwischen Deutschem Hygiene-Museum und NS-Regime," in *Gesundheit und Staat: Studien zur Geschichte der Gesundheitsämter in Deutschland, 1870–1950*, ed. Axel C. Hüntelmann, Johannes Vossen, and Herwig Czech (Husum: Matthiesen, 2006), 63–77.

71. The "archenemy of fertility" was used by a number of authors. See, for example, E. Finger, *Die Pathologie und Therapie der Sterilität beim Manne* (Leipzig: George, 1898), 3; Benzler, "Sterilität und Tripper," 47; and Ferdinand Schenk, *Die Pathologie und Therapie der Unfruchtbarkeit des Weibes* (Berlin: Karger, 1903), 59.

72. Gynecological handbooks stressed that in the past the inflammation of ovaries and tubes had all too easily been blamed on gonorrhea. They pointed to abortions, appendicitis, tuberculosis, and medical interventions as formerly neglected causes. See, for example, Fritz Engelmann, *Sterilität und Sterilisierung* (Munich: Bergmann, 1927), 45–46.

Chapter Eleven

Fecundity in a World of Scourges

Venereal Diseases, Criminal Abortion, and Acquired Infertility in France, circa 1880–1950

Fabrice Cahen and Adrien Minard

In developing their critical narrative of state control, biopower, and sexual repression, historians of venereal disease in France have been particularly attentive to the cultural meanings and symbolic issues surrounding these pathologies, from social representations of moral disorder to fears of "degeneration."[1] They have examined prostitution-regulation policies in detail and demonstrated their hypocrisy, pitfalls, and shortcomings.[2] But historians have been more reluctant to address what may seem a meaningless, archaically positivist question: the demographic extent of these multi-consequential venereal epidemics and the necessarily complex impact of public policy in this area. From a history of populations perspective, the consistency of this demographic and epidemiological phenomenon constitutes a major issue, especially if the prevalences of syphilis and gonorrhea were as high as some current historians suspect.

There are various, conflicting views on the extent and impact of venereal disease in the French past. In *A History of French Passions*, Theodore Zeldin asserted that in 1925 four million inhabitants—one-tenth of the French population—were infected with syphilis.[3] The demographer-historian Jean-Noël Biraben, drawing on a corpus of written and indirect sources, situated the peak in venereal disease in the late nineteenth century, after military service became compulsory, confirming nineteenth-century views that army service, prostitution, and sexually transmitted infections (STIs) were closely associated. He argued that syphilis was well and truly the cause of many miscarriages and stillbirths. According to Biraben, what produced a decrease in STIs over the twentieth century was the surveillance of prostitution and associated health policies, though gonorrhea did considerably reduce French fecundity until the postwar baby boom.[4] While many studies suggest that the prevalence of STIs remained high at least until the 1940s—that is, before sulfonamides and penicillin became part of the therapeutic armory—some researchers remain skeptical about quantitative claims of this incidence.[5] In fact, the problem is primarily one of methodology. What seems problematic in Zeldin's work, for instance, is not the magnitude of his figures per se, but the fact that he uncritically copied and pasted statistical byproducts of the state office in charge of antivenereal propaganda in the 1920s, the Service de prophylaxie des maladies vénériennes.[6] Our intent in this chapter is precisely to analyze the emergence of the statistical problematization of venereal disease (VD) in France and what it consisted in at a time when French natality had fallen to its lowest level ever.[7]

The poster reproduced here (fig. 11.1), which labels gonorrhea a "social scourge," helps us formulate our research questions. It depicts a barren woman (is she injured? sick? convalescent?) and recycles the classic metonymy of the "empty cradle." What knowledge tools and cognitive frame were used in studying the epidemiological dimension of STIs in France? Why were these diseases so seldom related to the issue of reproductive health? As Virginie De Luca Barrusse and Christian Benoît have shown, we have a massive quantity of medical writings and population statistics at our disposal.[8] Here we draw on a fraction of the available quantitative sources (published or archival), taking as our guide the Académie nationale de médecine (Academy of Medicine; the main French scholarly institution that actively discussed the relationship between population sciences and medicine in this period), and documents issued by the public health administration.[9] In contradistinction to the usual discourses on venereal disease prevalence in France, traditionally focused solely on the sphere of prostitution, we give priority to the content of contemporaneous demographic, medical, and epidemiological sources focused on the population at large.[10] This shift involves paying particular attention to gonorrhea, which was relatively neglected by physicians and health authorities. It

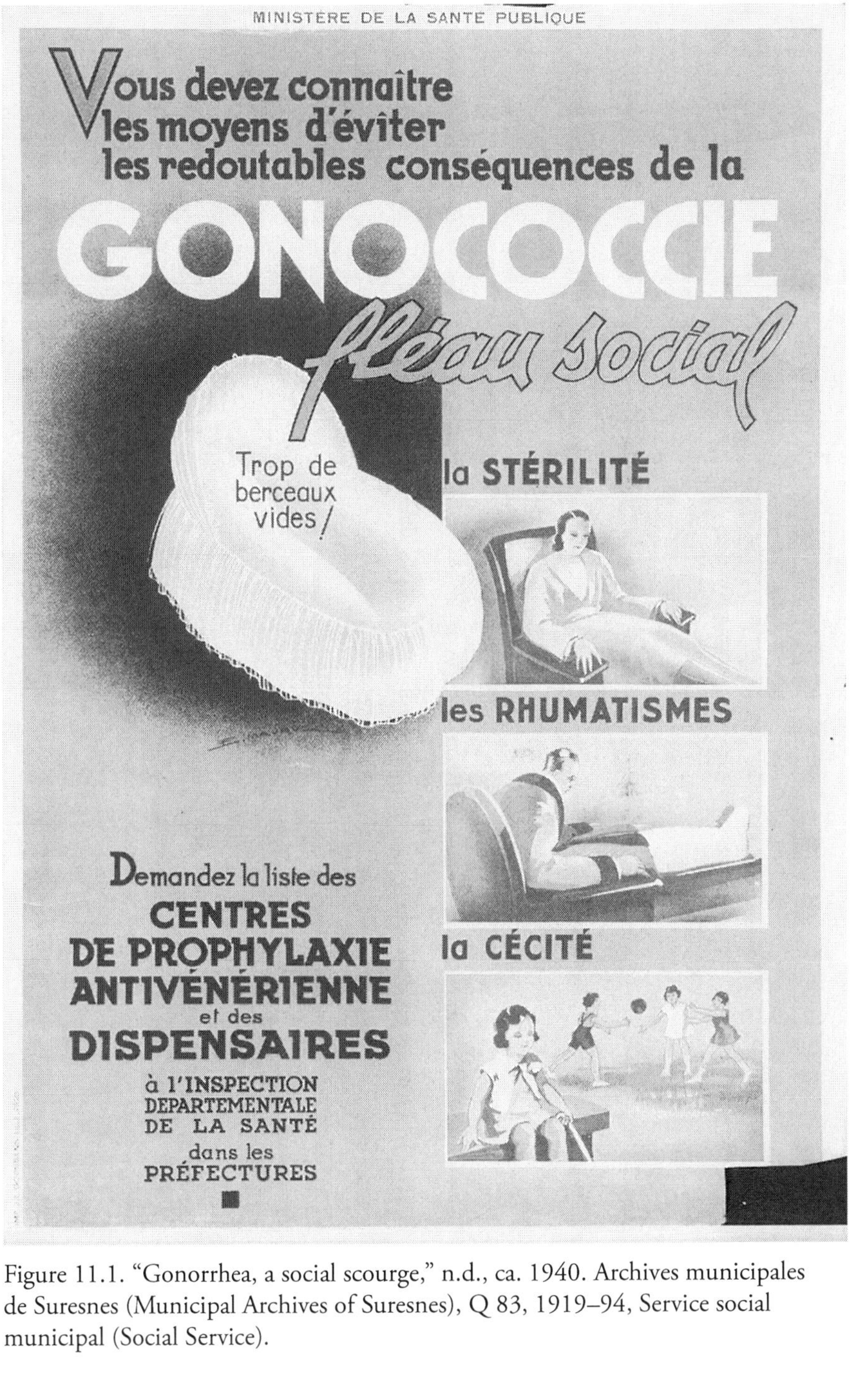

Figure 11.1. "Gonorrhea, a social scourge," n.d., ca. 1940. Archives municipales de Suresnes (Municipal Archives of Suresnes), Q 83, 1919–94, Service social municipal (Social Service).

also requires expanding our object of study by placing issues of sexual and reproductive health at the core of a cross-sectional analysis of these "social scourges."

In the first section we describe the institutional framework for knowledge about venereal diseases and infertility in the late nineteenth century. The aim is to understand the intellectual, political, medical, and statistical factors that led to what was quite a narrow representation of sexually transmitted diseases, one dominated by the haunting specter of syphilis. The second section analyzes the consequences of the Great War, which required the French authorities to manage a venereal disease crisis, from which it then developed an epidemiological monitoring system based on the circulation of medical data. We show how during the subsequent interwar decades wider medicalized concerns about the threat to the nation of failing rates of reproduction and of reproduction disorders put postvenereal sequelae in competition with other causal explanations of infertility, which were deemed to be of greater significance, notably that of criminal and incompetent abortions. The third and last part concentrates on the critical moment of World War II, bringing to light the stigmatization of certain social groups caused by the design of the administrative information system constructed to address venereal diseases, its blind spots, and the crucial issues that it in fact obscured, which primarily related to the real extent of the French population's exposure to STIs during the wartime period.

Medical Infertility in the Shadow

Dr. Alfred Fournier's Moment

Haunted primarily by syphilis, the "disease of Naples," the French were disinclined to attach equivalent importance to gonorrhea, despite claims for its effects on disease-induced sterility as a factor of birthrate decline. Neither public discourse nor public health policy proved receptive to an argument about the impact of venereal diseases on reproductive health. The intervention in the 1880s of Dr. Alfred Fournier, the country's most renowned VD specialist, in this medicodemographic debate can be used to examine the landscape of the practices and knowledge of the time. Of the various areas of French medical practice that dealt with sexual diseases in the nineteenth century—gynecology, urology, dermatology, puericulture, military medicine, and venereology—the last was mainly in the hands of "syphilologists" (*syphiligraphes*), especially after Fournier created the first university chair of dermatology and syphilis in 1879 at the Hôpital Saint-Louis in Paris.[11] "Syphilology" was a recognized specialty that generally meant (except for those who provided care for venereal disease in ordinary hospitals or private practice) rubbing shoulders with the underworld of prostitution, either as a prefecture physician (i.e., assigned to registered prostitutes) or as a doctor in a specialized institution such as the Dispensaire de salubrité, established under the authority of the Préfecture de police de Paris (Paris Prefecture of Police) in 1802, or the hospital-prison of Saint-Lazare, where sick prostitutes were treated from 1836 until the late 1920s.[12] The social problematization of sexual diseases and the medical scrutiny of prostitution were structurally intertwined.[13] The principal elements in this context—where sex workers, soldiers, and young men in military service were almost the only figures discussed—had already appeared in the influential research of Dr. Alexandre Parent-Duchâtelet in the 1830s.[14]

Between 1880 and 1890 the prestigious Academy of Medicine was the locus of important discussions. Alfred Fournier was offered several opportunities to present his ongoing quantitative research on the venereal plague. He revealed a mass of clinically detailed findings from his personal observation of hundreds of patients, selected from among his *own* middle- and upper-class private clientele.[15] This information gave insight into elements of the civil population, whereas usually quantitative studies of STIs were based on sources from the army and surveillance of sex workers, all dating back to a period when there was no compulsory notification of venereal infections and, above all, no serologic screening. The ritual accusation that "clandestine" (i.e., unregistered) prostitutes "sowed syphilis" rested on interpretations of military surveys focused on the role of garrison towns as sources of the disease, combined with the personal experiences of those specific doctors involved in overseeing prostitutes, most of whom were Parisians.[16] Profiling individual dramas, particularly striking case histories of women incapable of keeping their fetuses, Fournier intended above all to establish a link between VD (considered at the scale of the population at large using a numeric approach based on proportions and percentages) and the critical public issue of demographic slowdown.[17] In 1885 he claimed that at least 68 percent of several hundreds of pregnancies in syphilitic families (defined as one or both parents having syphilis) resulted in the death of the child. Through miscarriage and infant mortality, syphilis was definitely a substantial factor of "depopulation."[18] Subsequently, in 1901, Fournier estimated the frequency of syphilis among the male Parisian population at 13–16 percent.[19] Nevertheless "the pox" did not cause an inability to *conceive*: "If syphilis were a cause of sterility," Fournier lamented, "we would not have to deplore so many hereditary disasters."[20] This brings us to the demographers' perspective.

The relevance of medical physiology-based explanations of "depopulation" had been heavily debated throughout the nineteenth century. However, the category of biological infertility (*infertilité*) did not appear in the demographic literature, where the principal concern was instead childlessness (then called *stérilité*), regardless of its determinants, and referring in fact to the observed state of zero children present in the household when censuses were taken (until Lucien March's census of 1906 asked household heads how many children had ever been born).[21] When, in 1890, Arsène Dumont—whose thinking was a source of inspiration for Adolphe Landry's influential subsequent theory of "demographic revolution"—explicitly distinguished between "voluntary" and "involuntary" childlessness, he did so to eliminate the involuntary processes from his spectrum of analysis.[22] He and the other mainstream demographers agreed to consider *dénatalité* (birth decline) as a sociological and demographic matter instead of a biological one. In his belief that the continuous development of "civilization" was in conflict with instincts, Dumont had been influenced by Herbert Spencer's theory of a rivalry between the instincts of individuation and procreation; nevertheless, he rejected the idea that the problem could result from a decline in reproductive capacity, at least in terms of a possible weakening of spermatogenesis or ovulation.[23] Human will (*volonté*) was a brain mechanism that effectively contradicted the strength of instincts but that involved neither a pathological deficiency of any sort—physiological, anatomic, or anatomico-pathological—nor physiological degeneracy observable at the scale of the "race." Discomfort in dealing with intimate matters together with a dearth of statistics on birth control practices were some of the factors that led demographers toward alternative theories of "psychocultural" determinants of fertility change.[24] But these were not the only reasons; a combination of patriotic moralism, pronatalist utilitarianism, and an "accounting" style of reasoning was also important. The pronatalist leader Jacques Bertillon—the founder in 1896 of the powerful Alliance nationale pour l'accroissement de la population française (National Alliance for the Growth of the French Population)—argued that to limit the negative effects of French individualist "egoism" on the birthrate, the best solution was to devise efficient incentive policies.[25] Consequently, attending to statistically marginal phenomena, such as mere biological causes of sterility among a small minority of the population, was irrelevant, especially from a remedial national policy perspective.

Measuring Childlessness

The physician and anthropologist Gustave Lagneau was one of the members of the Academy of Medicine appointed to discuss Fournier's argument. In a report presented in 1890, Lagneau agreed that syphilis was a threat to the French race but refused to consider involuntary infertility as a major cause of the falling birthrate.[26] To substantiate this position he cited a comparative study on France and the other European countries conducted by Bertillon.[27] Based on the 1886 census, the first-ever French survey asking "heads of families" the number of their offspring in their households, this study apprehended the distribution of families by parity, to assess the weight of childlessness and above all to distinguish voluntary limits on family size from medical sterility.[28] Bertillon selected households of couples who had been married fifteen to twenty years to ensure that their reproductive life was over. As Adolphe Pinard and Charles Richet would do in 1903 with a comparable outcome, Bertillon adopted the postulate that nullparity (a marriage with "zero" children) was a convenient proxy for unwanted (involuntary) childlessness.[29] Bertillon found that 12.5 percent of households belonged to this category. Neither he, nor Richet and Pinard, could estimate the fraction of miscarriages, and they both ignored the problem of *secondary infertility* after a first living birth; in their minds a couple who had brought a first child into the world was necessarily able to conceive a second one—and was therefore guilty of voluntarily having not done so. Since their comparative studies showed that absolute childlessness in France, at a level of about 12.5 percent, was not much different from elsewhere, they both concluded that the real problem behind France's unusually low birthrate was the prevalence of voluntary restriction; on this point they were in line with Alliance nationale discourse that the only serious problem that had to be tackled was the excessive number of voluntarily *small* families. The dogma was in place.

In a subsequent 1917 survey Richet put forward an arbitrary appraisal of *postvenereal* childlessness, which, he estimated, afflicted half of their new figure of 10 percent of childless households, that is to say, 5 percent of French married couples. At that date, then, Richet did recognize the issue of infecundity due to disease, speculating that it was likely due to spouses practicing coitus interruptus, which he supposed would lead to sexual frustration and then to infidelity, resulting in STIs. Nevertheless, he supported and reinforced Bertillon's point of view, arguing that the chief priority was to combat *voluntary* limitation of births.[30] What is more, methodological differences in other sources at this time produced even lower estimates of childlessness. A 1912 report on "marriage productivity" used data from the

1906 census, in which the new head of the Statistique générale de la France (French Bureau of Statistics) office, Lucien March, had revised the definition of "childless households." Instead of being asked how many children currently resided in their household at the census date, heads of families (mainly men, including the divorced and widowed, but widowed women were also included) were now asked how many children they *had ever had* (i.e., including stillborn and children who had died), making it possible to estimate more reliably the proportion of couples who had *never* had a child. The resulting tables on "infertile married men" selected those who had been married at least twenty-five years. Employing this methodology, only 6.4 percent of them were considered sterile. Thirty years later the 1906 census was used again, but differently, by Landry.[31] He chose to concentrate on the data for coal miners, the occupational group that supposedly made the least use of birth control of any kind.[32] Their childlessness rate was found to be only 2.8 percent, a figure Landry used to suggest that "true" unwanted infertility (childlessness) accounted for no more than 4 percent of French households, so that even the 6.4 percent found by March's methodology was still excessive.[33]

No Room for Gonorrhea

In addition to their refusal to take into account factors that did not fit with the standard demographic model or were in their view statistically too small to deserve attention, belle epoque scholars worked to obscure the issue of infertility in another way—their obsession with syphilis. Although Fournier and his successors were aware of the problem of pregnancy disorders, they were primarily worried about "hereditary syphilis" and its so-called dysgenic consequences. Doctors somewhat complacently believed that improved preventive treatments for pregnant women would reduce the prevalence of such disorders.[34] The focus on syphilis as a cause of "defects," a disease that filled hospitals and asylums with "human waste," and the belief that the father could infect the fetus even if the mother was healthy, moved physicians to ignore gonorrhea. Because of its transmission pattern, "the clap" (*chaude pisse* [burning piss]) had been categorized as a venereal disease and was assigned mostly to dermatologist-syphilologists, despite the absence of cutaneous symptoms. Only a few physicians were specialized in it, and, significantly, this subspecialty had no name. Moreover, the primarily dermatologically focused specialists in France had resisted Emil Noeggerath's hypotheses on gonorrhea and procreation because of their main interest in the treatment of skin lesions and their mistrust of laboratory medicine, in which their specialty lacked any training.[35]

It was only in the late 1890s that two surgeons at Saint-Lazare, Drs. Fernand Verchère and Louis Jullien, proclaimed the accuracy of Noeggerath's "revolutionary" theses, fully demonstrated by microscopic observation and surgical interventions.[36] Validating the link between undetected gonorrhea, pelviperitonitis, salpingitis, and infertility, they made the case that this disease should be taken as seriously as syphilis.[37] Jullien and Verchère were among the founding members of the first French antivenereal league, the Société de prophylaxie sanitaire et morale, created by Alfred Fournier in 1901.[38] Yet this organization was always focused primarily on syphilis, and the internal dissymmetry in the importance accorded to the two diseases was never really contested. During the interwar period syphilis terrified people, but childlessness was played down; meanwhile *chaude-pisse* (gonorrhea's colloquial name) was a nonissue for many stakeholders.

The Venereal Risk Reconsidered?

The Great War and Epidemiological Information

When Dr. Fournier died in December 1914, the Société de prophylaxie had not reached its goal, inasmuch as neither civilian nor military authorities had devised the necessary measures to oversee the sexual health of the population. A very small number of syphilologists had improvised basic facilities to care for blatantly infected soldiers. In November 1915 a new debate revolving around VD and prostitution was held at the Academy of Medicine.[39] It exposed the division between those preaching sexual abstinence and more pragmatic observers who were of the opinion that the poilus could not be blamed for occasional moments of weakness. The academy timidly chose to recommend "individual prophylactic measures," an imprecise formula that probably referred to calomel ointment rather than condoms.

Some weeks later three heads of the Hôpital Saint-Louis, the syphilologists Louis Brocq, Georges Thibierge, and Ernest Gaucher, presented fresh figures in an attempt to shock public opinion and the government.[40] Gaucher claimed he had diagnosed eight hundred cases of syphilis in five thousand patients between August 1914 and December 1915: 15 percent of his consultations, as against 10 percent on the eve of the conflict.[41] In January 1916 Justin Godart, the head of the Service de santé des armées (Military Health Service), initiated a new large-scale policy calling for the creation of "dermatological-venereal centres," systematic hospitalization of contagious soldiers, and the deployment of prophylaxis propaganda. He also created specialized, free, and blameless outpatient clinics (*dispensaires* or *services annexes*) in large towns, hoping to promote screening campaigns within the civilian population.[42] In rural areas doctors in private practice were requested to collaborate through their private consulting activity.[43] Eventually, later in the war there ensued a system modeled on that of the US allies: several hundred prophylactic stations were opened across the country to provide soldiers with chemical prophylaxis after sexual intercourse.[44]

These new health provisions changed the economy of epidemiological information. Although it is extremely difficult to determine whether military clinic consultations give an accurate idea of the volume and trend of detected STIs, notably because the Wassermann test was seldom done (it had been introduced into clinical practice in 1910, though laboratory analyses remained exceptional due to the dearth of bacteriological facilities), several outcomes can hardly be doubted.[45] First, contagion occurred primarily behind the front lines and was therefore correlated to heavy use of clandestine and casual prostitution, either during periods of leave or when the troops traversed rural zones.[46] Second, though no one emphasized this, the proportion of known cases of gonorrhea—70 percent of the total amount of VD cases (gonorrhea plus syphilis)—was spectacular. We cannot with any certainty relate the 145,000 cases of gonorrhea detected between 1916 and 1919 to a reference population, as the disease was underdetected, but we can reasonably assume, given that underdetection, that a number of those who survived the war returned home with the infection and its effects. And to that unknown proportion we can add several fragmentary data on noncombatant populations, such as figures from the hospital annex of Issy-les-Moulineaux, which treated munitions factory workers from the Paris region.[47]

Eye-catching but unsubstantiated extrapolations were still being put forward in the 1920s. It was claimed that four million people in France were syphilitic (one-tenth of the population) and that this led to forty thousand miscarriages and twenty thousand stillbirths every year.[48] Furthermore, the practice of collecting statistics on sexual diseases, first undertaken during the war, was continued. A Service de prophylaxie des maladies vénériennes of the new ministère de l'Hygiène (Ministry of Hygiene; 1920) and a Rockefeller-funded Office national d'Hygiène sociale (National Office of Social Hygiene; 1924)—located in the same office—were established to gather health documentation and organize public campaigns on more rational grounds.[49]

Trends of the Venereal Evil

André Cavaillon, who headed the Service de prophylaxie and vice-chaired the Office national d'hygiène sociale; Marcel Moine, who ran the office's statistics commission; and Lucien Viborel and George Risler, who headed its propaganda commission, were four leaders in the field of social hygiene in the first half of the twentieth century. In addition to producing and distributing leaflets, posters, and propaganda films, they undertook to obtain better statistics by centralizing the local records of public VD facilities. A series of circular letters encouraged physicians to send regular and accurate information. Each venereal clinic or dispensary was called on to appoint a nurse to fill out the forms on individual patients containing an anonymous section with confidential medical details. The forms were then compiled in a nationwide register (see fig. 11.2).

There can be no doubt that these monitoring practices served direct political aims, especially those of justifying greater antivenereal disease subsidies and supporting the campaign of the time to institute a premarital certificate of health. Were they nevertheless more effective than prewar health policies, centered on prostitution, to capture empirically over time and space the

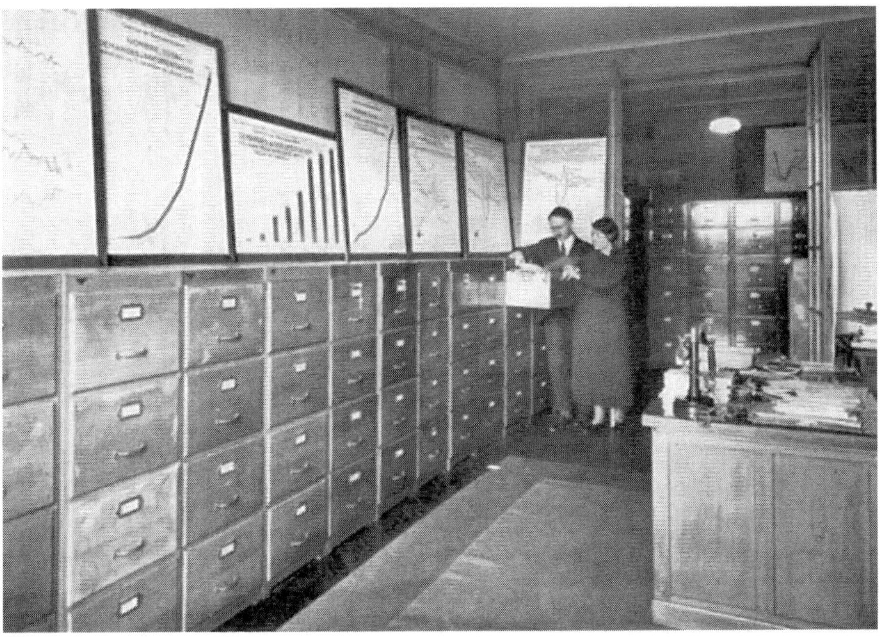

Figure 11.2. The statistics service of the Office national d'hygiène sociale. *L'Illustration*, May 19, 1934.

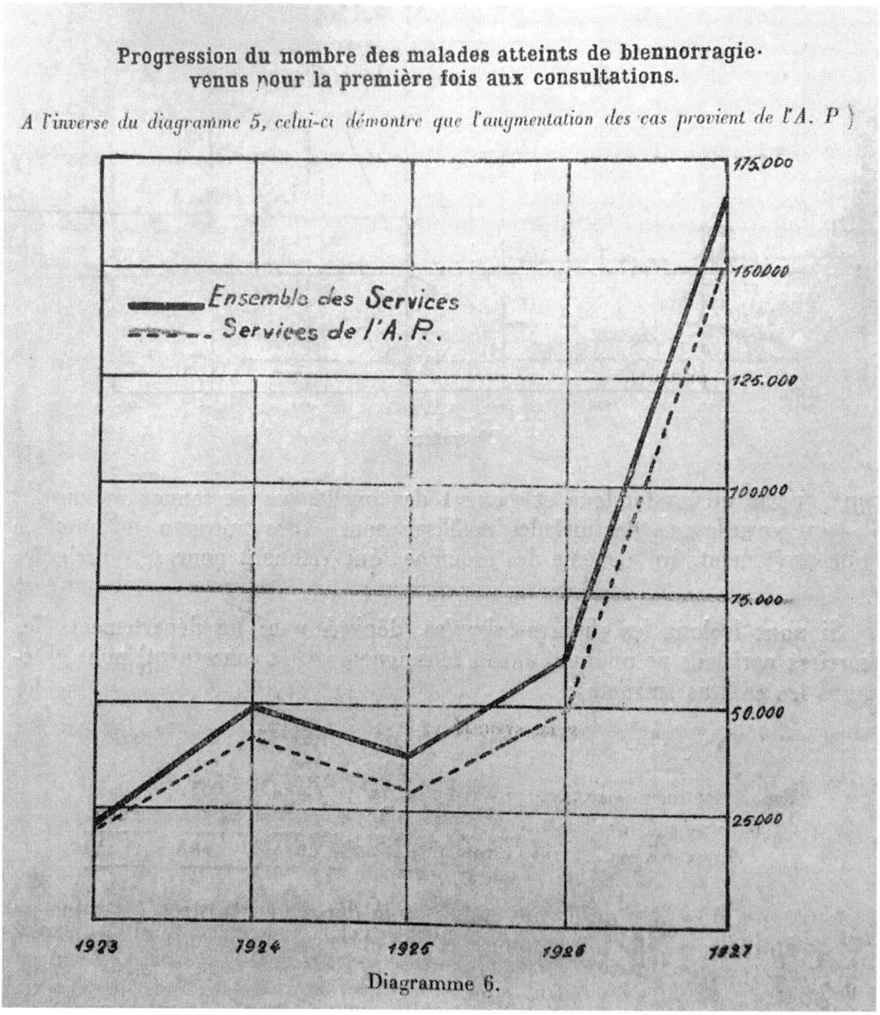

Figure 11.3 "Progression in the Number of Individual Initial Consultations for Gonorrhea," an erroneous curve. Cavaillon and Moine, *Étude statistique*, 22.

sexual and reproductive health of the French population? In 1928 Cavaillon and Moine, drawing on the statistical material collected on a quarterly basis by the Service de prophylaxie des maladies vénériennes, published the first comprehensive, periodic account of VD cases diagnosed in the antivenereal services since 1920.[50] Unavoidably, the system missed the segment of patients who preferred to consult private doctors, ordinary hospitals, or for-profit clinics instead of free dispensaries. According to the autobiography of a private, self-proclaimed "sex doctor," Georges Lévi-Valensin, such patients were not always confined to the well-off: several clinics in Paris had some relatively poor men among their clients who managed to pay for the expensive care, hoping their urethral stenosis would be treated with maximum discretion.[51] Generally, aggregated published statistics also ignored the sex variable, though gender information was collected on the individual forms.

In practice these statistical series fed sensationalists, who began decrying a syphilitic "outbreak" as soon as there seemed to be any slight rise anywhere rather than fueling a cautious epidemiological approach to monitoring VD.[52] What is more, they provided new opportunities to denounce the absence of compulsory hospitalization and to point fingers at clandestine prostitutes, immigrants, and workers from the French colonies—the last group being the target of an increasing number of accusations. Cavaillon and Moine occasionally used their more "comprehensive" statistics to play down these false arguments, perhaps because it was in their own interest to garner new subsidies by suggesting a correlation between the efficiency of the dispensary system and downward trends in the disease (even the decrease in infant mortality was used to make their case).[53] There is therefore no reason to suppose that the spectacular mistake they made in the line chart reproduced in figure 11.3 summarizing new detected gonorrhea—that is, a rising curve, which appears to be totally unjustifiable given the data in the table—was deliberate (and, so far as we can establish, this obvious mistake was neither pointed out at the time nor has it drawn comment subsequently).

While longitudinal observation was particularly problematic, the detailed information presented in the annual tables, especially for the well-documented year of 1928, deserves closer examination. Given that people were more likely to seek treatment for syphilis than gonorrhea, those figures may confirm that the ratio of syphilis to gonorrhea was about one to three, which is similar to the ratio found in other studies.[54] Supplementing these figures with a study on male wage earners with social insurance who consulted at public hospitals and clinics (especially civil servants and clerks), we find once again that stage 1 and 2 syphilis was relatively infrequent (0.35 percent of male patients were treated for it), while gonorrhea ranked third (3.7 percent), just behind tuberculosis (7.1 percent) and "asthenia."[55]

Competing Diseases, Limited Budgets

The previous figures and the poster at the head of this chapter must not let us think the importance of gonorrhea was eventually acknowledged by everybody. To gain the status of "scourge" in the Third Republic, a phenomenon had to be accorded the important status of a "major factor of depopulation." It therefore had at least to be quantitatively reckonable: its promoters had to be able to prove that by sowing death, spreading "defects," or preventing births, it affected the *whole population* and not just specific subgroups or groups on the margins of society. This was the precondition for treating or trying to treat a "problem" by means of cost-effective public action, in particular the expected outcome of the public effort needed to be quantified in *saved lives*. Another property facilitated the legitimization of a cause: the fact that it was potentially imputable to "guilty" parties, bad behaviors, or scapegoats.[56] In Fournier's wake syphilis had been personified not only as a new plague that damaged French offspring but also as a "great abortionist" that was undermining the future of the race: as a cause, it was no longer open to debate. In the 1930s syphilis was said to destroy 140,000 lives per year (80,000 "deaths," plus 20,000 "killed children"—meaning stillbirths—plus 40,000 abortions), while Cavaillon and Moine attributed at least 10,000 "saved lives" to the antisyphilis effort.[57]

By contrast, gonorrhea did not fit the grammar of social scourges as clearly. Although commonly known to be widespread and insidious, it continued to be considered benign, even by many skilled physicians.[58] What is more, doctors who were committed to combating gonorrhea and who called for a stronger effort to get prostitutes into medical facilities and to include systematic screening for gonorrhea made little use of the fecundity argument, and so it was not included as a prerequisite for the granting of the Vichy prenuptial certificate, which was instituted in 1942 (the section on venereal disease was limited to syphilis). This is not surprising, given the low degree of mobilization around the matter of involuntary childlessness. So when Dr. Léon Bizard and health-center heads such as Dr. André Demonchy succeeded in organizing the first Conférence de défense sociale contre la blennorragie (Social Preservation Conference against Gonorrhea) (supported by the Office national d'hygiène sociale and the ministère de la Santé publique (Ministry of Public Health) in 1933, it came as a surprise that gonorrhea was finally officially admitted into the small, privileged circle of social evils.[59] In one of the conference sessions, an official from the Ministry of Public Health straightforwardly asked participants if they were "sure that one can consider gonorrhea a social scourge?"[60] There were many good reasons for considering other priorities as more pressing in such a difficult financial context. The fact that gonorrhea threatened fecundity appeared only in a small handful of publications and a few isolated, and apparently not widely attended, public talks. Professor Pinard, a leading obstetrician and herald of "puericulture," who had cowritten a report on infertility two decades before, was one of these few. He published a leaflet in 1925 reminding young people of their duty to procreate and warning them about VD. Pinard expressed strong disapproval of anyone who found any humor in a disease that condemned those who had it to the "humiliation" and personal "decline" (*déchéance*) of infertility.[61]

Pinard's sermon fell into the category of propaganda. But, after 1925, more practitioners came to feel that the impact of syphilis might have been overestimated compared to gonorrhea.[62] It can be argued that a better understanding of the incidence of gonorrhea at that time resulted from developments in the medicine and physiology of reproduction. Over the interwar decades infertility consultations improved the quality of internal examination and turned medical attention toward "ordinary" women and couples as well.[63] Sperm was as yet rarely screened: reproductive medicine was practiced in France mostly by gynecologists-obstetricians, notably in women's outpatient clinics, and the husbands were usually absent and strongly reluctant to be examined, meaning that gonorrhea's impact on semen had not really been elucidated.[64] But the development of tubal insufflation and hysterosalpingography shed new light on female post-contagion disorders.[65] For gynecologists such as Claude Béclère, in practice in Couvelaire's infertility consultancy at the Hôpital Baudelocque), "the main factor" of infecundity, which explained 75 percent of cases of women unable to become pregnant, had thereby been unmasked.[66] Béclère was even convinced that a number of cases of *post-abortum* salpingitis were of gonococcal etiology, whereas *post-abortum* tubal infection was routinely attributed solely to streptococci.

But for many gynecologist-obstetricians, the main factor was not venereal; a more convincing explanation was the aftereffects of abortion. Overall, there was much greater consensus that "criminal abortion" was to be blamed for infertility—partly because it involved women's behavior more than men's. Once contraceptive devices were prohibited by law in 1920 (except condoms, which were tolerated specifically to prevent venereal transmission and therefore became even more closely associated with commercial, nonmarital sex), abortion became the pet peeve of the Alliance nationale, which had never ceased to emphasize *voluntary* infertility. Activists claimed that four hundred thousand abortions—and perhaps as many as one million—were performed every year. In the late 1920s their propaganda repertoire was reinforced by shrewd arguments on the damage caused by abortion to genital and reproductive health. As maternal deaths were decreasing and could less convincingly be used as a scare tactic, pronatalists and antiabortion crusaders cited the proceedings of a gynecologists' convention held in Kiev in 1927, after the legalization of abortion in the Soviet Union; they selected and tactically exploited the participants' most negative accounts. Then in 1935 the French Academy of Medicine produced its own highly pessimistic report on abortion and the damages it caused to the female reproductive system.[67] But conservative pronatalists were not the only ones to present the "crime" of abortion as a major cause of maternal mortality and a factor of tubal infertility: birth control activists also had reasons to emphasize abortion aftereffects.[68] Speaking from the standpoint of gynecology, they insisted that *post-abortum* disorders could be induced by unskilled uterine curettages. Sexual education and birth control—and, some members of the movement thought, legal, safe abortion—would be the best answers to the problem.

The Dead End of Health Policy

An Increase in Sexual Risk?

The period from the eve of World War II to its aftermath (roughly 1938 to 1947) was another decisive one for the long-term history of intimacy. After the French defeat of 1940 and the establishment of the dictatorial, reactionary Révolution nationale, a combination of factors—the fact that many men were in captivity (including under compulsory labor in Germany), the German occupation, and the high number of troop movements—dramatically aggravated the tension surrounding sexual life in a context of extreme moral order and social control, characterized in particular by the intensification of antiabortion policies.[69] This critical moment, abundantly documented, is a relevant—albeit somewhat distorting—lens with which to approach the interplay between objective risks, moral panics, and the governing of sexuality in the twentieth century.

It is clear from a wide array of documents that, as early as the *drôle de guerre* (the "phony war" of September 3, 1939 to May 10, 1940), the authorities were haunted by the specter of great social scourges: abortion, alcoholism, and VD. One source is a note on "antialcoholic and antivenereal prophylaxis," issued by the Service de santé des armées on September 13, 1939, which anticipated several later measures for protecting military human resources.[70] The fifth item recommended providing soldiers with means for "individual prophylaxis" "as far as possible." The reason this item deserves particular attention is that there are very few allusions to male contraceptive devices in the French historical sources. Condoms were a topic so seldom openly discussed that, regrettably, we know virtually nothing of their actual use over time. The issue may be of particular importance, as the reputedly high French consumption of commercial sex is undoubtedly a historical truth. On this matter we can cite the extremely valuable *Rapport sur le comportement sexuel des Français* (Report on the sexuality of the French people, 1972), in which Pierre Simon, a doctor and a major figure in France's family-planning movement, provides several findings that corroborate the central place of commercial sex in male sexual life in France.[71] The topic first appears in a chapter on sexual "initiation": 9 percent of male respondents reported they had been initiated by a prostitute (we could probably add a fraction of the 5 percent who did not answer the question), with the highest percentage found for the generation born before World War II. But the most spectacular figure is in the chapter on "extraconjugal sexual intercourse": 33 percent of men admitted resorting to sex workers during their married life (here again, 14 percent of male respondents did not answer the question). The average number of prostitutes visited by this category of respondents was 7.8.[72]

Moreover, most historians agree that the high price, poor quality (though latex was a notable improvement), and shameful connotation of the *capote anglaise* (French letter) still considerably limited its use in the first part of the twentieth century; they conclude that condoms were essentially used only in commercial sex.[73] The relevant question, then, is to what extent the policies or practices of the relevant French institutions were giving any encouragement to men to take personal responsibility to protect their own health (and therefore also that of their sexual partners) by adopting condoms. "Individual prophylaxis kits" were first tested in the army in 1922; between the wars it became common practice to hand out such kits to soldiers, consisting of a piece of soap, sheets of thin paper, and calomel ointment.[74] A particularly explicit document on a health experiment carried out in colonial Cochinchine (Vietnam) clarifies that though condoms may have been readily accessible, they were not necessarily used. When Dr. Gaston Muraz set out in the early 1930s to combat what he deemed as a disastrous epidemic situation in Saigon and Cholon brothels, he ordered that prophylactic kits—including condoms—be available in every place where prostitution was practiced. Yet European soldiers and marines willing to use ointments considered condoms superfluous. As a result, it was the prostitutes themselves who had to submit to extensive prophylaxis measures.[75]

After the fall of the Vichy regime, this issue was resparked when a rise in contagion was seen across the country: the disorders of the Liberation had made antivenereal activists and officials particularly alarmist and—as in their behavior regarding prostitution and abortion—highly sensitive to short-term variations in apparent epidemic prevalence.[76] Between February and April 1945 a conflict pitted the Ministry of Health and Population against the ministère de la Production industrielle (Ministry of Industrial Production). The former deemed it urgent to satisfy "the needs of the [French] army" for condoms: this time the word was uttered. Faced with a shortage of that item it requested the latter to import two tons of them from Great Britain.[77] This interministry bargaining confirms that the military hierarchy, supported by the public health administration, had eventually opted for regulated and safe sex rather than for stubborn, hypocritical encouragements on abstinence. The provisional government could not ignore the fact that the Germans had made condom use compulsory in the French brothels they controlled, to protect Aryans from the "venereal fifth column" and that, after June 1944, US GIs received a kit every month and had unlimited access to prophylactic stations.[78] On the other hand, the document of 1945 reveals that the number of available and technically satisfactory condoms was considered insufficient, leaving French soldiers at risk. The 1972 Simon report observed the extremely low degree of knowledge on STIs and the survival in high schools and barracks of a certain amount of male "folklore" and jocularity about gonorrhea, especially among older respondents, those sexually active around midcentury.[79] Finally, only 4 percent of male respondents reported that they used a condom during their first sexual experience, including with female prostitutes—a figure suggesting that commercial sexual relations were probably often unprotected.[80]

The Obstinate Quest for the "Contaminator"

Despite the promotion of individual prophylaxes in 1939, World War II was primarily a time for stepping up the effort to target "agents of contamination." French republican medical values had been undermined by changes in procedures for monitoring the health of the population pursuant to the decree of November 22, 1939, followed by a circular letter of December 31, 1940, and two years later the law of December 31, 1942 (passed under pressure from the Germans).[81] These measures required infected individuals and recalcitrant syphilitics to report to the authorities; they were called on to divulge the names of any presumed *agents contaminateurs* and to conduct "epidemiological inquiries" with the aid of social workers or police services to trace the "source" of the infection, force that person to get treatment, and prevent them from reintegrating the sex-work market before they had recovered.[82] These procedures were now compulsory, a situation that fueled the stigmatizing tendencies of social hygiene crusaders.

At the core of these institutional arrangements was each administration's duty to collect monthly reports on newly detected cases, not only in dispensaries but also in hospitals, prisons, and private practices.[83] In actual fact, the revised conditions were so authoritarian that the majority of physicians, including some dispensary practitioners, were reluctant to violate medical confidentiality, either on ethical or economic grounds.[84] Even after adding other information sources, such as serologic data from the Instituts Pasteur (Pasteur Institutes), the local and national authorities obtained only an incomplete overview of the epidemiological conditions. According to official reports, the proportion of identified "contagion agents" in the late 1940s and early 1950s consistently remained below 15 percent of notified cases.[85] Health administrators chose to proceed as if the lists and tables could serve as epidemiological indicators, arguing that the structural biases were not enough to make them unusable. But they did not try to correct or improve them. Consequently, they were pushed into focusing more exclusively still on the individuals or groups most frequently denounced, that is, the most vulnerable and stigmatized.

Even after the highly controversial law of 1946 abolished the regulatory system and closed brothels, a law that shifted medical-police surveillance to a role of "sociosanitary" support, sex workers remained prime targets.[86] But the war and immediate postwar context, and the law of 1946, probably blurred statistical differentiations between "official," "clandestine," or "casual" prostitutes and cases of extramarital sexual intercourse. In fact, the proportion of diseased men who mentioned "clandestine prostitution" as the origin of their infection (between 40 percent and 50 percent of registered cases) was approximately the same as those who reported an "open relationship" (*relation libre*).[87]

For the French authorities the temporary presence of GIs in France did not qualify as a major explanation of an upsurge in the disease. A report on the situation in the *département* of Nord attests to health observers' concern about a risk of venereal contamination from those they called "Black Americans."[88] The doctor who headed the department-level health authority mentioned that he had previously acquired data tables from the Public Health Service of Bethesda, Maryland, showing that the black subpopulation had a high infection rate.[89] But it was hoped that the GIs would go back home once their task was done, and public health administrators who claimed they could "observe" on their local tables several epidemic hotspots on the Americans' route through the region wagered that their venereal imprint would diminish quickly after they left.

By contrast, public health agencies found an ideal culprit in "North-Africans." Archival documents from the *département* of Nord help us to understand how they constructed and differentiated this group, supposedly overinfected by STIs. Despite the 1946 law, several "indigenous" military brothels, reserved exclusively for North African soldiers, where they could find prostitutes from the colonies, seem to have been set up in metropolitan areas in 1947.[90] Actually, it was useless to try to create de jure segregated houses of prostitution: down-market brothels (vividly referred to as *maisons d'abattage*, where prostitutes worked as on an assembly line) survived the 1946 ban, particularly in the district known as La Goutte d'Or in Paris, the city's poorest neighborhood, and the low prices there meant that only unskilled migrant workers used them. They were tolerated in accordance with the idea that the "indigenous" libido had to be channeled.[91] The figure of the filthy, instinct-driven, more or less deviant Maghrebin, a delinquent or procurer and, above all, the contaminator of French prostitutes or respectable women, was in place long before the Algerian Independence War. As early as the nineteenth century, "indigenous" men from Algeria had been designated syphilis carriers due to ethnic-cultural habits related to sexual hygiene or prostitution practices.[92] Historical research has shown that the apparently strong prevalence of "Arab syphilis" described by colonial physicians was often in fact, in rural areas at least, a *nonvenereal* dermatosis mistakenly identified as syphilis.[93] This belief was apparently corroborated by the great proportion of syphilitic Muslims consulting at urban free clinics.[94] On metropolitan soil the first wave of panic arose during the Great War and led Justin Godart to institute a compulsory medical examination.[95] But in the interwar period physicians and hygienists, wrestling with antidiscrimination resistance, never stopped calling for stricter control at boarding and arrival, if not for the expulsion of contagious migrants.[96]

Even the two most specialized studies of the 1940s—one of which was conducted by the great historian-demographer Louis Chevalier in 1947—remained prisoners to these ethnic-cultural stereotypes.[97] Yet they proved unable to demonstrate that Algerian Muslims were much more infected than "Europeans." Their data was classified according to civic status, but despite the fact that they often conflated persons consulting medical personnel with sick, if not diseased and contagious, persons, none of them put their numerator figures over the right denominator, that is, the raw number of each group (indigenes being six times more numerous), which would have significantly reduced the "ethnic" gap. In the data we have extracted from the Service de prophylaxie, the figures do not distinguish between "indigenes" and settlers (the latter probably less frequently treated in dispensaries) and do not take into account the unequal geographic distribution of facilities.[98]

The (late) endeavor to launch health campaigns in colonial Algeria and to facilitate access to prenatal and venereal care—a program in the self-interest properly understood of the metropolis—genuinely improved the situation in the interwar period, an example being the birth of many "injection children" (fetuses saved by treating the pregnant mother with penicillin).[99] But this did not remedy the poverty or poor living and housing conditions of Arabs and Kabyles in Algeria and above all in metropolitan France, whereas it is those conditions that primarily explain the possibility of the excessive prevalence of VD. In metropolitan industrial areas "Muslim" populations were casual workers, frequently moving and hard to control. Instead of consulting public health services in case of symptoms, they may have preferred to manage by themselves or seek out camp nurses.[100] They were overrepresented in heavily biased official data on VDs. Above all, they were more likely to be subjected to detailed medical examinations than native French in the official job-hiring centers, due to the relatively low-skilled occupations they typically applied for, and data from those centers was used to supplement official health reports. Furthermore, contrary to the temporary presence of US GIs, North Africans settled permanently in coal-mining and industrial areas and worked hard for what would later be called "Reconstruction." Many became permanent residents.

Did VD Statistics Shed Light or Add Shadow?

Our purpose in this chapter was to revisit the history of VD in France by studying the history of how it was cognitively framed and the material means by which its demographic consequences were understood. As we have pointed out, three factors tended to obscure the role of VD in sexual and especially reproductive health—including involuntary childlessness. The first was the repopulation ideology inherited from the late nineteenth century, which led observers to focus exclusively on the big parameters of demographic dynamics. The second was the plurality of scourges that could be implicated in fecundity disorders. Third, there was the difficulty of translating the venereal threat into national-scale prevalence, trends, or incidences, in spite of the gradually increased effort at statistical monitoring.

In the framework of the accounting paradigm that characterized the French pronatalist tradition in demography and due to the resulting narrow focus on voluntary demographic processes, the medical issue of infertility was excluded from that discipline's politically influential research and analyses. Moreover, French institutionalized medical traditions resulted in venereal diseases being considered the prerogative of physicians specialized in syphilology and dermatology, not gonorrhea and infertility. Even when attempts were made to assess infertility, the effort to estimate VD prevalence and demographic incidence ran up against marked underdeclaration and undervisibility. Demographers who managed to provide a proxy for childlessness considered that less than 15 percent of couples were infertile and less than 5 percent (one-third) of those couples were infertile due to a microbial disease.[101] This was deemed to be a relatively insignificant fraction of the nation's "missing" births and a low policy priority compared to trying to combat the much larger volume of voluntary restraint on fertility. Expressing these figures in such relative values was also somehow a way of concealing infertile people's sufferings and of masking some of the medical consequences of gonorrhea, especially as physicians and health authorities were primarily alarmed by and focused on so-called hereditary syphilis (which in fact proved to be a chimera, unlike the sterility that gonorrhea caused).

The Great War gave rise to new governing procedures and statistically informed attempts to conceptualize, manage, and treat these issues. The data enforced stereotypes and fueled stigmatization; officials often did not want to see some of the realities before their eyes—the apparent spread of gonorrhea, for instance. They preferred to focus attention on syphilitic "contagion agents" (which became an administrative category), particularly "clandestine" prostitutes, and, increasingly, the figure of the North African. The latter emphasis illustrates the dead end that policies based on stigmatization rather than collective and individual prevention ran into, focusing as they did on individual behaviors rather than socioeconomic contexts of poverty.[102]

Because it generated growing concern about human reproduction, World War I gave more visibility to genital disorders. The development of infertility consultations might have led to better prevention of gonorrheal infertility. But instead it induced competition between several causes and encouraged their champions to promote authoritarian policies that targeted specific categories, setting aside the complexity of the factors involved in the epidemiology of such diseases. "Criminal abortion" served as the ideal culprit for a large fraction of moral crusaders and pronatalists; their propaganda emphasized the dangers of postabortion infections. The priority given to postabortion damage was probably reinforced by the relative decline in VD after the 1940s. Furthermore, the statistical information defined and collected by the health administrations at the time were usually narrowly oriented to their policy goals, so the available data they generated does not enable historians today to disentangle and hierarchize the various factors involved in reproductive disorders. The sources, meanwhile, once reinterpreted, invite us to be cautious in formulating general statements on the prevalence of VD and its impact in France, since it seems most likely that its incidence varied significantly both socially and geographically.

Notes

1. Alain Corbin, "L'hérédosyphilis ou l'impossible rédemption: Contribution à l'histoire de l'hérédité morbide," *Romantisme*, no. 31 (1981): 131–49; Andrew Aisenberg, "Syphilis and Prostitution: A Regulatory Couplet in Nineteenth-Century France," in *Sex, Sin and Suffering: Venereal Disease and European Society since 1870*, ed. Roger Davidson and Lesley A. Hall (London: Routledge, 2001): 15–28.

2. Alain Corbin, *Women for Hire: Prostitution and Sexuality in France after 1850* (Cambridge: Harvard University Press, 1990); Jean-Marc Berlière, *La police des mœurs sous la IIIème République* (Paris: Seuil, 1992).

3. Theodore Zeldin, *A History of French Passions, 1848–1945*, vol. 1 (Oxford: Oxford University Press, 1993), 304.

4. Jean-Noël Biraben, "Le rôle des maladies sexuellement transmissibles en démographie historique," *Population*, nos. 4–5 (1996): 1041–57.

5. Claude Quétel, *Le mal de Naples: Histoire de la syphilis* (Paris: Seghers, 1986), 247.

6. Cf. Simon Szreter's computations based on a secondary reanalysis of the Royal Commission on Venereal Diseases figures (1916) and contemporary Wassermann test samples. "The Prevalence of Syphilis in England and Wales on the Eve of the Great War: Re-visiting the Estimates of the Royal Commission on Venereal Diseases, 1913–1916," *Social History of Medicine* 27 (2014): 508–29.

7. The historical-demographic side of this study, specifically to reconstruct plausible figures and evaluate the real impact of VD on fecundity over the twentieth century in France, has not been attempted in this chapter. It is intended that this will be undertaken in a subsequent research project.

8. Virginie De Luca Barrusse, *Population en danger! La lutte contre les fléaux sociaux sous la Troisième République* (Bern: Lang, 2013); Christian Benoît, *Le soldat et la putain: Histoire d'un couple inséparable* (Paris: Taillac, 2013).

9. Libby Schweber, *Disciplining Statistics: Demography and Vital Statistics in France and England, 1830–1885* (Durham, NC: Duke University Press, 2006).

10. For a contribution in this vein, see Yves Charbit, "The Prostitute as an Urban Savage (Paris 1830's–1900's): French XIXth-Century Premises of the Anthropological Demography of Health" (presented at the Anthropological Demography of Health Conference, Institute of Human Sciences, School of Anthropology, Oxford University, March 29–31, 2017). The author argues that prostitutes were perceived by dominant social groups as "urban savages."

11. Patrice Pinell, "Champ médical et processus de spécialisation," *Actes de la recherche en sciences sociales*, nos. 156–57 (2005): 4–36.

12. Sandie Servais, "L'infirmerie spéciale Saint-Lazare. Quand la maladie devient un délit: Prostitution et maladie vénérienne," in *Les maux et les soins: Médecins et malades dans les hôpitaux parisiens au XIXe siècle*, ed. Claire Barillé and Francis Demier (Paris: Action artistique de la Ville de Paris, 2007), 263–74.

13. Corbin, *Women for Hire*; Berlière, *Police des mœurs*; Clyde Plumauzille, *Prostitution et révolution: Les femmes publiques dans la cité républicaine (1789–1804)* (Paris: Champ Vallon, 2017).

14. Alexandre Parent-Duchâtelet, *De la prostitution dans la ville de Paris, considérée sous le rapport de l'hygiène publique, de la morale et de l'administration* (Paris: Baillière, 1836).

15. Alfred Fournier, "Sur la diminution de l'accroissement de la population de la France," *Bulletin de l'Académie de médecine* 14 (March 3, 1885): 281–99. Fournier had already presented a "Provisional outcomes" study in *Syphilis et mariage* (Paris: Masson, 1880).

16. Léon Le Fort, *Bulletin de l'Académie de médecine* 19 (February 21, 1888): 267; Louis Le Pileur, *Note sur un projet de statistique universelle concernant les maladies vénériennes* (Clermont: Daix Frères, 1901).

17. Fournier, *Syphilis et mariage* (Paris: Masson, 1880): 243–45. Fournier highlighted the case of a forty-year-old seamstress admitted to the Hôpital Lourcine in 1870. She had had ten pregnancies, three before she contracted syphilis that were brought to term and produced healthy children, seven after contracting the disease that ended in four premature births and three abortions.

18. Fournier, "Sur la diminution," 299.

19. "But et espérances de notre société," *Bulletin de la Société de prophylaxie sanitaire et morale*, no. 1 (1901): 5. Note that this figure is similar to, but a little above, the estimate of 11.4 percent cumulative incidence among males aged in their midthirties in London a decade later, in 1911–12. Szreter, "Prevalence of Syphilis," table 3.

20. Alfred Fournier, *Traité de la syphilis*, vol. 1 (Paris: Rueff, 1899), 748. The argument is classic among British eugenicists: Anne Hanley, "Changing Medical Knowledge and Practice: Diagnosing and Treating Gonorrheal and Syphilitic Infertility, 1880–1914," in *The Palgrave Handbook of Infertility in History: Approaches, Contexts, Perspectives*, ed. Gayle Davis and Tracey Loughran (Palgrave Macmillan, 2017): 335–58.

21. Readers should note that French and English terminology do not align in their usage of the terms for *fecundity* (the physiological capability of a woman, man, or couple to reproduce, meaning to produce a live birth) and *fertility* (the actual, or "achieved" reproductive output of an individual, couple, or group). This can cause confusion, especially given the change in conventions and usage over time. Fertility is *fécondité* in French, while fecundity translates into French as *fertilité*. Similarly, whereas the biological state of sterility in English corresponds to *infertilité* in French,

childlessness for any reason, including personal preference, was designated *stérilité* in the French historical sources used here. However, French biodemographic vocabulary has since been standardized so that *stérilité* is now commonly understood by French demographers to mean exclusively "absolute" *infertilité*, that is, the biological incapacity to conceive. Further potential for ambiguity lies in the fact that demographic social scientists have developed various measures to pursue their disciplinary goal of devising statistically reliable population measurements of various aspects of fecundity and fertility, which differ in their purpose and definition from medical professionals, who focus their attention on the treatment of individual patients and couples presenting with a range of "fertility" problems. In the French historical sources used in this chapter, the views of both medical professionals (engaged in treatments for venereal diseases) and (early) demographers are cited, along with various other items drawn from the public discourse of the period across several decades, during which understandings of the fertility-related effects of syphilis and gonorrhea were subject to change. For further clarification, see James Trussell's helpful entry, "Fecundity," in *Encyclopedia of Population*, ed. Paul Demeny and Geoffrey McNicoll, vol. 1 (New York: Macmillan Reference 2003), 397–99.

22. Dumont's original publication was Arsène Dumont, *Dépopulation et civilisation, étude démographique* (Paris: Lecrosnier et Babé, 1890); it was republished in 1990 as *Dépopulation et civilisation, étude démographique: Suivie d'extraits d'articles de l'auteur* (Paris: Economica, 1990). See also Adolphe Landry, *La révolution démographique: Études et essais sur les problèmes de la population* (1934; repr., Paris: Institut national d'études démographiques, 1982).

23. Arsène Dumont, *Natalité et démocratie: Conférences faites à l'École d'anthropologie de Paris* (Paris: Schleicher Frères, 1898), 62; André Béjin, "Arsène Dumont et la capillarité sociale," *Population* 44, no. 6 (1989): 1009–28.

24. On psychocultural reasons, see Joseph J. Spengler, "French Population Theory since 1800," *Journal of Political Economy* 44, no. 5 (1936): 577–611. See the chapters in this volume by Roy F. Scragg and by Tim Bayliss-Smith on Rivers's subsequent influence in propagating a primarily psychocultural view of infertility among Pacific Island communities in the English-language literature of the 1920s; and the chapter by Simon Szreter and Kevin Schürer on the similar exclusive focus by demographers in Britain after 1918 on sociocultural factors to account for falling marital fertility.

25. Jacques Bertillon, *La dépopulation de la France* (Paris: Alcan, 1911), 261–79.

26. Gustave Lagneau, "Des mesures propres à rendre moins faible l'accroissement de la population de la France en restreignant ses fâcheuses conditions démographiques," *Bulletin de l'Académie de médecine* 24 (July 22, 1890): 93–135.

27. This survey was published only in 1893; Jacques Bertillon, "La natalité en France et les moyens à employer pour la relever," *Revue internationale de sociologie* 1 (1893): 24–46.

28. Paul-André Rosental, *L'intelligence démographique: Sciences et politiques des populations en France (1930–1960)* (Paris: Jacob, 2003), 208–16.

29. Adolphe Pinard and Charles Richet, "Rapport sur les causes physiologiques de la diminution de la natalité en France," *Annales de gynécologie et d'obstétrique* 59 (1903): 15–24, 93–121. The authors used the 1896 census, with couples married for fifteen to twenty-four years, and concluded that 10–13 percent of such marriages had produced zero children.

30. Charles Richet, "Sur la dépopulation de la France," *Bulletin de l'Académie de médecine* 77 (May 15, 1917): 617–20.

31. Adolphe Landry, "Familles sans enfants," *Journal de la société statistique de Paris* 82 (September–October 1941): 232–33.

32. Landry's approach to the miners' fertility as providing a "natural fertility" baseline can be compared to the use made of the Hutterite population data by Ansley Coale and his colleagues in developing the Princeton fertility indices in the 1960s.

33. According to his own logic, Landry did not see that his calculations on miners could instead be interpreted as suggesting that out of the 6.4 percent national sterility, only 2.8 percent was due to completely unwanted natural infertility and that therefore as much as 3.6 percent might be attributed to venereal diseases. Landry did not interrogate this gap between the two percentages. He was not interested in exploring what today would be called the various proximate and intermediate determinants of fertility; rather, both politically and scientifically he chose to focus on psychocultural factors.

34. Dr. Henri Le Grand, *La syphilis cause d'avortement* (Paris: Davy, 1889).

35. On the speciality of dermatology and its training, see Gérard Tilles, *Dermatologie des XIXe et XXe siècles: Mutations et controverses* (Paris: Springer Verlag France, 2011), 75–79.

36. Louis Jullien, *Blennorragie et mariage* (Paris: Baillière et Fils, 1898), 132.

37. Fernand Verchère, *La blennorrhagie chez la femme*, vol. 2 (Paris: Rueff et Cie, 1894), 63–64, 212.

38. "Buts et espérance de notre société," *Société de prophylaxie sanitaire et morale* 1 (1901): 6.

39. Maurice Letulle, "Sur la distribution dans l'armée de Notices relatives à la prophylaxie des maladies évitables," *Bulletin de l'Académie de médecine* 74 (November 16, 23, 1915): 531–35, 557–71.

40. Jules Simonin, "Organisation de la lutte antivénérienne dans les milieux militaires et civils pendant la guerre (1914–1917)," n.d., Service historique de l'armée de terre (SHAT), GR 9 NN 7/1049.

41. Ernest Gaucher et Léon Bizard, "La syphilis après deux ans de guerre," *Paris médical* 23 (1917): 54–57.

42. Jean-Yves Le Naour, *Misères et tourments de la chair durant la Grande Guerre: Les mœurs sexuelles des Français, 1914–1918* (Paris: Aubier, 2002), 146–51.

43. Ministère du Travail, de l'hygiène, de l'assistance et de la prévoyance sociales, "Instructions générales concernant la lutte contre les maladies vénériennes," in *L'armement antivénérien en France*, ed. André Cavaillon (Paris, 1928), 108–27.

44. Michelle K. Rhoades, "Renegotiating French Masculinity: Medicine and Venereal Disease during the Great War," *French Historical Studies* 29 (2006): 293–327; Judith Surkis, *Sexing the Citizen: Morality and Masculinity in France, 1870–1920* (Ithaca: Cornell University Press, 2006), 230–38. The condom was sometimes mentioned as a possible prophylactic, but military physicians did not consider it sufficiently safe; cf. Jean-Yves Le Naour, "L'éducation sexuelle du soldat en 14–18," *Bulletin du Centre d'étude d'histoire de la médecine de Toulouse*, no. 32 (2000): 5.

45. In 1921 Lucien March (head of the Statistique générale de la France) noticed that the raw number of syphilis cases was never compared to the strength of the military unit. This made it difficult to calculate prevalence, which March thought could not exceed three or four per thousand; Lucien March to Dr. Lévy, December 2, 1921, SHAT, 9 N/989-2.

46. Emmanuelle Cronier, *Permissionnaires dans la Grande Guerre* (Paris: Belin, 2013).

47. Report on the military hospital annex of Issy-les-Moulineaux, n.d., ca. late 1916, Archives of the Service de santé des armées, Hôpital du Val-de-Grâce, Paris.

48. Edouard Jeanselme, *La syphilis, son aspect pathologique et social* (Paris: Gauthiers-Villars et Cie, 1925); Adolphe Pinard, *À la jeunesse, pour l'avenir de la race française* (Paris: Ligue nationale française contre le péril vénérien, 1925); Lucien-Marie Pautrier, *Sixième congrès de la natalité* (Strasbourg: Alsacienne, 1925).

49. Lion Murard, "Les médecins de la santé publique en France (1886–1945)," in *Médecins de santé publique*, ed. Pierre-Henri Bréchat, Emmanuelle Salines, and Christophe Segoin (Paris: École nationale de la santé publique, 2006), 70.

50. André Cavaillon and Marcel Moine, *Étude statistique sur l'activité antivénérienne enregistrée de 1920 à 1928 inclusivement* (Paris: Imprimerie Nationale, 1928).

51. Georges Lévi-Valensin, *Je suis un avorteur* (Paris: Filipacchi, 1974), 24.

52. Edouard Jeanselme and René Burnier, "La syphilis est-elle en décroissance dans la population ouvrière?," *Bulletin de l'Académie de médecine* 95 (March 9, 1926): 214–36; Albert Touraine and Mlle Chon, "Les sources de contamination syphilitique (statistique personnelle d'après deux dispensaires)," *Bulletin de la Société française de dermatologie et de syphiligraphie* 4 (1937): 1–13.

53. Cavaillon and Moine, *Étude statistique*, 22–23. On the difficulty of correlating medical data and public policies, see Roger Davidson, *Dangerous Liaisons: A Social History of Venereal Disease in Twentieth-Century Scotland* (Amsterdam: Rodopi, 2000), 237–58.

54. According to Cavaillon and Moine's compilation, 62,808 cases of gonorrhea were detected in 1928. To compare this number with the one for syphilis, we had to perform a series of operations, since the number of syphilis cases in the Institut prophylactique de Paris (Paris Prophylactic Institute) and in public hospitals overseen by the Administration générale de l'assistance publique à Paris (Public Assistance) in Paris was an overall amount that included "hereditary" cases (that is, among infants and children). It was then necessary to estimate this number by calculating the rate of stage 1 and 2 syphilis among all nonhereditary cases in the rest of metropolitan

France (that rate was 29 percent) and applying it to the Parisian institutions. The result is 22,986 cases of contagious syphilis. Consequently, gonorrhea seems to have been 2.7 times as frequent as syphilis. For Swedish data in this period, see Szreter, "Prevalence of Syphilis," notes 83 and 84.

55. M. Bernier and Norbert Marx, *Le service de statistique médicale de la Caisse interdépartementale des assurances sociales de la Seine et de la Seine-et-Oise* (no pagination, Imprimerie de Clairvivre, 1938). The reference population is unknown, since the number of assignees was likewise unknown.

56. Fabrice Cahen, *Gouverner les mœurs: La lutte contre l'avortement en France, 1890–1950* (Paris: Institut national d'études démographiques, 2016).

57. Ligue nationale française contre le péril vénérien, *Annuaire 1932: Compte-rendu de la neuvième assemblée générale du 10 décembre 1931* (Paris: LPV, 1932), 4; André Cavaillon and Marcel Moine, "Les résultats de la lutte antivénérienne en France en 1930," *La prophylaxie antivénérienne*, no. 1 (1932): 5–29.

58. Armand Siredey, "Discussion," *La prophylaxie antivénérienne*, no. 6 (June 1933): 265.

59. *Conférence de défense sociale contre la blennorragie* (Paris: Tancrède, 1933).

60. Serge Gas, in *Conférence de défense sociale*, 297–98.

61. Pinard, *Jeunesse*, 10–11.

62. Lucien Périn, "La syphilis, cause de stérilité," *Revue française de dermatologie et de vénéréologie* 7–8 (1927): 406–17; Henri Vignes, "Stérilité syphilitique," *La sage-femme et le puériculteur*, December 1932, 10–18.

63. Pr. Pierre Lereboullet, "Sur la dénatalité en France," *Bulletin de l'Académie de médecine* 119 (April 26, 1938): 427–35; Fabrice Cahen, "Obstacles to the Establishment of a Policy to Combat Infertility in France (1920–1950)," in Davis and Loughran, *Palgrave Handbook of Infertility*, 199–219.

64. François Lebeuf, "Contribution à l'étude des facteurs étiologiques de la stérilité masculine (d'après une statistique de 100 cas)," *Annales de biologie clinique* 8 (1950): 507–11; Raoul Palmer and Elisabeth Palmer, *La stérilité involontaire: Évaluation des méthodes de diagnostic et de traitement* (Paris: Masson, 1950). The studies on infertility also point to syphilis as a cause of azoospermia; cf. Emile Bertin and Ernest Schulmann, *La stérilité syphilitique* (Paris: Masson, 1924).

65. The *stérilité* entry of the *Larousse* medical dictionary stated that half of female (primary or secondary) cases of infertility were due to gonorrhea. *Larousse médical illustré* (Paris: Larousse, 1924).

66. Claude Béclère, "La blennorragie feminine, cause principale de stérilité secondaire," *Paris médical: La semaine du clinicien* 108 (1938): 422; Claude Béclère, "La gynécologie et son rôle social dans les consultations hospitalières, les centres de diagnostic et les dispensaires," *La prophylaxie antivénérienne*, no. 2 (1945): 96–106. In contrast, physicians usually agreed that one-third of cases of the incapacity to procreate were due to a female disorder.

67. Auguste Brindeau, "Sur la question de l'avortement légal en U.R.S.S.," *Bulletin de l'Académie de médecine* 113 (March 12, 1935): 345–46.

68. Jean Dalsace, “La stérilité,” *Marianne*, February 8, 1939.

69. Cyril Olivier, *Le vice ou la vertu: Vichy et les politiques de la sexualité* (Toulouse: Presses Universitaires du Mirail, 2005); Luc Capdevila, François Rouquet, Fabrice Virgili, and Danièle Voldman, *Sexes, genre et guerres (France, 1914–1945)* (Paris: Payot, 2010).

70. Head of the Service de santé des armées, note on “Antivenereal and antialcoholic prophylaxism,” September 13, 1939, Cour suprême de justice, Riom, Archives nationales, 2W/54.

71. Pierre Simon, Jean Gondonneau, Lucien Mironer, Anne-Marie, and Dourlen-Rollier, *Rapport sur le comportement sexuel des Français*, avec la collaboration de Claude Lévy (Paris: Julliard; Charron, 1972).

72. Simon et al., *Rapport sur le comportement*, 47–48.

73. Alain Corbin, “Les prostituées du XIXe siècle et le ‘vaste effort du néant,’” *Communications*, no. 44 (1986): 259–75; Anne-Claire Rebreyend, *Intimités amoureuses: France, 1920–1975* (Toulouse: Presses Universitaires du Mirail, 2008); Régis Revenin, *Une histoire des garçons et des filles: Amour, genre et sexualité dans la France d'après-guerre* (Paris: Vendémiaire, 2015).

74. Ministère de la Guerre, “De l'utilisation dans l'armée à titre d'essai des nécessaires prophylactiques individuels,” SHAT, GR 9 NN 7/1061.

75. Gaston Muraz, “Essai d'organisation de la lutte antivénérienne dans la région de Saigon-Cholon (Cochinchine),” Prix Monbinne, 1934, no. 3, Archives of the Académie nationale de médecine.

76. Report on the organization of antivenereal services in prisons, November 27, 1946, Archives départementales du Nord (ADN), 138 W 63324.

77. These two tons had to be withdrawn from a stock reserved for the production of baby-bottle nipples.

78. Insa Meinen, *Wehrmacht et prostitution sous l'Occupation (1940–1945)* (Paris: Payot, 2006); Mary Louise Roberts, *What Soldiers Do: Sex and the American GI in World War II France* (Chicago: University of Chicago Press, 2013). Penicillin treatment was first used in France in 1944 for US GIs, and it was then reserved for allied soldiers. Although a few physicians were authorized to test it on their patients and the new remedy began to be produced in France in April 1945, thereafter it was administered only in a few hospitals. Despite the enthusiasm of the general press, French syphililologists remained cautious about its long-term effects until the early 1950s. See Tilles, *Dermatologie*, 217–20.

79. Simon et al., *Rapport sur le comportement*, 124. There is considerable evidence that in French popular culture the *chaude pisse* was a common subject of jokes. An example is Georges Brassens's bawdy song (not quite on the mark scientifically): “Il n'a pas eu la chaude pisse” (He never had the clap), about a man who “wishes” to catch the disease, in fact to experience a homosexual relation.

80. Simon et al., *Rapport sur le comportement*, 60.

81. “Loi n°1073 du 31 décembre 1942 relative à la prophylaxie et à la lutte contre les maladies vénériennes,” *La prophylaxie antivénérienne*, no. 2 (1943): 34–36.

82. André Cavaillon, "Le médecin praticien et la lutte contre la syphilis," *La prophylaxie antivénérienne*, no. 2 (1943): 38–40. Even during the Great War, soldiers were expected to indicate the identity of their "contaminator." Current research on HIV has shown that it is very hard to be certain of this kind of information.

83. Circular letters, December 21, 1940, and January 14, 1941, mentioned in the report on antivenereal services, February 28, 1941, ADN, 138 W 63324; André Cavaillon, note on antivenereal service statistics, August 9, 1946, Office départemental d'hygiène sociale, ADN, 138 W 63323.

84. Jean-Robert Debray, "Ordre national des médecins: Commission des maladies vénériennes," *La prophylaxie antivénérienne*, no. 4 (1947): 234. The Ordre des médecins, the corporative structure created by the Vichy regime, denounced practitioners who did not follow the law. In the department of Seine, however, only 348 declarations out of 22,792 came from practitioners.

85. Institut prophylactique (Prophylactic Institute), report on medical activity (dispensaries and prisons), 1950, Archives nationales, 19760214/23. According to the July 1951 report of Dr. Bernard Le Bourdellès, head of the Départementale de la santé (Health Department) on antivenereal policy in the Nord, the epidemiological investigation to find the "contaminator" was successful in only 2 percent of cases (ADN, 138 W 63321).

86. Commission of Venereal Diseases, December 17, 1946, Office départemental d'hygiène sociale, ADN, 138 W 63321.

87. Le Bourdellès, report on the antivenereal policy in Nord, n.d., ca. 1947–48, Office départemental d'hygiène sociale, ADN, 138 W 63321. Data from the Institut national d'hygiène, created in 1941, show that among 37,768 cases of syphilis in 1945, 35 percent of men and 18 percent of women were contaminated through "open relationships." J. Renard, "Graphiques des modes de contagion des maladies vénériennes déclarées en 1945," *Bulletin de l'Institut national d'hygiène* 1 (1946): 313.

88. Bernard Le Bourdellès, report on the antivenereal policy in Nord, n.d., ca. 1947, ADN, 138 W 63321; Le Bourdellès and Dr. Gillot, "Épidémiologie des maladies vénériennes dans le département du Nord," *La prophylaxie antivénérienne*, no. 7–8 (July–August 1948): 532–38. The question of why African American soldiers drew peculiar attention is addressed in Roberts, *What Soldiers Do*.

89. Bethesda played a role in the "infamous" Tuskegee Syphilis Study; cf. Allan M. Brandt, "Racism and Research: The Case of the Tuskegee Syphilis Study," *Hastings Center Report* 8 (1978): 21–29.

90. Pr. Claude Huriez, Commission des maladies vénériennes (Commission of Venereal Diseases), October 19, 1948, Office départemental d'hygiène sociale, ADN, 138 W 63321. On these *bordels militaires de campagne* (mobile field brothels) for North Africans, see Todd Shepard, *Mâle décolonisation: L'homme arabe et la France, de l'indépendance algérienne à la révolution iranienne* (Paris: Payot, 2017), 169–74.

91. Emmanuel Blanchard, "Le mauvais genre des Algériens," *Clio: Histoire, femmes et sociétés*, no. 27 (2008): 209–24. After 1954 Algerian prostitutes were significant

contributors to the Front de libération nationale cause; see Amelia H. Lyons, *The Civilizing Mission in the Metropole: Algerian Families and the French Welfare State during Decolonization* (Stanford: Stanford University Press, 2013): 144–45.

92. Christelle Taraud, *La prostitution coloniale: Algérie, Tunisie, Maroc (1830–1962)* (Paris: Payot, 2003). For Louis Chevalier, "the *indigene* does not worry about the chancre" and is not compliant. *Le problème démographique nord-africain* (Paris: Institut national d'études démographiques/Presses universitaires de France, 1947), 164.

93. Adrien Minard, "Syphilis and Indigenous Skin Lesions through French Physicians' Eyes in the Colonial Maghreb, 1830–1930," in *A Medical History of Skin: Scratching the Surface*, ed. Jonathan Reinarz and Kevin Siena (London: Pickering and Chatto, 2013), 85–98.

94. In 1923 Victor Demontès, a teacher in Algiers, estimated that syphilis was the most frequently treated ailment in local clinics for natives, where almost a quarter of all patients had the disease; cf. Kamel Kateb, *Européens, "indigènes" et juifs en Algérie (1830–1962): Représentations et réalités des populations* (Paris: Institut national d'études démographiques, 2001), 130–31.

95. On French authorities' fear of seduction and promiscuity between colonial soldiers and French women, see Richard S. Fogarty, *Race and War in France: Colonial Subjects in the French Army, 1914–1918* (Baltimore: Johns Hopkins University Press, 2008), 202–29. Compulsory examinations were implemented because fifty North African men had been diagnosed with syphilis in a war factory. Cf. Lucien-Marie Pautrier, "Inspection des travailleurs indigènes" (Bourges: unpublished paper, 1916); "Examen dermato-vénéréologique des travailleurs coloniaux et étrangers à leur arrivée et pendant leur séjour dans les usines," circular 399 Ci/7, SHAT, GR 9 NN 7/1053.

96. Virginie De Luca Barrusse, "Foreign Bodies in the Nation: The 'Health Problem of Immigration' in France during the Interwar Period," *Hygiea Internationalis*, no. 11 (2015): 163–89. The situation can be compared with that in Australia, Britain, or the United States, where ethnic migrants and minorities were often perceived as contaminators and stigmatized as carriers of physical or social diseases; see Alan M. Kraut, *Silent Travelers: Germs, Genes, and the "Immigrant Menace"* (Baltimore: Johns Hopkins University Press, 1994); Lara Marks and Michael Worboys, eds., *Migrants, Minorities and Health: Historical and Contemporary Studies* (New York: Routledge, 1997); Howard Markel and Alexandra Minna Stern, "The Foreignness of Germs: The Persistent Association of Immigrants and Disease in American Society," in *Race and Immigration in the United States: New Histories*, ed. Paul Spickard (New York: Routledge, 2011): 203–29; and Alison Bashford, ed., *Medicine at the Border: Disease, Globalization and Security, 1850 to the Present* (London: Palgrave, 2006).

97. François-Georges Marill, "La fréquence de la syphilis dans la population européenne et indigène de l'Algérie," *Annales de dermatologie et de syphiligraphie*, nos. 5–6 (1943): 134–45; Chevalier, *Problème démographique nord-africain*.

98. Cavaillon and Moine, *Étude statistique*, 132–33.

99. In the 1920s health facilities were not yet widely accessible to indigenous inhabitants; the situation changed gradually. Kateb, *Européens, "indigènes" et juifs*, 130; Chevalier, *Problème démographique nord-africain*, 36.

100. Le Bourdèlles, report on the antivenereal policy in Nord, n.d., ca. 1951, Office départemental d'hygiène sociale, ADN, 138 W 63321.

101. The soundest postwar estimates tend to prove that all conjectures published, from Bertillon to Landry, were coherent. Paul Vincent, "La stérilité physiologique des populations," *Population* no. 1 (1950): 45–64; Laurent Toulemon, "Très peu de couples restent volontairement sans enfant," *Population* nos. 4–5 (1995): 1079–109; Sandra Brée, "Évolution de la taille des familles au fil des générations (France, 1850–1966)," *Population*, no. 2 (2017): 309–42. Nevertheless, all these studies are at the national scale; subnational comparison would be necessary to provide more interesting paths of reflection.

102. According to Lévi-Valensin, trained as a practitioner in a dispensary for Muslim prostitutes in Algiers (in 1927–29), sex workers were often infected, but they docilely followed regulatory policies; on the other hand, their (Muslim) clients often refused to use condoms (Lévi-Valensin, *Je suis un avorteur*, 9–11).

Chapter Twelve

Revealing the Hidden Affliction

How Much Infertility Was Due to Venereal Disease in England and Wales on the Eve of the Great War?

Simon Szreter and Kevin Schürer

The Decline of a Nation?

By the turn of the twentieth century the British nation's declining birth-rate was increasingly the subject of anxious public and scientific debate, as the Registrar General's annual reports continued to confirm a downward national trend, which had in fact commenced from the late 1870s. The secularist Malthusian League had positively promoted birth control, and now economists and eugenicists, feminists and Fabians, as well as leading figures in the church and in the medical profession, all agreed that this was a momentous matter.[1] Previously, human fecundity—the capacity to conceive and reproduce—had not been considered a significant social variable. While the fertility of individuals or couples might be subject to some variation, with the odd exception populations and nations had dependably high fertility.[2] Since Malthus—and even more so since Darwin's generalization of Malthus's proposition to all species—it was an accepted fact that nature was fecund to a fault. Fertility was too robust, not too frail. Consequently, one of the eternal human predicaments, both for the individual and for government, was how to rein in this exuberant fertility. So the dawning perception of the nation's flagging and apparently fragile vitality—and indeed that of several other urbanizing nations, too—was a serious shock, expressed not just in politics but also science and literature.[3]

The three decades before the outbreak of the Great War therefore saw an intensification of attention to the newly problematized issue of human fertility. Many competing theses and theories were advanced and publicly aired to account for the challenging new phenomenon. The diversity of speculation during these decades was fed by the rapidly changing state of both pure and applied knowledge within the biological and the medical sciences, concerning both evolutionary theory and germ theory.[4] Simultaneously, fraught social and political debates over sex and gender norms were intensifying into the crescendo of the militant suffragette campaign, which also raised the temperature further with the issue of infection of innocent wives by their sexually irresponsible male partners.[5] This intellectual ferment has left a considerable volume of primary source material, which includes several major official inquiries devoted to important aspects of understanding the problem of the falling birthrate in Britain: the Interdepartmental Commission on Physical Deterioration of 1903–4; the Royal Commission on the Care and Control of the Feeble-Minded, 1904–9; the 1911 census's Fertility of Marriage inquiry; and the Royal Commission on Venereal Diseases of 1913–16.[6]

These sources have been used productively by historians for a wide range of studies, including those which have provided accounts of the contested discourses of gender relations, sex, eugenics, and evolutionary theory in relation to nationalist and imperialist ideological and political themes of the period. The empirical studies of fertility and infertility conducted in this period of course all reflected these contemporary agendas. However, the value of the evidence they collected, classified, and presented to make their respective cases, or to confound their intellectual antagonists, is not necessarily exhausted by the terms of reference of those now-defunct discourses. It is also possible, with historicist care and attention both to the scientific context of the period and to the intentions and classificatory designs of the originators of the data, to revisit historical evidence, such as that collected in the early twentieth century, and subject it to a critical secondary analysis in a form that can be used to evaluate a different agenda, informed by our changed scientific and social scientific understandings today. In other words, demonstrating that demographic analysts and epidemiologists of various complexions in the past produced analyses that were ideologically constructed in various ways does not exhaust the potential value to historians of such research conducted in the past. We ignore to our impoverishment the treasure trove of evidence collected by those who demonstrably thought differently from us today. Elsewhere a combination of three such contemporary sources from the period 1910–12 has been reanalyzed to produce comparative estimates of the absolute prevalence at that time of syphilis infection rates in the national population of England and Wales and in various sections of the populations.[7]

In this chapter we pursue those sexually transmitted infection (STI) prevalence estimates for 1910–12 a little further and link them to the theme of this volume and also to both historical and current debates about the phenomenon of secular decline in the nation's fertility that so perplexed contemporaries, and whose understanding continues to pose a challenging puzzle for historians and social scientists today. In particular we examine how these sources can offer further insights into the possible relationship between STIs and aspects of infertility during this period, which has been somewhat overlooked by demographers ever since. It has been overlooked in part because the discourse of degeneration and disease, within which these contemporary researches were conducted, has been thoroughly—and rightly—deconstructed by intellectual and cultural historians.[8] It has also been overlooked because the possibility of STIs having significant influence on infertility has come to be associated, since the 1920s, exclusively with "other" populations in Oceania, sub-Saharan Africa, and among black Africans in the United States, but not among white Europeans wherever they settled in the world.[9]

To what extent might the imperial white Anglo-Saxon nation itself, including even the metropolitan middle-class professional and administrative elite, have suffered significant infertility due to STIs? The Royal Commission on Divorce, 1909–12, certainly exposed the fact that the guilty secret of middle-class males infecting their wives was in fact a reality for some, as campaigning doctors and feminists had been alleging.[10] However, the increasing proportion of very low-fertility marriages among the middle classes in the late Victorian and Edwardian decades could just as easily have been due to the private wishes of both partners to avoid too great a domestic burden, and it has been impossible so far for historical demographers to tease out the relative importance of these two influences. This is because such private intentions remained at this time unarticulated and inadmissible by the majority. Although birth control had been a subject of public discourse on and off throughout the nineteenth century, it had never achieved respectability in polite society. Throughout the decades of Victoria's long reign—and beyond, into the first two decades of the twentieth century—open acknowledgement of a desire by a couple to restrict their marital fertility continued to be deemed religiously disrespectful by conventional educated opinion, a debilitating problem for public articulation in a culture that remained respectful of religion as an arbiter of moral values. The Malthusian League, campaigning since the 1870s for public recognition of the rationale for birth control, was, in the eyes of the socially conservative majority, considered synonymous with morally dubious, godless secularists.[11] To want fewer children in a marriage blessed by Christian religion was at best "selfish," at worst hubristic in wishing to thwart the divine maker's plans. The various contraceptive devices required to bring about such plans were viewed by most as distasteful and unnatural and as the accoutrements of the sordid commercial sex trade and of libertines' attempts to avoid disease, not as something appropriate to the marriage bed. Yet it was evident by the 1900s that family sizes had been falling dramatically among the middle classes—and among certain other large social groups too, such as the factory workers in many textiles towns. All the possible suspected reasons for this were viewed as deeply problematic, as far as public moral discourse was concerned.

In many ways the most apocalyptic possibility—a feared general decline in biological fecundity—was most acceptable as a subject for inquiry and public debate because it implied no failings in the personal morality of the unfertile middle classes, and this may in part explain the capacity of the eugenics agenda to take the lead in public debate on the subject in the Edwardian period.[12] Thus, social Darwinist discourse of "degeneration" or "deterioration" licensed earnest and rational discussion, in the interests of science, of the feared possibility that certain worrying and still-unexplained diseases might be causes of the nation's flagging vitality, such as tuberculosis, alcoholism, feeble-mindedness, and of course syphilis (though it took the insistence of feminists to bring gonorrhea also within this sphere of discourse).[13] Eugenicists, who fondly entertained the notion that "inheritance" across the generations was the key to understanding everything, subscribed to the somewhat illogical and self-contradictory notion that any or all of these conditions were probably also heritable and might therefore help explain, with various contortions of reasoning, the decline in fertility of the race. The long-observed phenomenon of supposedly "congenital" syphilis was thought to demonstrate heritability of the disease. The new findings after 1900 that syphilis infection was capable of causing death from "general paralysis of the insane" (GPI) or other conditions into late middle age also seemed to confirm the horrifyingly long reach of the disease, apparently across generational time.[14] Meanwhile, voluntary limitation of family sizes—the other main possible cause of secular fertility decline—was only cautiously discussed in public and usually presented as an undesirable possibility, because few wanted to acknowledge that clandestine religious and moral hypocrisy could be occurring on a potentially widespread scale throughout the nation's upper and middle classes, the supposed moral paragons of the imperial civilizing nation. However, it was increasingly being seen—in the final few years before the Great War erupted—as an issue at least meriting dispassionate research, hence the government's sanctioning of the enormous nationwide survey represented by the fertility of marriage questions included for every coresident married couple to answer at the 1911 census.

It was the second part of the extensive official report by Dr. T. H. C. Stevenson, the General Register Office's Statistical Superintendent, on the data collected at this census, whose publication was delayed by the war until 1923, that finally seemed to refute conclusively the notion that some kind of biological causes of infertility were at work in reducing the nation's fertility.[15] In his own subsequent interpretative publications, Stevenson emphasized instead the importance of volitional, social, cultural, and economic motives as the causes of declining fertility.[16] All other interwar analysts broadly accepted these conclusions, which then remained the primary and formative focus of all subsequent research, not only on Britain's secular fertility decline but on that of most other populations, too.[17]

The Possible Role of STIs in Childless Marriages in the 1911 Census

It is therefore not surprising that despite all the effort that has been devoted by social scientists and historians over so many decades to elucidating the demographic patterns and diverse possible causes of the historical secular fertility declines that occurred in so many countries during the past two centuries, there has been no critical and systematic evaluation of the possible role of STIs—most notably gonorrhea and chlamydia, which form the multidisciplinary primary focus of this volume, *The Hidden Affliction*.[18] In closing the volume, this chapter attempts to offer a preliminary evaluation of the contribution of these two hidden afflictions to the fertility decline that occurred in England and Wales as recorded in the famous "Fertility of Marriage" Census of England and Wales in 1911. Specifically, this chapter provides a quantitative estimate of the likely effect that STIs had on one component of the emerging pattern of low marital fertility: childless marriages.

It is certainly the case that untreated gonorrhea and chlamydia would also have caused some secondary sterility in marriages after the birth of a first or subsequent child. On the one hand, men and women can—and did—become infected with STIs during, as well as before, marriage. On the other hand, many contemporaries believed that a prior gonorrhea infection could also account for "a one-child sterility," as Prince A. Morrow (professor of genitourinary diseases at New York University) explained in 1904: "A woman with gonorrhea of the cervix may readily conceive," but the process of parturition at the first pregnancy "opens the gates to the infection which may have been long installed in the external genital canal, the cervix, or uterus, and permits its ascension to the tubes, ovaries, and peritoneum."[19] However, given the intrinsic difficulties in working with the partial historical evidence that is available, the focus here is exclusively on the epidemiologically and demographically most straightforward relationship that can be empirically studied: that between rates of absolute marital sterility (a parity of zero births) of various subgroups of the population and estimates of the relevant age-specific rates of prior infection with STIs among different occupational groups with specified ages at marriage. But it should be borne in mind, that the results reported here represent a proportion, and not the sum total, of the likely impact of STIs in causing involuntary, very low fertility.

The topic of very small families in the British fertility decline before 1914 has rarely been the subject of investigation in historical demographic study. One exception is the work of Michael Anderson, who used tables from the Scottish 1911 census, where some parity distribution information was published, along with later evidence for England and Wales produced by the Royal Commission on Population of 1944–49. Anderson's is an excellent, wide-ranging study; however, it does not at any point discuss the possibility that STIs could be responsible, in part, for the patterns revealed by the occupational fertility data reviewed. This is entirely understandable, in that no robust, empirically based quantitative estimates of the extent of STIs among the British population before 1914 existed for Anderson to draw on. He was consequently constrained to conclude that such extremely low fertility as he found was mainly the product of volition, though he was clearly troubled by the paucity of cultural or literary evidence, pre-1914, which could provide explicit contemporary documentation acknowledging or valorizing this putatively novel form of volitional behavior resulting in "highly restricted" fertility in the upper and middle classes of society in the decades before 1914.[20]

This chapter presents a conservatively constructed model of the extent to which the overall level of STIs prevalent in the population of England and Wales during the decades prior to the 1911 census could have contributed to the degree of absolute childlessness enumerated at that census in marriages of completed fertility. In a previous publication contemporary primary sources from the period just prior to the outbreak of the Great War, notably including two quasi-random samples of the population administered with Wassermann tests, have been subjected to secondary analysis to yield an estimate that at the time of the 1911 census approximately 7.8 percent of men in England and Wales had incurred an infection with syphilis by the age of 33–35 years old.[21] With the addition of various further considerations, this figure can now be used as the basis to derive an estimate of the extent to which STIs were responsible for the overall proportion of childless marriages recorded at the 1911 census of England and Wales.

It is, of course, gonorrhea that causes sterility, and not syphilis. So it is first necessary to bring forward relevant information that can permit a known rate of prevalence of syphilis to act as a guide for the prevalence of gonorrhea in the population at this time. Second, we need to establish, by consulting the results of relevant modern clinical and epidemiological studies, the quantitative capacity of gonorrhea infections to cause sterility in either women or men. Third, this information needs to be articulated with what we know of the sexual mores and practices of the majority in British society at this time in relation to courtship and marriage so that we can form plausible sex-differential estimates of the opportunity for gonorrhea infections to result in the absolute sterility of marriages. Fourth, the likely contribution to marital sterility of another major STI, chlamydia, also needs to be carefully considered and incorporated into the model.

Since the ultimate objective of this chapter is to form a quantitative evaluation of the extent to which the prevailing incidence of STIs in 1911 was responsible for a proportion of the number of childless marriages enumerated at the census, it is also necessary to adapt the previous work of historical demographers of the early modern English population to produce an estimate of the extent of childlessness that would be expected in this population, regardless of the effect of any STIs. To produce such an estimate, results from the Cambridge Group for the History of Population's parish reconstitution data are used, with a correction factor added to take into account a newly published, empirically based figure to adjust for the extent to which those parish populations were themselves likely to have been subject to a moderate level of fertility-reducing STIs.[22]

Once the available evidence for all these components of the required model has been presented, weighed, and considered, the calculations can then be combined to offer an empirically based best estimate of the extent to which STIs accounted for a proportion of the completely childless marriages enumerated at the 1911 census. The proportion turns out to be far from insignificant.

A Model of the Impact of STIs on the Infertility of Marriages in 1911

In this section we first construct a model for male sterility due to gonorrhea, before producing an estimate for female sterility. Previous published work has established that in 1911 men in England and Wales (married and unmarried combined) accumulated approximately a 7.8 percent chance of having been infected with syphilis by the time they reached age thirty-three to thirty-five. If we make the simplifying assumption that for most males the chance of becoming infected in this era started after the teenage years, at age twenty, and was roughly equal per year, then we can estimate that 0.52 percent of new men (one in two hundred) were infected with syphilis at each year of age between twenty and age thirty-four inclusively.[23]

While syphilis infection has no direct implications for sterility, a robust indicator of its prevalence, such as this, can be useful to derive an estimate of the extent to which men were at this time infected with gonorrhea, the primary STI causing sterility. Gonorrhea (and chlamydia) are significantly more infectious (and reinfectious) than syphilis; this is partly because the spirochete is much more fragile and must access the bloodstream for transmission and also because a single inoculation with syphilis usually produces immunity to subsequent infection, which is not true of either gonorrhea or chlamydia. The key issue therefore is to provide a plausible estimate of how much more prevalent was infection with gonorrhea than with syphilis at this time in Britain. There is relevant contemporary evidence for the population of Sweden, where both syphilis and gonorrhea were compulsorily notified. This Swedish data for the two most comparable years, 1918 and 1919, indicates that the prevalence of gonorrhea among men was approximately four times greater than syphilis.[24]

If we know that the rate of infection with gonorrhea is likely to have been four times as great, this implies that approximately 2.08 percent of men (one in fifty) were infected with gonorrhea at each individual year of age from twenty to thirty-four (assuming an approximately equal risk of exposure over this age range). That in turn means that by age twenty-four 10.4 percent had been infected with gonorrhea at some point in their lives; by age twenty-nine the figure was 20.8 percent, and by age thirty-four the figure was 31.2 percent. Making the deliberately conservative and simplifying assumption that the chance of further infection of either partner more or less stopped around the point of marriage, this means that the chances of ever having had an infection with gonorrhea among men marrying at age twenty to twenty-four would have been about 5.2 percent (half of 10.4 percent, assuming an even distribution of marriage ages across this age range).[25] However, among those marrying at the more typical ages of twenty-five to twenty-nine, 15.6 percent would have had a gonorrheal infection at some point in their lives by the time they married (adding together the annual chance in all of the five years among those aged twenty to twenty-four, plus half of the five years between ages twenty-five to twenty-nine, again assuming an equal distribution of men marrying across each of those five years). Applying a similar logic produces a figure of 26.0 percent having had a prior infection among those males marrying at ages thirty to thirty-four.[26]

We now need to multiply these figures, for the rising proportion of males having had an infection at each marriage age, by an estimate of the chance of a gonorrhea infection causing male sterility. This happens through the complication of epididymitis (see figure 10.3, page 320) and, less frequently, prostatitis and secretory gland involvement.[27] About one-sixth (17 percent) of untreated cases of gonorrhea in men lead to epididymitis and, in turn, estimates vary between 23 and 41 percent of such individuals being rendered permanently sterile.[28] If we adhere to a conservative estimate of 29 percent, which is at the lower end of this range (being twice as near to the lower figure of 23 percent as to the upper figure of 41 percent), this would indicate that about 4.9 percent (just under one in twenty) of those males infected with untreated gonorrhea would be sterilized in consequence.[29]

To calculate the proportion of males marrying at ages twenty to twenty-four who were sterile at the beginning of their marriages due to gonorrhea we should multiply successively by 17 percent and by 29 percent the estimate that 5.2 percent of men aged twenty to twenty-four at marriage would have encountered an infection with gonorrhea before (or in the early stages of) marriage. This equates to 0.256 percent for men marrying at age twenty to twenty-four (5.2 percent × 0.0493, the product of 0.17 × 0.29). The comparable figure for men marrying at twenty-five to twenty-nine is 0.774 percent (equivalent to [10.4 + 5.2] × 0.0493). The comparable figure for men marrying at thirty to thirty-four is 1.282 percent (equivalent to [20.8 + 5.2] × 0.0493).

To these figures for the rising proportion of male STI sterility with later male age at marriage has to be added the chance at each female age at marriage of female sterility due to gonorrhea. Modern research has found that in a population of women generally experiencing repeated chances of conception and childbearing (i.e., a population in which it was the social norm for married women to experience more than one live birth), about 30 percent of those with gonorrhea usually progress to pelvic inflammatory disease (PID).[30] Furthermore, among those women contracting PID, if untreated for three days (as would have been the case for all women in Britain before 1914, in that even if they did come immediately under medical care—itself unlikely—there was no effective treatment to deploy), there is a further 30 percent chance that the occurrence of PID will result in TFI (tubal factor infertility, see above, figures 7.2, page 231, and 10.4, page 231).[31] This implies that one in eleven (9.09 percent) of all women who originally became infected with gonorrhea at any point before the development of effective treatments from the late 1930s onward were likely to have become sterile due to PID.

This estimate of STI impact on female sterility has to be further adjusted to take into account the additional effect of chlamydia. It is not justifiable to discount entirely the effects of chlamydia in the pre-1914 decades simply because of the unavailability of positive evidence for a disease that was at that time unknown. As the contribution to this volume by Ian N. Clarke and Hugh R. Taylor shows, it is inconceivable that the disease was not present, and, equally, as Michael Worboys's chapter carefully documents, a range of nonspecific, non-gonorrheal conditions were recognized by clinicians during the early twentieth century, though they did not identify them as what is now called chlamydia.[32] Untreated chlamydia, like gonorrhea, has a definite capacity to cause female sterility through PID and consequent tubal blockage in a proportion of those affected, as well as leading to some ectopic pregnancies. It is also known that *C. trachomatis* causes urethritis and epididymitis in males. However, the precise mechanisms through which chlamydia infections can produce infertility consequences appear to be extremely complex and variable, and the field is currently a highly dynamic one of ongoing research.[33] Early scares of chlamydia's gross sterilizing effects were clearly exaggerated, as pointed out in Worboys's chapter. Nevertheless, there is unanimity that untreated chlamydia is a cause of a nontrivial amount of infertility in women.[34] Given all the relevant considerations discussed in detail in appendix E, the proposal adopted here is to increase any estimate of the effect due to gonorrhea on female sterility by one-third, to take into account the likely scale of the additional effect of a known but unquantifiable presence of chlamydia in the pre-1914 population. In keeping with the conservative principles of estimation adopted throughout and consistent with the present state of knowledge, no additional sterility effect on male fertility will be attributed here to chlamydia.[35]

Thus, the chance of female sterility from any single episode of infection with gonorrhea is significantly higher than the male chance (one in eleven as against a one in twenty male chance), and there is also the added risk that female sterility can be caused by chlamydia infection (which we are assuming, following the latest scientific consensus, is unlikely to cause male infertility). However, assuming that most married women were not exposed to the chance of infection prior to marriage (except with their future spouse) or outside marriage, a major difference between the sexes is that whereas males may enter marriage already sterile from a premarriage infection with gonorrhea—and their chances of this being the case rise the later they marry—the female chances of becoming sterile due to exposure to STI infection (from her marriage partner) are invariant with respect to her age at marriage. In these circumstances, because they are a function only of her exposure just before or during the first year or so of her marriage regardless of her age, the probability of a wife being unable to conceive a first child would always relate to the chances of her male partner having acquired a transmissible infectious condition (of either gonorrhea or chlamydia) no more than six to twelve months before initiating intercourse with his spouse, or from him having acquired the infection from extramarital intercourse within six to twelve months of the marriage commencing. If acquired any later in the marriage, though its transmission to the wife might have curtailed subsequent fertility, it would have been unlikely to have resulted in her failure to conceive a first child and her complete childlessness.[36] The female chance of infection at any particular age at marriage is therefore set as being equal to approximately two years' worth of the chance of their husband having acquired either a gonorrheal or chlamydial infection in the period immediately before or during the early months of marriage.

The chance of female sterility at any age is therefore 1.04 percent (two years' worth of the male annual chance of gonorrhea infection) multiplied by 0.1212 (to reflect both the 0.909—one in eleven—chance of female sterility, inflated by a factor of one-third to take into account the additional sterilizing effect of chlamydia). This produces a value of 0.126 percent representing the chances of women at any single year of age being infected, which therefore needs to be multiplied by five to reflect the chance of sterility among a five-year age group of women, such as those marrying at twenty to twenty-four, twenty-five to twenty-nine, and thirty to thirty-four. This produces a final female sterility estimate of 0.63 percent for each age-at-marriage quinquennium grouping of married women.

Assuming that in the generality of the population of England and Wales, males and females were more or less of the same age as each other at marriage (males typically in fact were a couple of years older at marriage, which simply has the effect of again making the following estimated figures conservative or minimal estimates of the role of STIs), the overall chance of marital sterility having been caused by the prevailing rates of STIs in 1911, among both husband and wife combined, are as follows for different female ages at marriage:

20–24: 0.886 percent
25–29: 1.399 percent
30–34: 1.912 percent[37]

The reason these figures rise with age at marriage is primarily a function of the accumulating chance of male sterility. Although most doctors in Britain before the Great War were apparently quite unaware of the substantial male role in marital sterility, as Christina Benninghaus documents in chapter 10, this would have been no surprise at all to the medical community—or even to the wider, educated public—in Germany. There, several influential clinical studies incorporating sperm testing had shown about one-third or more of sterile marriages to be due to male infertility.[38]

These figures can now be compared with the actual proportions of marriages sterile (i.e., childless) at these ages in the population of England and Wales reported at the 1911 census (table 12.1, row 3), being, respectively, as follows: 6.0 percent; 11.8 percent, and 22.6 percent. However, when comparing the two sets of figures, it must be borne in mind that a very significant proportion of the latter was due to other natural causes not attributable either to STIs or to birth control, and this has to be subtracted before the truly additive effect of the prevailing rates of STIs in 1911 can be quantified.

The rates of childlessness in 1911 due solely to natural variability in fecundity and other natural sources of infertility can be estimated by comparison with a historical reference standard provided by the Family Reconstitution Files of the parishes collated by the Cambridge Group, as analyzed by James Trussel and Christopher Wilson (see appendix A on the choice of Trussel and Wilson's methodology for the analysis of sterility used in this chapter).[39] However, the rates of sterility found by Trussel and Wilson are themselves not entirely free from the effects of STIs, since it is unlikely to have been the case that these English rural and small-town parish populations were entirely immune from STIs in the period circa 1600–1800. Allowance can be made for this because there now exists an empirically based quantitative estimate, published in 2017, of the likely prevalence of syphilis in rural England and Wales in the 1770s. This estimate has been constructed in such a way as to be demographically comparable with the published figures available for the population of England and Wales in the period 1910–12. This study found that in the mid-1770s in rural Cheshire and North Wales 0.93 percent of both sexes had sought treatment for the pox by age thirty-five (as against about 8 percent of the city residents of Chester).[40] Most of the sixteen parish populations in the pre-1850 set of family reconstitutions analyzed by Trussel and Wilson related to small rural settlements of the kind found in the agricultural region of west Cheshire and northeast Wales surrounding Chester. The two exceptions are the market towns of Banbury and Gainsborough, though both of these were very much smaller than Chester in this period.[41] That would suggest that the parity patterns found in most of the pre-1850 parish populations analyzed by Trussel and Wilson most probably reflected a very moderate prevalence of STIs, similar to the low rate of 0.93 percent rate for the pox empirically established for rural Cheshire and North Wales.

There needs to be some further adjustment to take into account the higher incidence of STIs likely to have been found in the townships of Banbury and Gainsborough. Allowance can be made for this, first, by deriving an empirical estimate from the raw data of the Cambridge Group's Family Reconstitution Files (FRF) of how much greater was the age-adjusted prevalence of sterile marriages in Banbury and Gainsborough than in the aggregate of more rural parishes, given that the primary cause of such excess sterility (once age at marriage has been controlled for) is most likely to have been the differential incidence of STIs (there is no evidence for volitional birth control in this period).[42] Second, the two different subpopulations can be weighted by an estimate of the relative size of Banbury and Gainsborough against the other fourteen parishes in the Trussel and Wilson group of sixteen parishes.

This reanalysis of the FRF data using all marriages of completed fertility (i.e., corresponding to the Trussel and Wilson methodology) found that across all marriages where wives were aged fifteen to thirty-four at marriage (and weighted for the different numbers of couples in each quinquennium of marriage age), those in Banbury and Gainsborough were 1.387 times more likely to be sterile than those in the other fourteen smaller parishes, combined.[43] That tendency to a higher rate of sterility then needs to be weighted by the relative population size of these two parishes. The earliest reliable estimate of the relative sizes of all sixteen parish populations shows Banbury and Gainsborough with a combined size of 8,922, while the other fourteen parishes totaled 20,427.[44] Therefore, to allow fully both for the higher STI prevalence in the more urban pair of parishes and their proportionate size among the sixteen parishes, the figure of 0.93 percent pox prevalence for entirely rural parishes (derived from Cheshire) needs to be adjusted upward by a factor of 0.424.[45] This results in an estimate that the comparable pox-prevalence rate (by age thirty-five) in all sixteen parishes, combined, would have been 1.324 percent (0.93 + [0.93 × 0.424]). This double-corrected estimate takes into account the fact that the more urban parishes of Banbury and Gainsborough had higher rates of STI infection than the other rural parishes, and their relative population weighting within the total of all sixteen parishes in the Trussel and Wilson data.

Following the method detailed in appendix B for adjusting the parish populations to take account of STIs in affecting a proportion of marriages recording no live births, table 12.1 provides a summary of the key steps in this process. Row 1 reproduces the Trussel and Wilson figures for sterility (proportion of marriages with parity zero) at the three main female ages at marriage in their original unadjusted form. These are then adjusted for STIs in row 2, by modifying the estimated prevalence of STIs as indicated by the 0.93 percent rates for rural Cheshire and North Wales, further modified to a rate of 1.324 percent to reflect the most probable evidence-based estimate for these sixteen parishes. Thus, in effect, row 2 equates to a pre-1800 English population entirely free from STIs.

Rows 3–5 of table 12.1 then provide the proportion of sterile marriages derived from the I-CeM database version of the 1911 census for England and Wales, together with the underlying total number of couples these figures are based on (for details on I-CeM see the next section of this chapter and note 48). Following these, rows 6 and 7 indicate the percentage by which the proportion of sterile marriages observed for 1911 are in excess of, first, the Trussel and Wilson unadjusted rate for pre-1850 England (row 6), and, second, the Trussel and Wilson rate adjusted for STIs (row 7). Subtracting the Trussel and Wilson STI-adjusted rate (row 2) from the rates of sterility observed in 1911 at the census of England and Wales (row 3) provides the set of "excess" sterility rate figures given in row 8.

The figures in row 8 indicate the amount of childlessness at each of these three different female ages at marriage in the population of England and Wales at the 1911 census that is in excess of that which can be explained by the amounts of such sterility found in the FRF rural parish populations, adjusted to be free from STI effects (row 2). These, then, are the quantities of childlessness in 1911 that remain "unexplained" by any base rate of "natural" infertility and that are therefore due either to the prevailing STI rates or to voluntary restraint of fertility within marriage. We have no direct, quantifiable evidence on the latter, but we do have for the former, and so the approximate contributions of each can then be gauged.

This is done by bringing together these estimates of the amount of "excess" sterility in different female age-at-marriage groups shown in row 8, with the estimates, calculated previously (see top of page 384), for the proportions rendered sterile by the prevailing STI rates in the population of England and Wales in 1911, which are shown in row 9. Making, again, the conservative, minimizing assumption that males and females were more or less of the same age as each other at marriage, the bottom row (10) of table 12.1 shows the percentage of sterile marriages in 1911 most probably due to the effects of

Table 12.1 Marriages of completed fertility in England and Wales at 1911 census: estimates of proportion of childless marriages due to STIs. Female marriage ages: 20–24 (married 25–29 years); 25–29 (married 20–24 years); 30–34 (married 15–19 years).

Row		Age at marriage		
		20–24	**25–29**	**30–34**
1	Trussel and Wilson's pre-1850 unadjusted % zero parity	4.6	9.1	16.6
2	Trussel and Wilson's pre-1850 STI-adjusted % zero parity	4.3	8.4	15.8
3	England and Wales, 1911, % zero parity	6.0	11.8	22.6
4	England and Wales, 1911, total number of couples	236,815	149,338	63,154
5	England and Wales, 1911, total number of couples with zero parity	14,273	17,650	14,260
6	England and Wales, 1911, proportionate excess over Trussel and Wilson's unadjusted % zero parity ([row 3 minus row 1] divided by row 1)	30.4%	29.7%	36.1%
7	England and Wales, 1911, proportionate excess over Trussel and Wilson's STI-adjusted % zero parity ([row 3 – minus row 2] divided by row 2)	40.0%	39.8%	43.1%
8	England and Wales, 1911, % "excess" marital sterility (zero parity): row 3 minus row 2	1.7	3.4	6.8
9	England and Wales, 1911, sterility (% zero parity) attributable to STIs in 1911 population	0.886	1.399	1.912
10	England and Wales, 1911, proportion of "unexplained" childless marriages due to STIs (row 9 divided by row 8)	52.1%	41.1%	28.1%

Note: Rows 1, 2, 3, 8, and 9 report arithmetically comparable percentage figures; rows 6, 7, and 10 present derivative figures for analytic purposes discussed in the text. For use of Trussel and Wilson sterility estimates, see appendix A, and for the derivation of row 2 from row 1, see appendix B. Source for row 3: I-CeM. The Integrated Census Microdata Project.

STIs. These are as high as 52.1 percent at the younger-than-average female age at marriage of twenty to twenty-four, and 41.1 percent when wives were aged twenty-five to twenty-nine at marriage (the average female age at marriage in 1911 was twenty-six years[46]), falling to 28.1 percent among wives aged thirty to thirty-four at marriage.

Overall, taking into account the different numbers of couples marrying at these different ages (row 4), the conclusions that follow from this exercise are that STIs were most probably responsible for about 45 percent of all excess childless marriages at this time, after allowing for those attributable to natural variability in human fertility.[47] On the one hand, therefore, these calculations show that it is probable STIs did play a substantial role in accounting for childless marriages at the 1911 census. On the other hand, it can be argued that this exercise nevertheless confirms that voluntary restraint was apparently responsible for somewhat over half the overall excess in childless marriages and for slightly over two-thirds among that minority of society delaying marriage the most, where the wife was aged thirty or above at marriage.

Childlessness and STIs among the Professional Middle Classes in 1911

To pursue this issue a little further, it is possible to examine in somewhat more detail a selection of marriages recorded at the 1911 census drawn from the professional upper and middle classes. This is the section of society that tended to delay marriage the most. It is also predominantly from this section of society that the variety of contemporary views on the nation's infertility, mentioned at the beginning of this chapter, emanated. These views included the concern that venereal diseases could be significantly implicated in the falling fertility of the nation and, according to some feminists and medical observers, that this was the case even in relation to the low fertility of their own privileged section of the nation. Can we now begin to quantify how much truth there may have been in this?

The official published reports on fertility emanating from the 1911 census tabulated an interesting range of information, which has for instance made possible the analysis of national average fertility rates of male occupations. However, the individual-level records that underlie the published tables have only since 2011 been digitized and made available for research in the form of the I-CeM database.[48] As a result, detailed parity-specific fertility information from the 1911 census can now for the first time be calculated for individual male occupations. Moreover, this occupation-specific fertility information derived from the I-CeM data can also be analyzed alongside a near-contemporary set of statistics on the prevalence of syphilis-related causes of death: namely part 4 of the decennial supplement to the seventy-fifth *Annual Report of the Registrar General* (*ARRG*). This official publication tabulated for a range of selected occupations the extent (age-standardized) to which men aged twenty-five to sixty-five died during the years 1910–12 from various causes of death, including the three most closely associated with a previous infection with syphilis: general paralysis of the insane (GPI), locomotor ataxy, and aneurysm.[49] Combining the two contemporaneous official sources, the 1911 census and this information from the death registers, enables the propensity to die from these three "parasyphilitic" causes of death to be directly related to patterns of childlessness for certain occupational groups.

In his presentation to the Royal Commission on Venereal Diseases (1913–16), drawing on the occupation-specific mortality figures later published in the seventy-fifth *ARRG*, T. H. C. Stevenson showed that the mostly professional males who composed Social Class I of the new official social classification scheme (which he devised for application to the 1911 fertility census[50]) died as a result of these syphilitic causes of death at a rate higher than the national average. Indeed, only the unskilled laboring class (Social Class V), at the other end of the social spectrum, recorded a significantly higher rate.[51]

A small set of five professional middle-class occupations identifiable in both the 1911 I-CeM census data and the tables of the seventy-fifth *ARRG* have been selected for further analysis here: clergy, barristers and solicitors (often combined as "lawyers" in the ensuing analysis because of the relatively small numbers of barristers), medical practitioners, and bankers.[52] These were chosen for their typicality as professions and for the variability they display in their recorded parasyphilitic causes of death (for further details on the provenance and construction of the professional groups, see appendix C).

Combining the available data from the seventy-fifth *ARRG*, Stevenson's evidence to the Royal Commission on Venereal Diseases 1913–16 (which also included deaths from "Syphilis" itself) and the estimates presented earlier in this chapter, table 12.2 shows the imputed chances of contracting gonorrhea by age thirty-five among the males of the four listed professional categories. The principal "translation" device here is that the absolute figure of 8.3 percent at the head of the second column, expressing the chance of contracting syphilis by age thirty-five (which is the previously published estimate by Szreter for Social Class I) and the ratio relationship between each of the figures for each individual occupation and the figure for Social Class I at the head of the first column, permits each of the occupations to be assigned a corresponding absolute value in the second column, bearing the same ratio relationship to the figure of 8.3 percent at the head of the second column as its corresponding figure in the first column bears to the figure of 26 at its head.[53] Table 12.2 demonstrates that Registrar General's Social Class I was far from being a homogeneous group in terms of the prevalence of STIs. While lawyers and bankers recorded levels substantially above the average for the class as a whole, the rate for physicians was around half of their rates and the rate for clergy, as might be expected, was significantly lower than the other selected occupations.

Table 12.2. Occupation-specific estimates of contracting gonorrhea

	Age-standardized mortality rate from parasyphilitic causes of death	**Accumulative chance of contracting syphilis by age 35 (%)**	**Accumulative chance of contracting gonorrhea by age 35 (%)**
Social Class I	26	8.3	33.2
Lawyers	31	9.9	39.5
Clergy	6	1.9	7.7
Physicians	16	5.1	20.4
Bankers	33	10.5	42.1

Note: The occupational specific figures cited in the first column are taken from column 11 of the main table of the supplement to the seventy-fifth *ARRG*: Registrar General, 1901–12, England and Wales Supplement to Registrar-General's Seventy-Fifth Annual Report: Part IV; Mortality of Men in Certain Occupations in the Three Years, 1910, 1911 and 1912, *Online Historical Population Reports*, 1901–12, accessed February 22, 2019, www.histpop.org, pp. 2–96. They are age-standardized rates of mortality that accurately express the relative extent to which different male occupational categories of the population died from the three parasyphilitic causes of death in the age range of 25–65 years old during the years 1910–12. The figures in themselves represent the number of deaths from these three causes combined that would have occurred if the occupational death rates recorded in 1910–12 had been operating on a sample of the general male population enumerated at the 1901 census, which had a particular age structure. The reason for standardizing on the 1901 age structure and not that of 1911 was that Stevenson was using this exercise to also compare occupational rates between 1900–1902 and 1910–12. It does not affect the validity of the comparative measures cited here for 1910–12, so long as they have all been standardized against the same population age structure. Using lawyers as an example, the figures for individual occupations in the second column of this table are calculated with reference to the figure of 8.3% at the top of the second column (for social class I as a whole) as follows: 8.3 × (31 / 26), producing the figure of 9.9% in this case. This is then multiplied by 4, reflecting the greater infectiousness of gonorrhea, to produce the figure of 33.2% in the third column. In contrast to the figures given in the first column, which are relative ratio figures, those in the two other columns are absolute measures.

Having established the estimated rates of contracting gonorrhea for each of the selected middle-class occupations shown in table 12.2, we can now turn to the proportion of marriages for each occupation producing zero live births to evaluate the evidence for a relationship between the two. However, before proceeding to that aspect of the analysis, we should first consider whether, or to what extent, there is evidence for an association between the chances by age thirty-five of each occupational category accumulating STI infections and the proportions of men remaining unmarried in their twenties and thirties in each occupation. Such a relationship would imply that the higher STI rates disproportionately afflicted the unmarried within each occupation and could not therefore be adduced as a necessary influence on marital sterility. That consideration is somewhat protracted and therefore is undertaken in appendix D, which finds no consistent evidence to support the hypothesis that STI infections before age thirty-five were confined disproportionately to the never-married sections of each of the professional occupations studied here.

Table 12.3 therefore shows for each of the selected professional occupations the proportion of marriages with no live births, by age at marriage of the wife (same marriage durations as table 12.1), relative to the comparable national figures for England and Wales in 1911; and the excess over the Trussel and Wilson adjusted (STI-free) estimates of sterility for English FRF parish populations as presented in table 12.1. Among the four categories of selected professional occupations, table 12.3 shows that the excess childlessness was over 50 percent greater than the national average of 39.8 percent among the professionals' modal female age-at-marriage group (wives marrying aged twenty-five to twenty-nine) and nearly twice as high specifically among the lawyers. The effect was even more pronounced where marriages had been contracted with relatively younger brides (aged twenty to twenty-four), and again this was marked particularly among lawyers. The excess was more muted—and little different from the national average—for marriages where the bride was relatively older (aged thirty to thirty-four). Overall, these findings confirm that the much greater proportions of childless marriages found in professional marriages indicate a more pronounced role for volitional causes than was the case in the general population. However, by contrast in the case of bankers marrying wives aged 30–34 very few marriages were childless because of birth control. Row 7A shows that almost three-quarters of the excess sterility among this older-marrying group was due to STIs.

Indeed, we know from table 12.2 that some of these professional occupations, notably lawyers and bankers, exhibited an incidence of parasyphilitic mortality about 25 percent higher than the national average, while physicians

Table 12.3. Sterility estimates, percentage excess over Trussel and Wilson's figures (in pre-1850 English parish populations) and proportion due to STIs in selected professional occupations by age of wife at marriage (completed marriages), 1911.

Row		Age at marriage		
		20–24	**25–29**	**30–34**
1	Clergy (% childless marriages)	9.1	13.6	22.2
2	Physicians (% childless marriages)	9.3	13.7	22.9
3	Lawyers (% childless marriages)	10.7	15.6	23.9
4	Bankers (% childless marriages)	7.8	13.5	18.2
	England and Wales 1911 % excess over Trussel and Wilson's STI-adjusted % zero parity (table 12.1, row 2)	40.0	39.8	43.1
5	Clergy: % excess over T&W STI-adjusted % zero	112.3	61.1	40.6
5A	Proportion of excess due to STIs	3.9%	3.6%	4.9%
6	Physicians: % excess over T&W STI-adjusted % zero	116.9	62.3	45.0
6A	Proportion of excess due to STIs	9.9%	9.4%	11.7%
7	Lawyers: % excess over T&W STI-adjusted % zero	149.6	84.8	51.4
7A	Proportion of excess due to STIs	14.9%	13.4%	19.9%
8	Bankers: % excess over T&W STI-adjusted % zero	81.9	60.0	15.3
8A	Proportion of excess due to STIs	29.1%	20.2%	71.6%

Source: The Integrated Census Microdata Project (I-CeM), http://doi.org/10.5255/UKDA-SN-7481-1

Note: England and Wales figures (between rows 4 and 5) taken from table 12.1, row 7. Figures in rows 5, 6, 7, 8 express rows 1–4 as excess values over those of table 12.1, row 2.

were roughly a third below this average, and clergy were way below the national average—by more than three-quarters. This points to very different sources of marital infertility among these professional occupations. Rows 5A, 6A, 7A, and 8A of table 12.3 show the proportion of sterile marriages in each five-year female age at marriage group attributable to each occupation's STI rates (shown in the third column of table 12.2). These estimates were calculated utilizing exactly the same method described above in detail on pages 380–87, which ultimately produced the figures in row 10 of table 12.3, but, of course, now using the relevant, occupation-specific STI figures. On the one hand, it seems that almost all of the high level of "excess sterility" among religious ministers and their wives was due only to deliberate fertility-restricting behavior (even though the clergy didn't marry quite so late as the other three professions). Among bankers in particular, although they tended to exhibit somewhat fewer sterile marriages than the other three professional categories, a larger proportion of the amount of childlessness that they did experience was due to the relatively high susceptibility of their occupation to STIs. Table 12.2 indicates that lawyers also contracted STIs at almost the same, relatively high, rates as bankers. But table 12.3 shows that, in addition to this, lawyers must also have practiced a much higher degree of volitional birth control than bankers, resulting in their significantly lower figures in row 7A, compared with row 8A.

Thus, the implications of the analysis in this chapter are thought-provoking in terms of wider theories concerning the springs and motivations of family limitation in this period. Table 12.3 indicates that the country's leaders of religious faith, widely regarded as the most stalwart objectors to atheistic contraptions of birth control, may have been among the most thoroughgoing family planners in the entire populace at this time. Putting these two characteristics together suggests a strong role for abstinence, especially in this section of society. On the other hand, very low fertility in the banking profession, supposed bastion of secular prudence, was due less to deliberate birth control and more to the risky behavior that resulted in STIs, particularly among those supposedly the most "prudential," who postponed marriage for longest.

The Hidden Affliction and the Quiet Revolution of Secular Fertility Decline

This exercise in the historical reconstruction of the scale of the hidden affliction of infertility due to venereal diseases in pre–Great War Britain has demonstrated the need for the impact of STIs to be taken into account when attempting to understand the scale and the incidence of extremely restricted fertility among married couples in the late nineteenth and early twentieth century. Table 12.1, row 10, indicates that among the vast majority of the population who married at one of the two most common female ages at marriage of twenty to twenty-four and twenty-five to twenty-nine years of age, STIs were in fact potentially responsible for over 45 percent of the excess number of childless marriages (relative to a population with no STIs). If, however, we focus on that section of the general population delaying marriage to a most unusual extent, where wives were aged thirty to thirty-four at marriage, STIs were responsible for a lower proportion of just over a quarter of the excess childless marriages, despite the fact that in absolute terms the chances of husbands entering marriage sterile, due to a previous infection with gonorrhea, were higher at this age than when they married younger. This study has confirmed therefore that the major role in the fertility decline was played by increasing volitional birth-controlling behavior. However, it is of importance to observe that, apart from the notable exception of bankers, such volitional control seems to have been generally positively correlated with delayed marriage as a closely associated form of behavior, which, as has been previously argued, indicates the likely importance of a regime of attempted abstinence from sexual intercourse within marriage, rather than the employment of contraceptive devices.[54]

Another conclusion from this exercise is that students of Britain's modern historical fertility decline need to pay far greater attention to involuntary sterility as a potentially contributory factor. The secular decline in national fertility rates has been referred to before as the silent or quiet revolution, in part signifying the acknowledged difficulty all students of the phenomenon have encountered when trying to offer convincing accounts for its causation that fully engage with all the evidence of social and geographic diversity.[55] It seems that one part of our collective difficulties may be due to the substantial but diverse role played by another dimension of historical silence—the "hidden affliction" of this book's title. Furthermore, the focus here, for simplicity's sake, has been only on the proportion of childlessness—zero parity marriages as reported at the 1911 census—that can be attributed to this form of involuntary infertility. In view of the phenomenon of "one-child sterility," particularly in relation to postpartum puerperal fever (which Irvine Loudon has found to have been particularly a problem afflicting upper- and middle-class women, who were disproportionately subject at their first births to the attendance of medical professionals lacking in proper antisepsis procedures), it seems likely that a considerable proportion of wives of professional men reporting having had a single birth, only, in 1911 would also be reporting the consequences of involuntary, rather than necessarily volitional, infertility.[56]

There is no reason to think that the importance of involuntary sources of infertility would only have been a feature of Britain's fertility decline, as the chapters in this volume on France and Germany in this period confirm. Though, as shown here, it is difficult rigorously and quantitatively to demonstrate the likely scale of effects involved, at least one French demographer has considered STIs and their infertility effects to have likely been of significance in accounting in part for France's low fertility throughout the modern period until the arrival of antibiotics in the 1940s.[57]

For the past one hundred years or so, studies by demographers and historians have almost completely discounted something that certain contemporaries, themselves drawn mostly from the professional middle classes, drew attention to and so feared. In their heightened state of concern, some contemporary feminists and medical specialists in the first two decades of the twentieth century undoubtedly overestimated the scale of effects due to syphilis and gonorrhea. However, the evidence presented in this chapter indicates that STIs—notably gonorrhea and chlamydia—probably did play a significant role in the secular fertility decline. This needs to be fully acknowledged and reintegrated into our efforts to understand this epochal transformation in the reproductive beliefs and behaviors of British society.

Appendixes

Appendix A: Trussel and Wilson's and E. A. Wrigley and Colleagues' Estimates of Sterility

There exist two different variants of published estimates of the sterility rates that can be derived from the FRFs of parish populations held by the Cambridge Group for the History of Population and Social Structure.[58] The difference between the two estimates is due to three independent sources of variation in the way they were each calculated, the first two of which have substantive effects. The Trussel and Wilson estimate was drawn from a different permutation of parishes from those used by Wrigley and colleagues, notably excluding the township of Birstall (over twice as large by 1789 as the next two largest parishes in the sample: Gainsborough and Banbury). Birstall was used in the more complex chronological grouping system by Wrigley and colleagues for the period 1600–1789. This is relevant, as it is the only parish that was both urban and fast growing across the eighteenth century, both factors likely to have raised the propensity of its population to suffer from STIs, relative to smaller and more stable rural or market-town communities.[59] Second, Trussel and Wilson based their calculations on all marriages, whereas Wrigley and colleagues based theirs on first-time marriages for both partners. Third, Trussel and Wilson experimented with a weighting device for allocating marriage ages within each quinquennium age of wife at marriage grouping—though they concluded from this exercise that "substantive results are unlikely to be affected."[60]

Despite the inclusion of Birstall, which might be supposed to inflate the proportion of sterile marriages in the Wrigley and colleagues series—if it is likely to have been a parish more prone to STIs than any other—it is the Trussel and Wilson estimates that produce significantly higher (by about

20 percent) proportions of sterility at all female ages at marriage, except the very oldest. This suggests that Trussel and Wilson's inclusion of all marriages may have admixed a certain amount of secondary sterility into their samples through the inclusion of widowers and, especially, widows (divorce in this period was virtually unknown outside the aristocracy), who may have already experienced pregnancy in previous marriages but who had since become sterile. This aspect of their calculations is fully acknowledged by Trussel and Wilson, and it was part of the aim of the subsequent work by Wrigley and colleagues, *English Population History from Family Reconstitution, 1580–1837*, to eliminate this influence.[61]

In a sense, the difference between the two sets of figures represents a more "pure" estimate of age-related biological sterility of couples in the case of Wrigley and colleagues' *English Population* estimates, whereas the Trussel and Wilson figures represent a schedule that includes the normal admixture of second and third marriages due to death or marital separation and remarriage that would be found in an actual population of the sort surveyed at the 1911 census, where the fertility questions related to the wife's current marriage, not to any previous marriages.

It has been concluded that, *provided* the combined effects of rates of spouse bereavement and marital separation were not dramatically different between those marrying in the seventeenth and eighteenth centuries and those marrying in the 1870s and 1880s, it is most justifiable to adopt the higher values of the schedule of rates of sterility published by Trussel and Wilson rather than the slightly lower "pure" estimates produced by Wrigley and colleagues, as being most appropriate for the specific comparative purposes of the exercise being conducted at this point in this chapter. This is to establish how much of the sterility found at the 1911 census among those marrying in the 1870s and 1880s can be attributed to voluntary limitation or to STIs. The conditions of this *proviso* seem to be met, in that while rates of spouse bereavement by 1911 would have been slightly lower for those marrying in the late Victorian decades (life expectancies were slightly higher on average than in the seventeenth and eighteenth centuries), this would have been offset by the fact that rates of marital separation were probably somewhat higher in the decades prior to 1911. Divorce remained rare, but from 1878 the Matrimonial Causes Act permitted magistrates courts to issue maintenance and separation orders, and by the 1900s there were about ten thousand per annum issued.[62]

Appendix B: Adjustments to the Trussel and Wilson Estimates of Sterility to Allow for the Influence of STIs

The likely scale of the contribution of STIs to the sterility rates found in the pre-1850 parish populations analyzed by Trussel and Wilson can be calculated as a derivative from the empirically based estimate that about 1.324 percent of the population of both sexes had probably been infected by syphilis by age thirty-five. There is direct evidence from the 1770s Chester Infirmary records that the two sexes were infected with pox at approximately equal rates, and this gender equality of incidence is broadly borne out also by Kevin Siena's study of the more extensive primary sources for London during the eighteenth century.[63] This indicates that the two sexes were also therefore approximately equally at risk to contract the much more infectious and potentially sterilizing STIs of gonorrhea and chlamydia. Gonorrhea has been found to be typically about four times more prevalent in populations lacking effective treatment for STIs, according to the most appropriate historical evidence available for making this comparison.[64] However, the modal age at marriage for both sexes during these centuries was approximately twenty-five years.[65] To calculate the likely general effect of STIs in accounting for sterile marriages, we therefore need to know the average chances at this time of contracting an STI by age twenty-five, not by age thirty-five. Fortunately, the research done on the Chester Infirmary registers can provide such an estimate, and this indicates that just under three-quarters of the overall chance of infection by age thirty-five in rural Cheshire and northeast Wales had occurred by age twenty-five.[66]

The precise working out of the estimates are as follows. It can be deduced from tables 7A and 7B of Szreter "Treatment Rates for the Pox" that those marrying at age twenty-five in Cheshire in the 1770s had a 73.28 percent chance of having contracted the pox relative to those aged thirty-five (this is the mean chance for both sexes combined), and so the estimated figure of 1.324 percent infection among the Trussel and Wilson English parish register population should be reduced to 0.970 percent (1.324 × 0.7328). Multiplied by 4 (to reflect the higher infectivity of gonorrhea), this equates to a 3.881 percent chance of infection with gonorrhea. Using the sex-differential formulas for the chances of this leading to sterility developed in the text of this chapter, a gonorrhea infection rate of 3.881 percent by age twenty-five implies that 0.19 percent of men would have entered marriage sterile (3.881 percent multiplied by a 4.9 percent chance of sterility). The female marital sterility rate due to STIs (including the effect of chlamydia) would have been 0.47 percent (3.881 percent multiplied by the 12.12 percent chance of sterility due to the sequlae of both diseases combined). This totals 0.66 percent, both sexes combined, thus reducing the Trussel and Wilson figure of 9.1 percent to 8.44 percent. The equivalent figures, adjusted by reference to the Chester schedule of the age incidence of pox exposure, can also be calculated in the same way for those marrying at twenty to twenty-four and thirty to thirty-four, producing estimates that the Trussel and Wilson figure of 4.6 percent sterile for those marrying wives at ages twenty to twenty-four would have been 4.287 percent in the absence of all STIs, and the figure of 16.6 percent for those marrying wives aged thirty to thirty-four would have been 15.79 percent.[67]

Appendix C: Constructing the Five Male Occupational Groups, Utilizing Both the 1911 Census I-CeM Data and the Seventy-Fifth *ARRG*.

Professionals are well-suited to this exercise as occupational identity tended not to change with age. Some 6,078 couples have been identified from the I-CeM database, where the husband was enumerated with one of the five selected professional occupations and where their wives were aged forty-five and over in 1911 and married at ages twenty to twenty-four, twenty-five to twenty-nine, and thirty to thirty-four, with a respective duration of marriage between twenty-five to twenty-nine, twenty to twenty-four, and fifteen to nineteen years, respectively (so as to ensure a completed fertility record).

The figure of 6,078 couples compares to that of 6,308 from the published table: Census of England and Wales, 1911, Vol. XIII: Fertility of Marriage, Part II (HMSO 1923), Cd 8491, Table 35. Marriages where the wife's age exceeded 45 years at census. Families and mortality therein, classified by occupation of the husband, duration of marriage, and age of wife at marriage (100–102, 108). There are multiple reasons why a discrepancy between what might be called the "observed" (the aggregate figure of the published 1911 census reports) and the "expected" (the figures calculated from the I-CeM database) will occur. First, some of the records of the original census manuscript appear to have been lost and are therefore not in the digital version; hence the population of England and Wales is reported in the published census as 36,070,492, while the comparable I-CeM figure is 36,031,749. Second, the original census document was handwritten, and because this is the first British census for which the householders' schedules themselves form the "original" census record, rather than a set of officially compiled census enumerators' books, the handwriting varies with each household and can sometimes be difficult to interpret. Thus, even though every best effort was taken to minimize "error" in the transcription, differences of interpretation will inevitably occur. Detailed checking of the data by hand, including verification against the original census records, confirmed that the transcription of the Hollerith occupation code (a three-digit number written in green ink by officials against each married male householder to assign the marriage's fertility to a single officially defined occupation) was extremely accurate. Given that the I-CeM project coded the occupation textual strings (derived directly from the written statement by the householder on the census document itself), independently of the assigned Hollerith code, a detailed check on this type of transcription error was undertaken and mistranscribed codes corrected (and miscoded occupations also corrected). The fertility information itself (number of years married, number of children ever born, number of children died, and number of children still living) can be cross-correlated. The Census Office eliminated 122,286 couples from the total of 6,136,605 from their analyses on the basis of invalid information, rejecting some 2 percent of all couple records.[68] For the I-CeM data this rejection rate is higher (4.01 percent), due largely to cases where the transcribers left blank the "years married" answer on the original schedule. Thus, it is impossible to replicate the figures published in the census tables precisely. However, more important is not the shortfall of valid fertility records but rather if those that are "missing" display significantly different fertility histories to the valid "observed" records. In this regard the difference is extremely slight: an observed number of births per couple of 2.93 against an expected 2.95. This, alongside all the manual checking on the records analyzed here, indicates that there is no evidence to suggest a substantial parity-specific bias of the sort that would invalidate the analyses of this chapter.

To these 6,078 couples it was necessary to add a further 627 couples. This is because the total numbers of deaths recorded in the seventy-fifth *ARRG*, which is being used here for the parasyphilitic death rates it reveals, were usually classified by the individual's *previous* occupation if he died postretirement (or out of work).[69] Thus, those from the selected occupations but identified as retired in the I-CeM database by self-attribution—many of whom were considerably less than age sixty-five—were also included in the analysis here to ensure comparability between the two sources. Aggregating the retired and active together is also important since, as table 12.4 illustrates, the retired exhibit a disproportionate tendency to childless marriages. In each of the selected occupations, the retired subset record both lower births per couple and higher percentage zero parity than their "active" counterparts, a tendency especially marked in the case of both lawyers (barristers and solicitors combined) and physicians.

Table 12.4. Children born per couple and parity among selected occupations: retired and active.

			Active			Retired			Difference	
Occupation	**Age of wife at marriage**	**Duration of marriage**	**Births per couple**	**% of couples with no births**	**Couples (n)**	**Births per couple**	**% of couples with no births**	**Couples (n)**	**Births per couple**	**% of couples with no births**
Bankers	20–24	25–29	3.60	7.4	367	3.52	10.3	126	-0.08	3.0
	25–29	20–24	2.51	13.0	539	2.28	17.1	111	-0.23	4.1
	30–34	15–19	1.99	18.2	231	1.41	40.5	37	-0.58	22.4
Clergy	20–24	25–29	4.17	8.8	772	3.28	19.4	36	-0.89	10.6
	25–29	20–24	3.16	13.3	992	1.73	34.6	26	-1.43	21.3
	30–34	15–19	2.24	22.2	640	1.36	21.4	14	-0.88	-0.8
Lawyers	20–24	25–29	3.42	10.1	436	2.84	18.8	64	-0.58	8.7
	25–29	20–24	2.68	13.7	526	1.73	45.5	66	-0.95	31.8
	30–34	15–19	1.92	23.9	284	1.57	23.8	21	-0.35	-0.1
Surgeons	20–24	25–29	3.60	7.4	367	2.31	31.3	48	-1.29	23.9
	25–29	20–24	2.51	13.0	540	2.10	23.8	63	-0.41	10.9
	30–34	15–19	1.99	22.9	384	1.67	26.7	15	-0.32	3.8
Bankers			2.76	12.3	1137	2.73	17.2	274	-0.02	4.9
Clergy			3.24	14.2	2404	2.40	25.0	76	-2.38	4.0
Lawyers			2.76	14.8	1246	2.18	31.1	151	-0.59	16.4
Surgeons			2.67	14.3	1291	2.13	27.0	126	-0.54	12.7

Source: The Integrated Census Microdata Project (I-CeM), http://doi.org/10.5255/UKDA-SN-7481-1

The association with sterility among those retiring relatively young could be due to various factors, none of which are mutually exclusive: selection for poor health generally or for the specific ill-effects on health as well as fertility of STIs; it could also be partly a reverse social selection effect that those restricting their fertility most rigorously—either voluntarily or involuntarily—could afford to retire relatively early. In relation to this latter point, it is also the case that the selected occupations we are studying exhibit greatly varying propensities to retire, as shown in table 12.5. Bankers, many of whom may have had a company superannuation policy, retired earlier and almost universally by age seventy. In contrast, clergy, the majority of whom would not have had any formal pension, seldom retired.[70] Three-quarters of lawyers and nearly two-thirds of physicians were still recorded as active at age sixty-five, yet it may have been that many of these were in reality part-time or practiced only when they wished to. Overall, these patterns and considerations tend to suggest the predominance of social, over morbidity, factors in the decision to retire.

Table 12.5. Proportions retired by age for selected occupational categories

	Percentage retired by age			
Age	**Bankers**	**Lawyers**	**Clergy**	**Physicians**
55	18	13	3	7
60	43	16	3	26
65	75	24	13	36
70	90	35	16	40

Source: The Integrated Census Microdata Project (I-CeM), http://doi.org/10.5255/UKDA-SN-7481-1

Note: These figures are based on the couples where wives were aged 45 and over in 1911 and married at ages 20–24, 25–29, and 30–34, with respective durations of marriage 25–29, 20–24, and 15–19 years.

Appendix D: Evaluation of the Possible Effect of Differences in Marital Status among Males Pursuing Professional Occupations on STI Rates by Age Thirty-Five

Before the widely differing occupational rates of implied infection with syphilis recorded in the supplement to the seventy-fifth *ARRG* can be confidently assigned any possible influence over marital fertility patterns through derivative estimates of STI infection by age thirty-five, it is first necessary to consider the possible effect due to the fact that these rates published in the seventy-fifth *ARRG* refer to married, widowed, and never-married men pursuing these various occupations. Unless only very small proportions of men pursuing these occupations never married, it is theoretically possible that a disproportionate number of those recorded in the nation's death registers as dying from parasyphilitic causes were drawn from among the unmarried in each occupation. This could be either because having knowledge of a prior infection deterred them from entering marriage or because it was those men within each occupation who had either failed or opted not to marry who were most at risk to contract an STI, if for instance it was the case that they were more likely, on average, to be exposed to the risks that followed from engaging in commercial sex than were married men.

While there is no directly relevant evidence with which to evaluate this possibility systematically (since the death registers of England and Wales cannot be searched systematically, unlike those of Scotland), it is nevertheless possible to assess this factor indirectly with evidence from the I-CeM database, from which can be derived statistics of the extent to which men pursuing these occupations in 1911 remained unmarried at different ages. Utilizing the I-CeM database, table 12.6 confirms that men in all these professional occupations tended to be significantly less likely to be married than the national average at all ages in 1911. The second row of table 12.6 shows that just over 50 percent of men had married before age thirty in the general population, as against less than 25 percent in these professional occupations. Just over three-quarters of men aged thirty to thirty-nine in the general population at the 1911 census were ever married, whereas this was the case for only five out of eight of these professional men. However, part of this is clearly related to the distinctive and different age distribution of men recorded in professional occupations at the census as can be seen by comparing columns (h) and (j). There were barely half the proportion of these occupations' totals engaged in their professional occupations at age twenty to twenty-four, compared to the national average (8 percent as against 14.6 percent) and still about one-fifth less at ages twenty-five to twenty-nine.

Furthermore, the detail on display in table 12.6 offers no evidence of a consistent correlation among these four occupational categories in this respect, particularly where the two most important age groups, twenty-five to twenty-nine and thirty to thirty-nine, are concerned. These two age groups are the most important, partly because, unlike ages twenty to twenty-four or higher ages above age thirty-nine, they each contain proportionately the largest number of individuals (11.8 percent per five-year age group) as can be seen from column (h). Second, and even more important, the differential behavior of older age-at-marriage groups cannot have exerted influence on

Table 12.6. Proportions of ever-married males by age in selected professional occupations and England and Wales, 1911.

(a)	(b)	(c)	(d)	(e)	(f)	(g)	(h)	(j)
		Proportions of ever-married men by age group					Age distribution (%)	
Age	All England and Wales	Bankers	Lawyers	Physicians	Clergy	Four professions combined	Four professions combined	England and Wales
20–24	14.6	2.0	4.9	3.2	5.3	2.3	8.0	14.6
25–29	50.8	24.1	22.1	22.0	19.5	22.6	11.8	14.2
30–39	76.9	62.5	59.1	62.9	64.5	62.5	23.6	25.7
40–49	86.0	79.2	78.6	82.0	81.2	80.5	22.8	19.5
50–59	89.2	83.4	83.2	87.0	86.9	85.4	17.4	13.4
60–69	90.4	88.9	85.7	90.1	90.3	89.1	10.5	8.3
70–79	92.0	92.5	89.0	89.7	91.2	90.9	4.7	3.6
80+	93.0	96.8	90.1	91.4	92.0	92.7	1.3	0.8

Source: The Integrated Census Microdata Project (I-CeM), http://doi.org/10.5255/UKDA-SN-7481-1

Note: Columns (h) and (j) each sum to 100 percent and give the percentage size of each male age group for the four professional categories combined (h) and for all men in England and Wales (j), regardless of marital status (ever married and never married combined).

the chances of acquiring a syphilitic infection by age thirty-five, which is the key "dependent variable" in this discussion of whether marriage propensities could have influenced STI differentials. At ages twenty-five to twenty-nine, it is in fact the clergy who are the least likely to be married, and the bankers who are most likely to be married among these professional occupations; yet they are at the opposite extremes in table 12.2, with bankers over five times more prone to have had a syphilitic infection by age thirty-five than clergy. The marriage patterns at the second most important age range, age thirty to thirty-nine, are also far from convincing in differentiating these four occupational categories according to their propensity to die from para-syphilitic causes of death. Bankers exhibit exactly the average proportion of unmarried men among this set of four professional categories, very similar to that of doctors, even though bankers' STI rate was the highest and over twice as high as doctors. At this age group it is the lawyers who are least likely to be married, rather than the bankers, yet table 12.2 shows that it was the latter who had a somewhat higher likelihood of contracting syphilis by age thirty-five. It is concluded therefore that there is no evidence here of a systematic relationship among these professional occupational categories between proportions of males remaining unmarried and propensities to die from syphilitic causes of death.

Appendix E: Considerations in Setting an Estimate for the Extent of Additional Marital Infertility Due to Chlamydia in Populations in England and Wales prior to 1914

A major review of 2013 that provides an international survey of eighty clinical epidemiological studies—including many conducted in India and other countries where population health and lack of comprehensive health service conditions are somewhat more akin to those prevailing in Britain's past before 1914 than can be the case for studies conducted among the populations of the OECD countries today—concludes, "Chlamydial PID is the single most important preventable cause of infertility. Approximately, three per cent of women with chlamydial genital tract infection develop infertility."[71]

However, the most rigorous attempt to evaluate the relationship between chlamydia infection and infertility in the British population today has produced a much lower overall headline figure, finding that the chance of a single chlamydia infection, either symptomatic or not, resulting in PID is as high as 17.1 percent but that only one in thirty-four infections (0.51 percent) then result in sterility (TFI).[72] This is of course a far lower rate of progression from PID to sterilization than the three in ten chance from a gonorrheal PID episode found in the Lund cohort study 1964–88, cited in the chapter's main text. But note the following point about the enhanced effectiveness of treatment for PID in the United Kingdom today, compared with Swedish populations recruited from the mid-1960s onward, which is partly contributing to this much lower progression rate. There are additionally a number of other important considerations, which need to be taken into account when comparing this 0.51 percent figure with the 3 percent figure from the 2013 international survey and when assessing these different estimates as a guide to likely sterility outcomes in pre-1914 British populations—which perhaps suggest that they are not quite as far apart as they may initially seem.

First, while the 0.51 percent estimate did, very helpfully, take into account the absence of treatment for the 76 percent of cases estimated to be asymptomatic, it should be mechanically inflated when applied to a pre-1914 populace to allow for the 24 percent of symptomatic cases in the contemporary United Kingdom that did receive treatment before the onset of PID. Therefore, for comparability to a pre-1914 population, the 0.51 percent figure should be adjusted upward by 31.58 percent (24/76) to a value of 0.671 percent. Second, this figure relates to a population enjoying modern Western treatment even before onset of PID. The authors estimate that 42 percent of all PID is in fact diagnosed and treated in the general population today before it can progress to TFI. The Lund study showed that women treated for TFI within three days of diagnosis had a 280 percent reduction in their risk of infertility, indicating that the complete absence of treatment for chlamydia in the pre-1914 population must have very significantly raised—indeed multiplied by a factor of about 2.8—the 0.671 percent figure, which is derived from modern populations generally receiving extensive treatment. This produces a figure in the region of 1.88 percent.

Third, a range of untreated coinfections, most notably gonorrhea itself but also the many other STI and non-STI conditions suffered by the pre-1914 populations, are likely to have exerted an additional multiplicative risk on the chance of any single chlamydia infection resulting in both PID and TFI, though exact research findings on the statistical scale of these effects are lacking.

Fourth, in an entirely untreated population of married couples, which is the focus of this chapter's analysis, it is not at all clear that infection with chlamydia can be treated as a sequence of discrete events, as has been possible in the contemporary methodology used by Malcolm Price and colleagues, and which is indeed fundamental to the way in which its findings are presented. With no treatment available to either partner, the risks of female infection leading to sterility in such circumstances are more akin to a compounded sequence of several infectious events, within the terminology of the Price and colleagues' study, "The Natural History of Chlamydia trachomatis." In these circumstances a woman exposed to unrestricted sex with a *C. trachoma*–positive partner (who would not have known of his typically asymptomatic condition relating to a disease at that time unknown) is most likely to have been exposed to an excess risk of the infection progressing to salpingitis and TFI for one of two reasons, according to the current models of the different processes that lead to variability in individual susceptibility to TFI, reviewed by Shruti Menon and colleagues.[73] One possibility is that such women would have been susceptible to a relatively rapid onset form of PID due to accumulating a high vaginal loading with multiple chlamydial inoculations from their individual partner before any immunity had developed in their own bodies and would then be at a high risk of developing PID once the immune response did react strongly to this high load (the tissue damage that causes PID and ultimately TFI is a byproduct of the body's immune response to the presence of chlamydia). Another possibility is that chlamydia can also produce PID from a more indolent pattern of repeat reinfection over a prolonged period due to a chlamydia-positive male partner in a stable relationship, since it has been shown in 2017 that male asymptomatic chlamydia infections can persist for over two years if untreated.[74] Katy Turner and colleagues have shown that, even with the levels of treatment available today, partners are chlamydia-positive in 60 percent of cases.[75]

In the present state of research, these factors are not amenable to calibrating in mathematical form to offer precise adjustments to the figure of 0.671 percent or that of 1.88 percent, but it is clear that they each have the effect of significantly increasing that figure and so indicate far less discrepancy with the figure of 3 percent offered in the 2013 international review than would appear to be the case at first sight. Consequently, the empirically based figure of 3 percent, equal to almost exactly one-third of the female infertility rate attributed to untreated gonorrhea, is adopted here as probably an appropriate approximation, in the current state of knowledge, of the risks of female sterility that applied in the epidemiological and health care conditions prevailing among the British married populations at any time before the Great War, when general disease and bodily hygiene conditions were so different than they are today among early twenty-first-century OECD populations.

Notes

1. Richard Soloway, *Birth Control and the Population Question in England, 1877–1930* (Chapel Hill: University of North Carolina Press, 1982); Susan Kent, *Sex and Suffrage in Britain, 1860–1914* (Princeton: Princeton University Press, 1987); Timothy Jones, *Sexual Politics in the Church of England, 1857–1957* (Oxford: Oxford University Press, 2013), esp. chap. 5.

2. For a pioneering medical and scientific examination of these issues, see James Matthews Duncan, *Fecundity, Fertility, Sterility and Allied Topics* (Edinburgh: A and C. Black, 1866; rev. ed. 1871).

3. Émile Zola's 1885 novel, *Germinal*, is of course a celebrated literary example, and see Fabrice Cahen and Adrien Minard, chap. 11, in this volume, on persistent French fears. On relevant literature in Britain, see Angelique Richardson, *Love and Eugenics in the Late Nineteenth Century: Rational Reproduction and the New Woman* (Oxford: Oxford University Press, 2003).

4. The literature is legion. For an early highly relevant contribution, see William Bynum, "Darwin and the Doctors: Evolution, Diathesis, and Germs in Nineteenth-Century Britain," *Gesnerus* 40 (1983): 43–53; for an overview, see Peter Bowler, *Evolution: The History of an Idea*, 3rd ed. (Berkeley: University of California, 2003); on germ theory, see Michael Worboys, *Spreading Germs: Disease Theories and Medical Practice in Britain, 1865–1900* (Cambridge: Cambridge University Press, 2000).

5. Louisa Martindale's *Under the Surface* (London: National Union of Women's Suffrage Societies, 1908) may have been the first to do so. See Lucy Bland, "Marriage Laid Bare: Middle-Class Women and Marital Sex, c. 1800–1914," in *Labour and Love: Women's Experience of Home and Family, 1850–1940*, ed. Jane Lewis (Oxford: Basil Blackwell, 1986), 123–46; and, more generally, Bland, *Banishing the Beast: English Feminism and Sexual Morality, 1885–1914* (London: Penguin Books, 1995).

6. On the first and the third of these inquiries, see Simon Szreter, *Fertility, Class and Gender in Britain, 1860–1940* (Cambridge: Cambridge University Press, 1996), chaps. 4, 5; on the second, see Harvey Simmons, "Explaining Social Policy: The English Mental Deficiency Act of 1913," *Journal of Social History* 11, (1978): 387–403; and Leon Radzinowicz and Roger Hood, *The Emergence of Penal Policy in Victorian and Edwardian England* (Oxford: Clarendon, 1990); on the fourth, see John M. Eyler, *Sir Arthur Newsholme and State Medicine 1885–1935* (Cambridge: Cambridge University Press, 1997), 277–94. The Royal Commission on the Poor Laws, 1905–9 and the Royal Commission on Divorce and Matrimonial Causes of 1909–12 were also major inquiries hearing relevant evidence. On the former, see Alan Marne McBriar, *Edwardian Mixed Doubles: The Bosanquets Versus the Webbs, a Study in British Social Policy, 1890–1929* (Oxford: Clarendon, 1987); on the latter, see Lucy Owen, "Divorce: 'Disease or Remedy'? Medical Witnesses before the Royal Commission on Divorce and Matrimonial Causes, 1900–1912" (PhD diss., University of Oxford, 1996).

7. Simon Szreter, "The Prevalence of Syphilis in England and Wales on the Eve of the Great War: Re-visiting the Estimates of the Royal Commission on Venereal Diseases, 1913–1916," *Social History of Medicine* 27 (2014): 508–29.

8. For instance, see Daniel Pick, *Faces of Degeneration: Aspects of a European Disorder c. 1848–c. 1918* (Cambridge: Cambridge University Press, 1989); and Richard Soloway, *Demography and Degeneration: Eugenics and the Declining Birthrate in Twentieth-Century Britain* (Chapel Hill: University of North Carolina Press, 1990).

9. See also Simon Szreter, "Fertility Transitions and Sexually Transmitted Infections," in *Reproduction: Antiquity to the Present Day*, ed. Nick Hopwood, Rebecca Flemming, and Lauren Kasssel (Cambridge: Cambridge University Press, 2018), 443–56; and Tim Bayliss-Smith, chap. 6; Roy Scragg, chap. 7; and Shane Doyle, chap. 8, all in this volume. On interwar claims in regard to black US Americans, see Stewart E. Tolnay, "A New Look at the Effect of Venereal Disease on Black Fertility: The Deep South in 1940," *Demography* 26 (1989): 679–90, 679.

10. Owen, "Divorce"; Kent, *Sex and Suffrage*.

11. Joseph Banks, *Victorian Values: Secularism and the Size of Families* (London: Routledge, 1981), esp. chap. 3.

12. Arguably, it was the eugenicists and their claims that resulted in the interdepartmental inquiry of 1904 and—following from its conclusions—the 1911 census inquiry and the Royal Commission on the Feeble-Minded of 1904–9. See Szreter, *Fertility, Class and Gender*, 238–82.

13. Michael Worboys, "Unsexing Gonorrhoea: Bacteriologists, Gynaecologists, and Suffragists in Britain, 1860–1920," *Social History of Medicine* 17 (2004): 41–59.

14. Juliet Hurn, "History of General Paralysis of the Insane in Britain, 1830 to 1950" (PhD diss., University of London, 1998); Sharon Matthews, "Matter over Mind: The Contributions of the Neuropathologist Sir Frederick Mott to British Psychiatry, 1895–1926" (PhD diss., University of Manchester, 2006).

15. Census of England and Wales, 1911, Vol. XIII: Fertility of Marriage, Part II (HMSO 1923), Cd 8491, xix–xlvii.

16. T. H. C. Stevenson, "The Laws Governing Population," *Journal of the Royal Statistical Society* 88 (1925): 63–90; Stevenson, "The Vital Statistics of Wealth and Poverty," *Journal of the Royal Statistical Society* 91 (1928): 207–30.

17. For a review of this literature, see Szreter, *Fertility, Class and Gender*, 9–66. See Cahen and Minard, chap. 11, in this volume, for a discussion of a similar trajectory toward a scientific consensus to focus exclusively on volitional forms of birth control among demographers in France.

18. There is one partial exception to this statement, which is a series of studies by US demographers in the 1970s and 1980s with the specific aim of estimating what proportion of the recorded fall in black fertility in the United States, circa 1880–1940, could be attributed to the impact of gonorrhea and syphilis. Commencing with Reynolds Farley, *Growth of the Black Population: A Study of Demographic Trends* (Chicago: Markham, 1970) and including Joseph McFalls and Marguerite McFalls,

Disease and Fertility (Orlando: Academic Press, 1984), chap. 19, this culminated in the multivariate statistical treatment by Tolnay, "New Look," in 1989. However, all these studies assumed in common a relatively low level of STIs at the baseline date in the 1880s, without offering any sound reason or evidence for making such an implausible assumption.

19. Prince A. Morrow, *Social Disease and Marriage: Social Prophylaxis* (New York: Lea Brothers, 1904), 106. Morrow also referred to "the expressive German phrase *ein kinde sterilität*" (sic). While *Einkindsterilität* was, indeed, associated with gonorrhea, it was also associated with other sequlae and infections following a first birth, notably puerpereal fever, all of which were also subsumed under the terms "secondary sterility" and "acquired sterility"—for instance, in the discussion in Enoch Heinrich Kisch, *Die Sterilität des Weibes*, 2nd ed. (Vienna: Urban und Schwarzenberg, 1895), 302–4. A subsequent 1910 summary in an authoritative German handbook for medical students pointed out that, while an infection with gonorrhea did not necessarily lead to sterility, as was proven by the gonorrheal eye infections of newborns, the opportunity for gonococci to ascend beyond the cervix in the postpartum period when lochia was produced could result in *Einkindsterilität*; and this was something that could also be provoked by unwise medical "interference" in the postpartum period (an oblique reference to other dangers, such as puerperal fever). Albert Döderlein, "Die Gonorrhoischen Erkrankungen der Weiblichen Geschlechtsorgane," in *Kurzes Lehrbuch der Gynäkologie*, ed. Otto Küstner, 4th ed. (Jena: Fischer, 1910), 436 and 443. We are grateful to Christina Benninghaus for information on these German sources (pers. email comm., February 2, 2019). The exact way in which, in women who had never had a birth, gonorrhea so often gained access from the cervical area to the fallopian tubes, without typically infecting the intervening endometrium, continued to puzzle medicine for decades. In his subsequent handbook, Pelouze cogently argued that since it could be shown that blood commonly retrofluxes through the fallopian tubes at menstruation, that this would carry the gonococcus upwards within the uterine system, explaining why salpingitis could be common even in 'nulliparae' women who had never given birth. Percy S. Pelouze, *Gonorrhea in the Male and Female: A Book for Practitioners*, 3rd ed. (Philadelphia: Saunders, 1941), 313–25.

20. Michael Anderson, "Highly Restricted Fertility: Very Small Families in the British Fertility Decline," *Population Studies* 52 (1998): 177–99, 193, 196. Anderson has returned to this theme but has not presented any substantial body of additional literature from the pre–Great War period: Michael Anderson, *Scotland's Populations: From the 1850s to Today* (Oxford: Oxford University Press, 2018), 292–93. He has added a citation from Beatrice Webb expressing conflicted attitudes about childlessness, though of course in her own case she did not marry Sidney Webb until she was thirty-four, following a long, unconsummated infatuation with Joseph Chamberlain: Pat Jalland, *Women, Marriage and Politics, 1860–1914* (Oxford: Oxford University Press, 1986), 221. As has been noted, as late as 1938, a whole generation later, there was still active concern being expressed in the *British Medical Journal* over

the undesirability of forms of contraception resulting in the possibility of sterility of marriage; see Caroline Rusterholz, "Testing the Gräfenberg Ring in Interwar Britain: Norman Haire, Helena Wright, and the Debate over Statistical Evidence, Side Effects, and Intra-uterine Contraception," *Journal of the History of Medicine and Allied Sciences* 72 (2017): 448–67, who shows that the concern that contraception could lead to sterility was still common in medical circles at that time, citing the debate in the *British Medical Journal* in 1938 between George H. Alabaster, Joan Malleson, and Margaret C. N. Jackson.

21. Szreter, "The Prevalence," 525, tables 2, 3.

22. The Cambridge Group's parish family reconstitution files are described in full and extensively analyzed in E. A. Wrigley et al., *English Population History from Family Reconstitution, 1580–1837* (Cambridge: Cambridge University Press, 1997). See also Simon Szreter, "Treatment Rates for the Pox in Early Modern England: A Comparative Estimate of the Prevalence of Syphilis in the City of Chester and Its Rural Vicinity in the 1770s," *Continuity and Change* 32 (2017): 1–41.

23. There is no known information for ascertaining age at first sexual intercourse for men in this period, beyond that of the age at marriage. The assumption made here is consistent with the findings of the first relevant national survey, which was conducted by interview in 1990–91 and which found that the oldest males interviewed (aged forty-five to fifty-nine, born 1931–45 and therefore nineteen years old between 1950 and 1964) had a median age at first intercourse of nineteen years (a figure that fell a further two years to age seventeen among those aged sixteen to thirty-four at the time of the interviews); see Kaye Wellings et al., *Sexual Behaviour in Britain: The National Survey of Sexual Attitudes and Lifestyles* (London: Penguin, 1994), 41, table 2.2. Median age at first intercourse for men born five decades earlier, 1881–95, is extremely likely to have been several years older than nineteen, since the historically low illegitimacy rates in the Edwardian period indicate that for most of the population premarital intercourse was not an extensive practice and the average male age at marriage was as high as twenty-seven years. It was the period 1945–60 that witnessed a sharp rise in the proportion of younger men (age twenty to twenty-four) entering marriage; see B. Jane Elliott, "Demographic Trends in Domestic Life," in *Marriage, Domestic Life and Social Change*, ed. David Clark (London: Routledge, 1991), 85–108, fig. 4.2a. There is no evidence for a widespread norm of sexual initiation for young men before marriage with commercial sex workers, as appears to have been the case in France (see Cahen and Minard, chap. 11, in this volume). Clearly, this was a distinct possibility for some young men, despite the lack of social approval for it, and certainly studies both of prostitution and of the military in this period indicate that such premarital sexual activity did occur at least in these sections of the population, though it remains too opaque to evaluate its quantitative extent; see Julia Laite, *Common Prostitutes and Ordinary Citizens: Commercial Sex in London, 1885–1960* (Basingstoke: Palgrave Macmillan, 2011); and Alan Skelley, *The Victorian Army at Home: The Recruitment and Terms and Conditions of the British Regular, 1859–1899* (London: Croom Helm, 1977).

The assumption made here that the male risk of contracting STIs began on average from age twenty onward (initially, of course, at age twenty, relating to only a fraction of the male population, and thereafter growing in numbers year by year) is made in light of the knowledge that it is approximately six years before the average male age at marriage at this time and five years after the minimum age for entering service in the Royal Navy, with entry in the army supposed to be age eighteen minimum, while entry into the merchant navy was less regulated and could be even younger. Of course, in the absence of national service or conscription, these age markers for military service apply only to minorities of the population, not to all young men, as in some continental European populations at this time.

24. For the Swedish data for 1918–19, see Gunnar Dahlberg, "Venereal Diseases in Sweden, 1913 to 1937," *American Journal of Hygiene* 33 (1941): 51–63, sec. A, table 1 and Szreter, "Prevalence," pp.526–27, including notes 77, 78, and 79. These two years are most comparable in the sense that salvarsan treatments had not yet become a widespread practice among any populace and so would not have affected the relative incidence of syphilis. McFalls and McFalls, *Disease and Fertility*, 473, argues that the number of persons infected with gonorrhea, relative to syphilis, might be only half the four to one observed infection rates, because people could be infected multiple times with gonorrhea, and only once with syphilis. However, this fails to acknowledge the massive under-reporting of gonorrhea because it is asymptomatic in 75 percent of female and 45 percent of males: Richard Pattman et al., eds., *Oxford Handbook of Genitourinary Medicine, HIV, and Sexual Health*, 2nd ed. (Oxford: Oxford University Press, 2010), 150. Previously Szreter, "The Prevalence," p. 528, suggested a rate of male gonorrhea 3.25 times the syphilis rate. However, given the scale of asymptomatic gonorrhea, this would more than offset any multiple visits in the Swedish data (it appears no record was kept of this) and so we propose here a fourfold ratio.

25. This assumption is conservative for at least two reasons. First, it would have been possible for husbands and wives in a number of cases to keep reinfecting each other for a time with a gonorrhea (or chlamydia) infection originally brought into the marriage by the husband. Second, some husbands, and indeed some wives, would have engaged in commercial or adulterous extramarital sex after marriage. Both these factors are potential sources for increasing the risks of STI infection, relative to the estimates offered here. They are being deliberately ignored, partly for lack of reliable quantifiable evidence in either case, partly for the sake of simplicity of the model, and partly to ensure the estimates offered here of the impact of STIs on sterility remain conservative, minimal estimates.

26. These estimates are extremely simplified but, overall, robust. Strictly speaking, the empirical pattern of male ages at marriage should be taken into account. For men in England and Wales at this time the average age at first marriage was approximately twenty-seven years, a figure that falls exactly halfway between age twenty and age thirty-four. This means that halving the 10.4 percent estimate down to 5.2 percent for men marrying at age twenty to twenty-four will produce a significant

underestimate of their risks of sterility, since more than half of them were unmarried at all these ages. The figure for age twenty-five to twenty-nine would also be a (more moderate) underestimate, since it also incorporates the underestimate for ages twenty to twenty-four within its construction. The half-and-half assumption (married, unmarried) is a reasonably accurate assumption for this age group, twenty-five to twenty-nine, which evenly straddles the average male marriage age figure of twenty-seven years. Finally, the figure for age thirty to thirty-four would appear to be something of an overestimate, since a majority of men would have been married in this age range, as it is entirely above the national average age at marriage. However, this overestimation effect is partly offset by several factors. First, arithmetically, it also incorporates, as components of its 26 percent figure, both the underestimated figures for ages twenty to twenty-four and twenty-five to twenty-nine. Second, it is more likely that the remaining minority of men delaying their marriages into their thirties would have been greater users of commercial sex than men who married at younger ages, and the chances of any individual becoming infertile was a function of the accumulating absolute number of times they were exposed to a possible gonorrhea infection, not the relative number of exposures per unit of time. Third, although the male singulate mean age-at-marriage average was twenty-seven, a very considerable proportion of those aged thirty to thirty-four were still unmarried, probably at least 25 percent. This is a guesstimate, but it is informed by the fact that we do know that even when they were fifteen to twenty years older, as many as 11.66 percent of men forty-five to fifty-four years old were recorded as still never married at the 1911 census.

A robust estimate of the national average male singulate mean age at marriage (SMAM) can be derived from the data for the slightly over two thousand subregistration districts published on the Cambridge Group's atlas website: "Populations Past: Atlas of Victorian and Edwardian Population," University of Cambridge, accessed February 22, 2019, www.populationspast.org. For the two most relevant dates, the census years of 1891 and 1901, this data produces an overall national average (summing the singulate mean age at marriage values for each Registration Sub-District and weighting them by their population sizes) of 26.96 for 1891 and 27.22 for 1901. The same weighting procedure was used to produce the estimate of 11.6 percent males never married at age forty-five to fifty-four in 1911.

27. A clinical review from 2012 concludes, "Major problems for male fertility may arise particularly in patients with epididymitis as this disease appears to have a greater influence on semen quality and male fertility than an infection/inflammation of the prostate or seminal vesicle. In addition, in quite a number of patients, the diagnosis of chronic epididymitis is extremely difficult as these patients do not feel discomfort and their health is not compromised. Due to a silent nature of the infection/inflammation, epididymitis will only be diagnosed once these patients appear in an andrological clinic consulting for infertility." See Ralf Henkel, "Infection in Infertility," in *Male Infertility: Contemporary Clinical Approaches, Andrology, ART and*

Antioxidants, ed. Sijo J. Parekattil and Ashok Agarwal (New York: Springer Science + Business Media, 2012), 261–72.

28. Percy S. Pelouze, *Gonorrhea*, 240; and McFalls and McFalls, *Disease and Fertility*, 298, citing Stephen Kraus, "Complications of Gonococcal Infection," *Medical Clinics of North America* 56, no. 5 (1972): 1115–25; see 1115 for the figure of 17 percent.

29. Men in the decades prior to 1911—certainly those of a class who could afford it, such as professionals—were significantly more likely to seek treatment for gonorrhea than women, because they were more likely to experience symptoms; however, lacking sulfa drugs or antibiotics, the treatment available was not especially effective and could be both excruciating and itself damaging of fertility due to strictures and other consequences, treatments consisting, as they did, of urethral flushing, dilators, and application of a heated bougie. See J. David Oriel, *The Scars of Venus: A History of Venereology* (London: Springer, 1994), 140–42.

30. Richard Sweet and Harold Wiesenfeld, eds., *Pelvic Inflammatory Disease* (London: Taylor and Francis, 2006), 21.

31. The Lund twenty-four-year prospective cohort study, 1964–88, generated numerous research reports, which are accessibly summarized by Sweet and Wiesenfeld, *Pelvic Inflammatory Disease*, 69–71.

32. Ian N. Clarke and Hugh R. Taylor, chap. 4; Michael Worboys, chap. 5, both in this volume. As Worboys has also observed (pers. email comm. with Simon Szreter, May 19, 2017) of the first decades of the twentieth century, "Only in hindsight can we link inclusion bodies found in genital smears in the 1900s to chlamydia now." At that time "finding inclusion bodies in the genital tract of females and males didn't equate with any disease." But the fact that they were found by the leading scientists of the day confirms that what has since been identified as chlamydia was there in a number of cases examined where gonorrhea-like symptoms were presented. Drawing from page 7 of Phillips Thygeson, "Trachoma Virus: Historical Background and Review of Isolates," *Annals of New York Academy of Sciences* 98 (1962): 6–13, Worboys observes, "In 1910 Ludwig Halberstaedter and Stanislaus Prowazek first found inclusions in female genital epithelium, and in the same year Karl Lindner found them in three cases of nongonorrheal urethritis of men. . . . He postulated that trachoma and 'inclusion blennorrhea' ('genital trachoma' or 'paratrachoma') were caused by the same agent but suggested later that the two diseases might have a relationship like that of variola and vaccinia." Halberstaedter and Prowazek did use the German term *Chlamydozoen* (from the Greek for a type of cloak) in their article title because they observed the nucleus of the affected cells appeared to be cloaked by the affecting agent, which they assumed to be a protozoan, like other high-profile tropical diseases that had then been discovered, such as malaria and sleeping sickness.

33. An in-depth review of the field has identified as many as four "distinct mechanisms or processes of host-pathogen interaction that are commonly referred to in the field to explain the process that underlies the development of infertility following

Chlamydia infection. The processes are not exclusive of each other, and there is evidence for and against a role for each process." Shruti Menon et al., "Human and Pathogen Factors Associated with *Chlamydia trachomatis*–Related Infertility in Women," *Clinical Microbiology Review* 28, no. 4 (2015): 969–85, 977, https://doi.org/10.1128/CMR.00035-15. Such researches have shown, for instance, that at the individual level the pathway from infection to infertility can be dependent on many factors, including which of the dozen or so serovars is involved and what kind of immune response it elicits, the genotype of the host, the presence of coinfections, and the general state of hygiene of the infected host.

34. The most recent US literature metareview is Danielle G. Tsevat et al., "Sexually Transmitted Diseases and Infertility," *American Journal of Obsteteric Gynecology* 216 (2017): 1–9, https://doi.org/10.1016/j.ajog.2016.08.008. The most recent major National Health Service review, which also reevaluated the high-quality data available from the Netherlands study by Land and colleagues, concluded that even with current screening and treatment regimes, chlamydia is probably responsible today for about 29 percent of all tubal infertility (a reduction from the 45 percent figure found in the Dutch retrospective study, due to the superior prospective methodology adopted): Malcolm J. Price et al., "The Natural History of *Chlamydia trachomatis* Infection in Women: A Multi-parameter Evidence Synthesis," *Health Technology Assessment* 20 (2016): chap. 11, esp. 138. The original Dutch study was J. A. Land et al., "Performance of Five Serological Chlamydia Antibody Tests in Subfertile Women," *Human Reproduction* 18, no. 12 (2003): 2621–27, http://dx.doi.org/ 10.1093/humrep/deg479.

35. The 2013 international review Malhotra Meenakshi et al., "Genital Chlamydia Trachomatis: An Update," *Indian Journal of Medical Research* 138, no. 3 (2013): appendix E, concluded in the section titled "*Chlamydia trachomatis* and Infertility" that in the present state of documented knowledge "the role of *C. trachomatis* in male infertility is not yet proven." This is despite the fact that Allan Pacey and colleagues have shown that a chlamydial infection can damage and kill sperm: Adrian Eley, Allan A Pacey, Massimiliano Galdiero, Marilena Galdiero, Francesco Galdiero, "Can *Chlamydia trachomatis* Directly Damage Your Sperm?," *Lancet Infectious Diseases* 5, no. 1 (2005): 53–57. The negative finding that there continues to be no convincing evidence that the damage to either sperm or epididymis in men caused by chlamydia is sufficient to cause sterility has been confirmed by Paddy Horner, coauthor of Price et al., "Natural History of Chlamydia" (pers. email comm. with Szreter, September 6, 2017). On the likely reasons for this, see the discussion in Simon Szreter's introduction to this volume, p. 15.

36. Note that we are talking here only about the chances of infertility due to STIs among the married female population, which are purely a function of exposure to transmission of a "live" infectious episode from her husband. We are not talking about the husband's chances of STI-induced sterility, which follow an entirely different schedule of probability and which are posited to increase with his age at marriage because of the accumulation of exposure to separate risk incidents, any one of which

may result in his infertility. Note also that the chances of a husband passing on an infection of either gonorrhea or chlamydia remain the same, regardless of his age and even regardless of whether or not he himself has already been rendered sterile by a previous episode of gonorrhea infection. One of the few high-quality studies available, based on using large numbers, interviewing named contacts, and bacteriological testing of infections, confirmed very high rates of infectiousness of gonorrhea, particularly from male to female, in the order of 90 percent (and 74 percent from female to male). A. H. Pedersen and W. D. Harrah, "Follow-Up of Male and Female Contacts of Patients with Gonorrhea" *Public Health Reports* 85, no. 11 (1970): 997–1000. Furthermore, it is relevant that this study included many casual contacts. Even higher rates, approaching 100 percent, would be expected where repeated and regular exposures occur with the infected partner, as in a marriage; see P. V. Marcussen, "Variations in the Stability of Sexual Relations as Explanation of Differences in the Spread of Syphilis and Gonorrhea," *American Journal of Syphilis, Gonorrhea, and Venereal Diseases* 37 (1953): 355–61.

37. To take the example of the group of women marrying at age twenty to twenty-four, the estimate of a 0.886 percent chance of a childless marriage is arrived at in the following way. The female chance is 0.63 percent, while the additional male chance at ages twenty to twenty-four is 0.256 percent, summing to 0.886 percent. The female component remains at 0.63 percent among the two older female age groups, but the added male chance rises to 0.769 percent at ages twenty-five to twenty-nine and to 1.282 percent at ages thirty to thirty-four.

38. On Britain, see Anne Hanley, "'The Great Foe to the Reproduction of the Race': Changing Medical Knowledge and Practice; Diagnosing and Treating Infertility Caused by Venereal Diseases, 1880–1914," in *The Palgrave Handbook of Infertility in History: Approaches, Contexts, Perspectives*, ed. Gayle Davis and Tracey Loughran (London: Palgrave Macmillan, 2017), 335–58; on Germany, see Christina Benninghaus, chap. 10, in this volume.

39. James Trussel and Christopher Wilson, "Sterility in a Population with Natural Fertility," *Population Studies* 39 (1985): 269–86.

40. Szreter, "Treatment Rates," 26.

41. Chester's population in 1774 was 14,713; Gainsborough and Banbury reached 5,112 and 3,810, respectively, in 1801. For the sixteen parishes, see Trussel and Wilson, "Sterility in a Population," 278n18.

42. The family reconstitutions of all twenty-six English parishes compiled at the Cambridge Group for the History of Population and Social Structure, including both the sixteen parishes used by Trussel and Wilson, "Sterility in a Population" and the larger number used by Wrigley et al., *English Population History*, were kindly supplied to the authors by Gillian Newton of the Cambridge Group.

43. The multiplier is calculated as follows. First, the English family reconstitution data were selected by parish and period in accordance with the groupings given in table 2.2, on page 26, of Wrigley et al., *English Population History*. This differs from those selected in Trussel and Wilson, "Sterility in a Population," since Wrigley

and colleagues include the additional parishes of Austrey, Birstall, Bridford, Dawlish, Great Oakley, Ipplepen, Lowestoft, March, and Morchard Bishop, while at the same time excluding data from certain parishes for given periods on the grounds of reliability. Note that Wrigley and colleagues exclude the small parish of Hawkshead, included by Trussel and Wilson, "Sterility in a Population," in its entirety, on the basis that "the level of childlessness among married women was suspiciously high" (29) together with (unspecified) "other reasons for doubt" (30). Following the selection of data, rates for marriage with parity zero (childless) were calculated for completed marriages (but in line with Trussel and Wilson, "Sterility in a Population," allowing for remarriages), where the wife was aged, respectively, fifteen to nineteen, twenty to twenty-four, twenty-five to twenty-nine, or thirty to thirty-four at marriage. Rates were calculated for all parishes combined and for Banbury and Gainsborough separately. The ratio between each set of rates was then calculated, producing the result that for the four age-at-marriage groups, the rate of childless marriages in Banbury and Gainsborough was higher than that observed for all reconstitution parishes, combined, by a factor of 1.73, 1.16., 1.47, and 1.31. The final figure of 1.387 is the average of these four rates weighted, respectively, by the number of observations in each age-at-marriage group.

44. This estimate is from the 1801 census reproduced in Wrigley et at., *English Population History*, 22–23, table 2.1.

45. The figure of 0.424 is the product of the following computation, which weights the ratio of how much more sterility there was in Banbury and Gainsborough (1.387 times more) by the relative population size of these two parishes (8,922), expressed as a proportion of the total population of all sixteen parishes (29,169): 1.387 × (8,922 / [20,247 + 8,922]). This is 1.387 × (8,922 / 29,169)—that is, 1.387 × 0.3059 = 0.424.

46. See note 26 on derivation of this figure from "Populations Past."

47. This is the product of this sum (row 10 of table 12.1, weighted by row 4): [(236.8 × 52.1) + (149.3 × 41.1) + (63.2 × 28.1)] / (236.8 + 149.3 + 63.2) = (12337.3 + 6136.2 + 1775.9) / 449.3 = 20249.4 / 449.3 = 45.07 percent.

48. Kevin Schürer and Edward Higgs, Integrated Census Microdata (I-CeM), 1851–1911[data collection]. UK Data Service, 2014 SN 7481, http://doi.org/10.5255/UKDA-SN-7481-1; see also Edward Higgs et al., *The Integrated Census Microdata (I-CeM) Guide* (Colchester: University of Essex, 2013). Further details on the I-CeM database, along with related resources, are available from the I-CeM website at "I-CeM: Introduction," Integrated Census Microdata Project, University of Essex, accessed February 27, 2019, https://www1.essex.ac.uk/history/research/icem/. The creation of the I-CEM database was made possible through funding from the UK Economic and Social Research Council, grant number RES-062-23-1629.

49. Registrar General, 1901–12, "England and Wales Supplement to Registrar-General's Seventy-Fifth Annual Report: Part IV; Mortality of Men in Certain Occupations in the Three Years, 1910, 1911 and 1912," *Online Historical Population*

Reports, 1901–12, accessed February 22, 2019, www.histpop.org. About 130 occupations were separately tabulated.

50. On the origins and limitations of this official scheme, see Szreter, *Fertility, Class and Gender*, 67–282; and Simon Szreter, "Fertility, Social Class, Gender and the Professional Model: Statistical Explanation and Historical Significance," *Economic History Review* 68 (2015): 707–22.

51. Final Report of the Commissioners, *Royal Commission on Venereal Diseases*, Cd. 8189, 1916. Stevenson did not rely on the cause-of-death category of "syphilis" because of the widely known reluctance on the part of physicians to imperil their commercial and confidential relationship with their paying clients by placing this obscenity on the death certificate of a beloved *paterfamilias*. Instead, Stevenson relied primarily on the evidence of age-standardized death rates from "general paralysis of the insane," locomotor ataxy, and aneurysm, each of which had only recently come to be understood as being due primarily to tertiary syphilis and so as yet carried no widespread stigma. See Szreter, "The Prevalence," 511.

52. Clergy include clergymen in the established church, as well as ministers and priests of other religious bodies (excluding Catholics), but excludes itinerant preachers, scripture readers, missionaries, and lay clerics. Barristers and solicitors exclude law clerks and other legal assistants. Attorneys are included with barristers. Medical practitioners include physicians, surgeons, and other registered practitioners but exclude dentists, pharmacists, dispensers, and herbalists. Bankers include bank managers and other bank officials and clerks. See Higgs et al., *Integrated Census Microdata*, 194–205.

53. Szreter, "The Prevalence," 525, table 2.

54. Szreter, *Fertility, Class and Gender*, 365–440. For other evidence on the importance of attempted abstinence, see Simon Szreter and Kate Fisher, *Sex before the Sexual Revolution* (Cambridge: Cambridge University Press, 2010), 229–65.

55. David Levine, John Gillis, and Louise Tilley, *The European Experience of Declining Fertility, 1850–1970: The Quiet Revolution* (Oxford: Blackwell, 1992). This diversity is further explored as part of the ESRC-funded Atlas of Victorian Fertility Decline project, ES/L015463/1, at the Cambridge Group for the History of Population and Social Structure, Department of Geography, University of Cambridge. For further details, see "An Atlas of Fertility Decline in England and Wales," Cambridge Group for the History of Population and Social Structure, accessed September 12, 2017, www.geog.cam.ac.uk/research/projects/victorianfertilitydecline/.

56. For postpuerperal sterility, see Maeve Kenny's work reported in Worboys, chap. 5, in this volume. See also Irvine Loudon, *Death in Childbirth: An International Study of Maternal Care and Maternal Mortality, 1800–1950* (Oxford: Clarendon, 1992), chaps. 12–15. Additionally, in note 19, above in this chapter, see the warning in the German medical textbook of 1910 against unwise medical 'interference' in the postpartum process, in relation to the risks of provoking *Einkindsterilität*.

57. Jean-Noël Biraben, "Le rôle des maladies sexuellement transmissibles en démographie historique," *Population*, (1996): 1041–57.

58. Trussel and Wilson, "Sterility in a Population"; Wrigley et al., *English Population History*, 384, table 7.11.

59. Compare Trussel and Wilson, "Sterility in a Population," 278n18, with Wrigley et al., *English Population History*, 22–39, esp. 26, table 2.2, and note that Wrigley explained (pers. comm., March 24, 2017) that a note on page 578, which states that Birstall originally lacked FRFs in the case of childless families, can be ignored since these were subsequently supplied and incorporated before the parish was used. Wrigley and colleagues draw on twenty-six separate parish reconstitutions. Trussel and Wilson draw on sixteen parishes listed in note 18 of their article (though this note lists in order of individuals who carried out reconstitution work, and so several parishes are listed twice).

60. Trussel and Wilson, "Sterility in a Population," 278.

61. Trussel and Wilson, "Sterility in a Population," 278.

62. Szreter, *Fertility, Class and Gender*, 290.

63. Kevin Siena, *Venereal Disease, Hospitals, and the Urban Poor: London's "Foul Wards," 1600–1800* (Rochester: University of Rochester Press, 2004), chap. 4, 135–80.

64. Dahlberg, "Venereal Diseases in Sweden," table 1, for data for the years 1918–19, before effective treatment for syphilis became increasingly widespread in the civilian population. For use of this source, see above p. 380 and note 24.

65. Wrigley et al., *English Population History*, 135, table 5.3.

66. Szreter, "Treatment Rates," tables 7A, 7B. Note that both the age incidence and the pattern of broad gender equality of infection among the surrounding rural population was similar to that of the Chester resident populace.

67. Szreter, "Treatment Rates," tables 7A, 7B. Those marrying at age twenty had on average only a 34.74 percent chance of having sought treatment for the pox, relative to those aged thirty-five, and so the figures of 1.324 percent infection should be reduced to 0.460 percent. Multiplied by 4 this equates to 1.84 percent infected with gonorrhea and therefore 0.223 percent of women and 0.090 percent of men sterile at marriage, totaling 0.313 percent, both sexes combined, thus reducing the Trussel and Wilson figure of 4.6 percent to 4.287 percent. Those marrying at age thirty to thirty-four had 89.94 percent of the chance of infection of those aged thirty-five, and so the 1.324 percent infection rate should be reduced to 1.191 percent. Multiplied by 4 (to estimate the gonorrhea rate), this equates to 4.763 percent infected with gonorrhea and therefore 0.577 percent of women (4.763 × 0.1212) and 0.233 percent of men (4.763 × 0.049), totaling 0.810 percent, both sexes combined, sterile at marriage; so the Trussel and Wilson figure of 16.6 percent would be reduced to 15.79 percent.

68. Census of England and Wales, 1911, vol. XIII, *Fertility of Marriage*, v.

69. Supplement to the seventy-fifth *ARRG*, pt. 4, p. vii, states that "throughout, the tables and figures refer to the occupied and the retired in the aggregate."

In fact, this was a new departure by Stevenson, as the "unoccupied" (including in that designation the retired) had previously been separated out in the corresponding occupational morality supplements to the sixty-fifth and the fifty-fifth *ARRGs*, relating to deaths registered in 1900–1902 and 1890–92, respectively. We can be sure that, to the contrary, those recorded in the census of 1911 stating they had retired from a named previous occupation were not included in any occupational fertility tables relating to the separate census exercise. This is because we know that with the new Hollerith punch-card system for analyzing the fertility census, all those stating they were retired (with the exception of the armed services and old-age pensioners (OAPs) specifically, which were each coded separately) were given the Hollerith code of 350 ("Retired from Business [Not Army or Navy]"), regardless of any other occupational information they included.

70. A voluntary pension scheme, the Clergy Pensions Institution was created in 1886 and had some 4,000 members by the late 1890s. In 1927 the Church of England Pension Board was created to provide a compulsory pension scheme and the institution was amalgamated into the new scheme. Alan Haig, *Victorian Clergy* (Basingstoke: Croom Helm, 1984), 324–25. In 1911 in England and Wales there were about 36,000 Anglican and nonconformist priests enumerated and about 3,300 Catholic priests.

71. Meenakshi et al., "Genital Chlamydia Trachomatis," 303–16, second sentence in section titled "Chlamydia Trachomatis and Infertility." This is broadly consistent with the results of a Cochrane review (also published in 2013), which found that "chlamydia ascends to the upper genital tract in approximately 10 percent of cases to cause symptomatic pelvic inflammatory disease" while "the probability of tubal infertility in women who have had chlamydia is estimated to be only 1% to 4%"; see Nicola Low et al., "Screening for Genital Chlamydia Infection," *Cochrane Database Systemic Review* 23, no. 12 (2013): 1–15.

72. Price et al., "Natural History of Chlamydia," xxvi. We would like to acknowledge the ready advice and assistance given by Prof. Malcolm Price, Dr. Paddy Horner, and Prof. Tony Ades when they were each consulted on the interpretation of the findings of their 2016 study. Responsibility for the use made of their advice and the judgements made here about historical applications remains of course that of the authors of this chapter.

73. Menon et al., "Human and Pathogen Factors," 969, 985, 977, fig. 1. Thanks go to Paddy Horner for additional interpretative assistance for this appendix.

74. Joanna Lewis et al., "Genital Chlamydia Trachomatis Infections Clear More Slowly in Men Than Women, but Are Less Likely to Become Established," *Journal of Infectious Diseases* 216 (2017): 237–44.

75. Katy Turner et al., "Costs and Cost Effectiveness of Different Strategies for Chlamydia Screening and Partner Notification: An Economic and Mathematical Modelling Study," *BMJ Research* 342, no. 7789 (2011): c7250, https://doi.org/10.1136/bmj.c7250.

Contributors

TIM BAYLISS-SMITH is Emeritus Professor of Pacific Geography at the University of Cambridge and a fellow of St. John's College, Cambridge.

CHRISTINA BENNINGHAUS is Deutscher Akademischer Austauschdienst (DAAD) Fellow in Modern History at Wadham College and University of Oxford.

FABRICE CAHEN is Researcher at the Institut National d'Études Démographiques (INED), Paris.

IAN N. CLARKE is Professor of Molecular Biology and Virology at the University of Southampton.

SHANE DOYLE is Professor of African History and Director of the Centre for African Studies, University of Leeds.

REBECCA FLEMMING is Senior Lecturer in Classics at the University of Cambridge and a fellow of Jesus College, Cambridge.

REBECCA KIPPEN is Associate Professor of Demography at the School of Rural Health, Monash University.

JANET MCCALMAN is Distinguished Professor of History at the School of Population and Global Health, University of Melbourne.

ADRIEN MINARD is an independent researcher.

REBECCA REDFERN is Curator of Human Osteology at the Centre for Human Bioarcheology, Museum of London.

CHARLOTTE ROBERTS is Professor of Archaeology at the University of Durham.

ROY F. R. SCRAGG, OBE, was Foundation Professor of Social and Preventive Medicine at the University of Papua New Guinea from 1970 to 1974.

KEVIN SCHÜRER is Professor of English Local History at the University of Leicester.

SIMON SZRETER is Professor of History and Public Policy at the University of Cambridge and a fellow of St. John's College, Cambridge.

HUGH R. TAYLOR is Melbourne Laureate Professor and Harold Mitchell Chair of Indigenous Eye Health at the University of Melbourne.

OLIVIA WEISSER is Associate Professor of History at the University of Massachusetts, Boston.

MICHAEL WORBOYS is emeritus Professor of the History of Medicine, at the Centre for the History of Science, Technology and Medicine, University of Manchester.

Index

An italicized page number indicates a figure or table